Martin Vogel, Gitta Turowski (Eds.)
Clinical Pathology of the Placenta

Martin Vogel, Gitta Turowski (Eds.)

Clinical Pathology of the Placenta

—

DE GRUYTER

Editors

Gitta Turowski
Oslo University Hospital
Dept. of Pathology, Center for Pediatric
and Pregnancy rel. Pathology
Kirkeveien 166
0450 Oslo
and Faculty of Medicine, University in Oslo (UiO)
e-mail: UXTUGI@ous-hf.no

Prof. em. Dr. Martin Vogel
Gänseblümchenweg 35
04158 Leipzig
e-mail: prof.m.vogel@t-online.de

With contribution of

Prof. Dr. Lars Christian Horn
Universitätsklinikum Leipzig
Institut für Pathologie
Liebigstr. 26
04103 Leipzig
e-mail: Lars-Christian.Horn@medizin.uni-
leipzig.de

ISBN 978-3-11-044997-6
e-ISBN (PDF) 978-3-11-045260-0
e-ISBN (EPUB) 978-3-11-045106-1

Library of Congress Control Number: 2019938235

Bibliographic information published by the Deutsche Nationalbibliothek
The Deutsche Nationalbibliothek lists this publication in the Deutsche Nationalbibliografie; detailed
bibliographic data are available in the Internet at http://dnb.dnb.de.

© 2019 Walter de Gruyter GmbH, Berlin/Boston
Cover image: Gitta Turowski
Typesetting: L42 AG, Berlin
Printing and binding: CPI books GmbH, Leck

www.degruyter.com

Preface

The morphological and functional development of the placenta is decisive for the development of the fetus. Many disorders and diseases of the fetus with possible lifelong consequences can be explained by disorders of placental function.

Against this background, the presentation of the clinical pathology of the placenta, umbilical cord and membranes is of extraordinary importance. Above all, this knowledge is the basis for a prenatal functional diagnosis of the placenta and thus for changes in fetal development due to placental disorders. The special field of perinatal pathology in the large field of pathology of medicine has a preventive significance. The result of morphological findings is important for the monitoring and counseling of parents in subsequent pregnancies. The knowledge of placental pathology must be integrated into the clinical practice of obstetrics. In addition, this knowledge results in an innovative research landscape. Furthermore, the correlation of morphological findings with prenatal examination results is a quality feature of prenatal and obstetric work.

The epicritic assessment of the course of pregnancy and birth on the basis of morphological placental findings is not sufficiently exercised in everyday clinical practice. In addition, it is a concern of the authors to propagate a standardized examination method of the placenta and also to standardize the nomenclature of placental diseases.

As an obstetrician, I congratulate the authors on this book, in which the existing possibilities of morphological placenta diagnosis for the benefit of mother and child are consistently demonstrated.

Joachim W. Dudenhausen
Berlin, February 2019

https://doi.org/10.1515/9783110452600-201

Acknowledgment

Proper pathological-anatomical examination of the placenta can be a valuable tool in assessing the child's well-being in utero, the obstetric situation, the fetal outcome and the post-natal development of the newborn. It may also indicate possible causes of fetal placental disorders due to maternal diseases during the current pregnancy and the risk of subsequent pregnancies.

However, this assistance is still far too rarely used at national and international level. There is a lack of a consistent standard of placental examination and a common nomenclature in placental morphology and pathology. Many thanks to Gitta Turowski for motivating me to introduce our many years of experience in abortion and placenta pathology in Berlin and Germany to a broad readership for discussion by means of an English-written book. The emphasis in the writing of this book has been given by the importance of an ongoing exchange of information between the experience of the elder and the unfulfilled curiosity of the younger colleague, with a view to possible solutions to many more open questions. In addition, our thanks to Ronan M. Doyle, Oslo University Hospital, who checked for linguistic correctness and reading fluency. Many other helpers were involved in the genesis of the manuscript. We thank Prof. Dr. med. L.-Ch. Horn, University of Leipzig, for taking over the chapter on gestational trophoblastic diseases. We owe numerous illustrations to Mrs. A. Schotte, graphic designer, Berlin, and one illustration by K. Berg-Eriksen, Oslo. For the majority of the ultrasound pictures we thank Prof. Dr. T. Braun, Charité Berlin, Prof. Dr. R. Chaoui Prenatal Diagnostics Berlin, Dr. D. Brückmann, Perinatal Diagnostics, Erfurt-Thüringen. We thank PD Dr. C. Tenstedt-Schenk, Institute of Pathology Mühlhausen for cooperation and provision of macroscopic and microscopic pictures, as well as Dr. N. Sarioglu, Charité, Berlin, Dr. Myriam Haab, Saarland University Hospital, Prof. Dr. M. Ratschek, University of Graz, Prof. Dr. Anne Cathrine Staff, Oslo University Hospital, Dr. Debra S. Heller, Newark, NJ and all colleagues at the Department of Pathology, Oslo University Hospital (OUS) Ullevål. We thank Springer-Verlag, Heidelberg, Berlin for provision of microscopic pictures in chapter eleven.

Last but not least we thank the de Gruyter publishing house, in particular Mrs. Vieweg, Mrs. Noto and Mrs. Kischke, who accompanied the creation and growth of the manuscript and provided for a good equipment of the book.

Special thanks to our families for their patience in sluggish phases.

https://doi.org/10.1515/9783110452600-202

Content

List of abbreviations

ADAM	Amniotic-Deformities-Adhesions-Mutilations
AE	Amniotic Epithelium
AT	Amniotic collagenous Tissue
AVM	Arrest of Villous Maturation
CH I	Chorangiosis Type I
CH II	Chorangiosis Type II
CHM	Complete Hydatidiform Mole
CK	Cytokeratin
CMV	Cyto Megalo Virus
CRL	Crown-Rump-Length
CT	Chorionic connective Tissue
CTG	Cardiotocography
De	Decidua basalis
DIC	Disseminated Intravasal Coagulation
DIV	Deficiency of the Intermediate Villi
DNA	Deoxyribonucleic Acid
eTr	Extravillous Trophoblast
EvITr	Extravillous Intermediate Trophoblast
EviTr	Extravillous invasive interstitial Trophoblasts
EvTr	Endovascular Trophoblasts
FGR	Fetal Growth Restriction
Fi	Langhans-Fibrinoid
FP	Fetal-placental (ratio)
GA	Gestational Age
GC	Giant Cells
GD	Growth Disorganization
GDM	Gestational Diabetes Mellitus
GTD	Gestational Trophoblastic diseases
GW	Gestational Week
HCG	Humane Chorion-Gonadotropin
HE	Hematoxylin-Eosin
HELLP	H = Hemolysis, EL = Elevated Liver enzymes, LP = Low Platelet counts
HPF	High Power Field
HPL	Human Placental Lactogen
HSV	Herpes Simplex Virus
IH-hydrops	Immunological Hemolytic Hydrops
IUD	Intrauterine Device
IUFD	Intrauterine Fetal Death
IUGR	Intrauterine Growth Restriction
IV ce	Intermediate Villi of the immature central type
IV pe	Intermediate Villi of the mature peripheral type
JL	Junctional Layer
LPF	Low Power Field
MPA	Monocytosis Producing Antigen
MPF	Medium Power Field
NiFi	Nitabuch-Fibrinoid
NIH	Non Immunological Hydrops

PAS	Periodic Acid-Schiff (reaction)
PCR	Polymerase Chain Reaction
PF	Placental-Fetal (ratio)
PHM	Partial Hydatidiform Mole
PROM	Premature Rupture Of Membranes
PVI	Peripheral Villous Immaturity
RNA	Ribonucleic Acid
RoFi	Rohr-Fibrinoid
RVM	Retardation of Villous Maturation
SGA	Small for Gestational Age
SP	Spiral arteries
SP	Pregnancy specific
SSL	Scheitel-Steiß-Länge
STAN	Strecken Analyse
sTr	Syncytio Trophoblast
StV	Stem Villi
SUA	Single Umbilical Artery
SZ	Solution Zone
TNF	Tumor Necrosis Factor
TTTS	Twin-Twin-Transfusion Syndrome
TV	Terminal Villi
UCI	Umbilical Cord Insertion
VUE	Villitis of Unknown Etiology
YS	Yolk Sac

1 Normal anatomy and maturation

1.1 Anatomy and morphology

The placenta is a discoid organ formed when the chorion level, the tissue free membranes separate from the chorion frondosum in gestational week 13 to 14. It reaches a diameter between 17 and 19 cm and has a net weight of ca. 500 g prior to term. The placental net weight corresponds only to the weight of the placental disc, to which most reference values refer, whereas the gross weight includes the umbilical cord, membranes and often amniotic fluid and blood; all of which can increase the weight to 600 g or more. The maternal/basal plate area, analogous to a stylized circle, should normally reach 250 cm^2 at term and can be calculated using the formula a$\frac{1}{2}$ × b$\frac{1}{2}$ × π. The placental thickness at term is between 20 and 25 mm.

   The fetal/chorionic plate is the part of the placenta adjoining the amniotic sac, and the maternal/decidual basal plate lies adjacent to the uterus (Fig. 1.1). Both meet in the marginal zone. The placental tissue between the fetal/chorionic and maternal/basal plates form the grossly visible cotyledons, which are comprised of villi and the intervillous space (ca. 58 % villi and 42 % intervillous space)

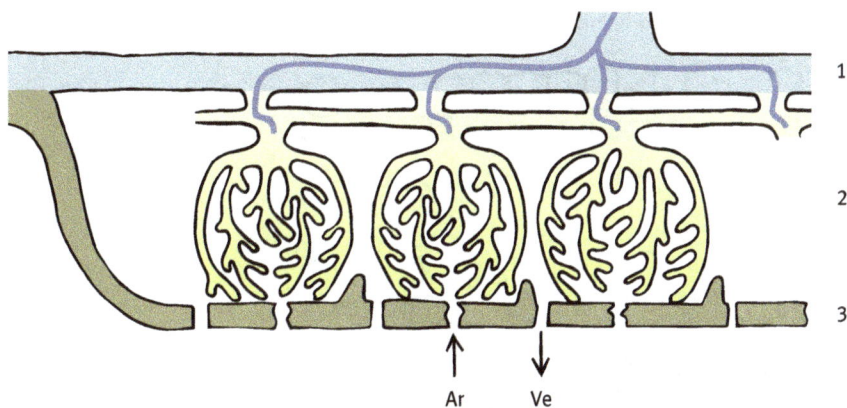

Fig. 1.1: Illustration. Structure of the human placenta: (1) Fetal/chorionic plate with umbilical cord vessels branching into the cotyledons, (2) cotyledons formed by villi and the intervening intervillous space, (3) maternal/basal plate with septa and interseptal spaces that enable maternal Arterial inflow (Ar) and maternal Venous outflow (Ve).

https://doi.org/10.1515/9783110452600-001

1.1.1 Chorionic plate

The chorionic plate consists of several layers that are easy to differentiate in early pregnancy.
- The *Amniotic Epithelium* (AE) layer covers the chorionic plate and forms the border of the amniotic sac.
- The *Amniotic collagenous Tissue* (AT) layer differs in density depending on gestational age and contains collagenous fibers.
- The *Junctional Layer* (JL) is a cell and fiber poor layer between the amniotic and chorionic connective tissue layers.
- The *Chorionic connective Tissue* (CT) layer is fiber rich and cell poor. Embedded here are the chorionic plate vessel branches (V) which arise from the umbilical cord vessels and supply the stem villi.
- The subchorionic layer of the *Langhans-Fibrinoid* (Fi) consists mainly of *matrix-type* fibrinoid and invasive cells of the extravillous trophoblast. The lamellar layer close to the intervillous space consists of fibrin-type fibrinoid.
- Focal aggregates of *extravillous Trophoblast cells* (eTr) are seen at the base of the chorionic connective tissue layer and in the Langhans-fibrinoid layer. *Syncytiotrophoblast cells* (sTr) can be focally detected at the junction to the intervillous space.

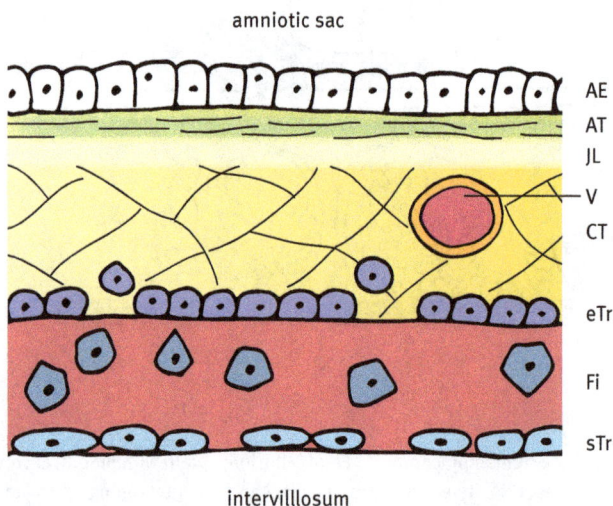

Fig. 1.2: Illustration. Chorionic plate tissue layers between the amniotic sac on one side and intervillous space (intervillosum) on the other side: Amniotic Epithelium (AE), Amniotic Tissue (AT), Junctional Layer (JL), fetal vessel branches (V), Chorionic Tissue (CT), extravillous Trophoblast (eTr), Langhans-Fibrinoid (Fi) and syncytiotrophoblast (sTr).

1.1.2 Basal plate

The basal plate defines the border to the uterine wall and consists of:
1. The extravillous trophoblast.
2. The maternal cells of the decidua basalis, soft tissue cells and leucocytes.
3. Fibrinoid.

Generally two types of fibrinoid can be differentiated [1,2]:
– *Fibrin-type fibrinoid* originating from coagulation processes and containing fibrin rich depositions and other maternal proteins.
– *Matrix-type fibrinoid* secreted from extravillous trophoblast cells and containing fetal proteins.

In early pregnancy the placenta is limited by the implantation bed and forms a zone-like structure (ch. 11). In middle pregnancy, several tissue layers form into a single basal plate of varying thickness. These different layers are not identifiable histologically.

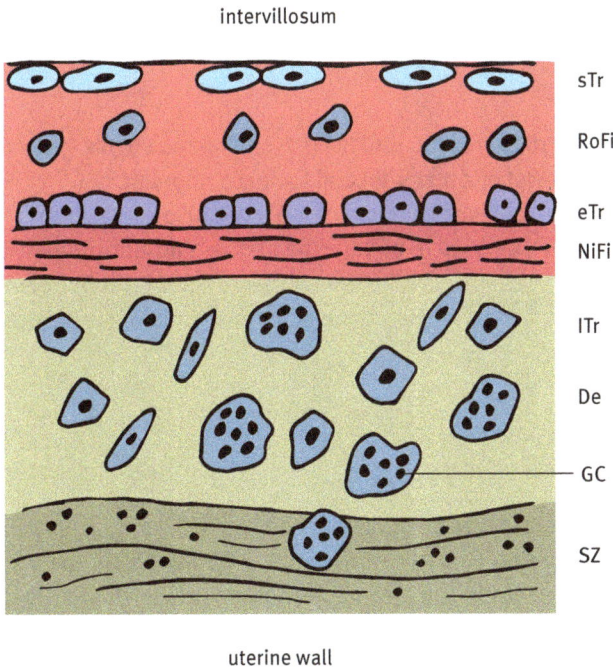

Fig. 1.3: Illustration. Maternal / basal plate structure between the intervillous space (intervillosum) on one side and the uterine wall on the other side: Syncytiotrophoblast (sTr), Rohr-Fibrinoid (RoFi), extravillous Trophoblast (eTr), Nitabuch-Fibrinoid (NiFi), Decidua basalis (De) containing Intermediate Trophoblasts (ITr) and Giant Cells (GC), and Solution Zone (SZ).

As in the layers of the chorionic plate, syncytiotrophoblast cells (sTr) can be focally seen at the junction to the intervillous space.

– The *Rohr-Fibrinoid* (RoFi) is seen next to the intervillous space and is infiltrated by non-proliferating trophoblast cells. A dense cell layer of basophilic Trophoblast cells (eTr) is seen underneath.

– The *Nitabuch-Fibrinoid* (NiFi) layer is the point at which placental separation occurs at birth. This layer has a heterogeneous appearance and is comprised of connective tissue fibers, endometrial stromal cells and macrophages.

– The *Decidua basalis* (De) contains stromal cells, macrophages, leucocytes and multinucleated Giant Cells (GC) of the extravillous and Intermediate trophoblast (Itr) types. Rudimentary fetal cells of the connecting stalk trophoblasts can also be found.

– The *Solution Zone* (SZ) demarcates the uterus from the basal plate and contains the mucous decidual membrane that remains in the uterus following birth.

– Vessel branches of the Spiral arteries (SP) transverse and branch within the basal plate and end in the intervillous space. One artery can have several fountain like openings in the central part of the fetal cotyledon [3]. Veins are extremely thin walled and often show sinusoidal dilatation.

1.1.3 Septa and islands

The septa arise from the basal plate, extend into the placental parenchyma (partly up to the chorionic plate) and consist of a maternal and foetal component.

The islands mainly contain extravillous trophoblast cells but also contain some decidua cells. Usually they are fibrinoid rich, of both the matrix- and fibrin-types. The central portion of the septa and islands can be pseudocystic, filled with fluid due to the fibrinolytic and proteolytic activity of the trophoblast cells, and large cysts can be seen macroscopically.

1.1.4 Villous compartment

The space between the chorionic and basal plates is filled with villi that are organized in villous bundles, each measuring 2 cm in diameter; these bundles form the cotyledons of the placental lobes. Data regarding the number and size of the villous bundles varies but there are between 40 and 60 villous bundles, measuring up to several cm in size, that are subdivided into ca. 300 sub-cotyledons [4–7].

Fetal cotyledons consist of a villous trunk and its ramifications. The 1st order of the villous trunk develops from the chorionic plate and subdivides into the 2nd and 3rd order villous trunks of each cotyledon (5). A single cotyledon consists of one 3rd order villous trunk arising from a 2nd order villous trunk [8].

The villous bundles are firmly attached to the basal plate by the 3rd order stem villi which, partly, form the anchoring villi.

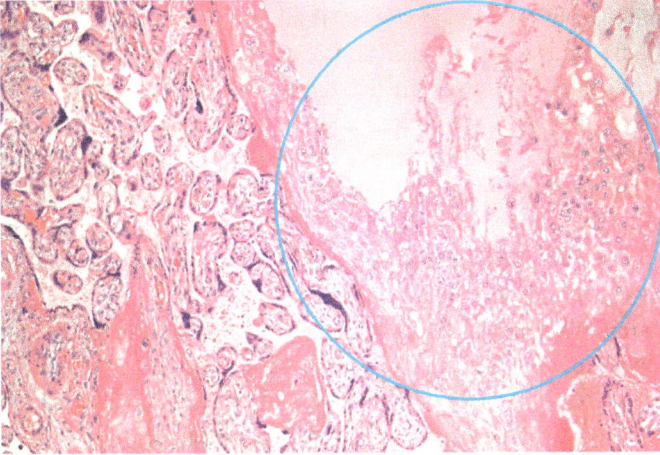

Fig. 1.4: Pseudocystic lesion lined by extravillous trophoblast cells with a fibrinoid matrix, decidua cells in the wall and filled with eosinophilic material centrally (circled). Placenta in gestational age 35 + 5, uncomplicated delivery.

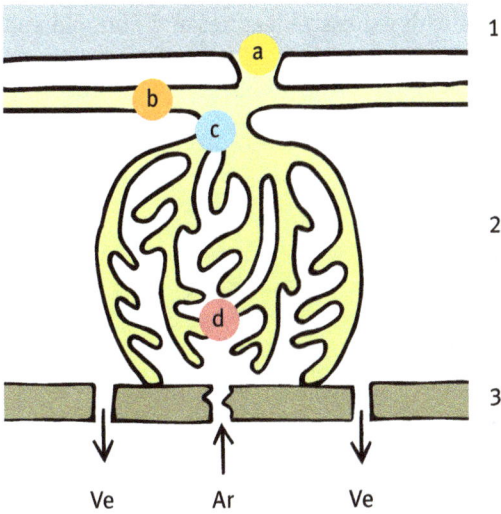

Fig. 1.5: Illustration. Fetal cotyledon: (1) Chorionic plate, (2) intervillous space, (3) basal plate, (a) 1st order villous trunk arising from the chorionic plate, (b) 2nd order villous trunk arising from (a), (c) 3rd order villous trunk arising from (b), (d) peripheral branching. (Ar) Maternal Arterial inflow and (Ve) Maternal Venous outflow.

1.1.5 Arrangement of the villous tree

The villous tree is anatomically and functionally differentiated into several subtypes of villis [9]:

– *Stem villi* are characterized by fetal blood vessels, branches of the chorionic plate vessels, which contain a tunica media. Their tunica adventitia merges almost imperceptibly into a concentric and collagen rich connective tissue that contains cells demonstrating an intense positivity for vimentin and α-smooth muscle actin on immunohistochemistry. This connective tissue extends from the umbilical cord, through the chorionic plate and into the peripheral stem villi. Their immunohistochemical profile verifies these cells as myofibroblasts. These cells originate from the chorionic plate and are identifiable from gestational week 8 onwards. The stem villi of the early fetal period already show a characteristic circular formation around larger vessels and the cells within these circular formations are considered to belong to the para/extravascular contractile system [10]. This contractile system is assumed to provide architectural stability to the tissue, facilitate blood flow to the stem villi and to regulate maternal blood circulation in the intervillous space by longitudinal villous contraction. Alongside the large vessels there coexists a subepithelial and paravascular capillary network [11]. This network is especially well developed in the small peripheral stem villi. In the early fetal period the villous trophoblast is predominantly double-layered and poorly differentiated, whereas in later pregnancy it differentiates into a single-layer with syncytial knots, nuclei with regressive features and fibrinoid and fibrin depositions on the stem villous surface.

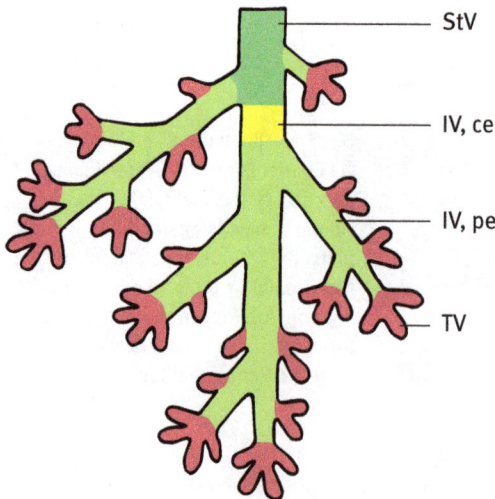

StV

IV, ce

IV, pe

TV

Fig. 1.6: Illustration. Structure of the villous tree in late pregnancy: (StV) Stem Villi; (IV.ce) Intermediate Villi of the immature central type; (IV.pe) Intermediate Villi of the mature peripheral type, (TV) Terminal Villi.

- *Intermediate villi of the (immature) central type* are located between the stem villi and the peripheral villi. They contain a loose embryonic stroma with cells displaying vimentin and desmin positivity but are negative for α-smooth muscle actin. Desmin and actin positive myofibroblasts are only located in the central transitional part, between the stem and intermediate villi, and along the larger tunica media containing vessels. Hofbauer cells are present in the stroma and surface antigens characterize them as a macrophage subpopulation. The majority of these cells are assumed to originate directly from fetal blood and they migrate into the villous vessels [12]; these cells retain their mitotic ability [13]. Vessels are irregularly distributed in the villous stroma and are predominantly thin walled capillaries.
Only exceptionally do the capillary branches reach the villous surface; at areas such as the vasculosyncytial membranes where the barrier between the fetal and maternal circulations is at its thinnest.
The villous epithelium is predominantly double-layered, has prominent nuclei and well defined cytotrophoblast cells. At the surface syncytial knots with cytotrophoblast nuclei can develop.
Function: The intermediate villi serve as the growth zone of the villous tree, from which centrifugal longitudinal growth and villous ramification progresses. Centripetally they are transformed into stem villi by the proliferation of tunica media containing fetal vessels and by condensation and differentiation of paravascular cells and fibers until gestational week 12. Blood flow transforms autochthonous capillaries into arteries and veins.
In early pregnancy the villous ramifications develop as sprouts of pure cytotrophoblast cells 'villous sprouts' from the villous surface. These sprouts transport mesenchyme via proliferating tissue cells and form the primitive mesenchymal villi [2,9].
- *Mesenchymal villi* have a thick chorionic epithelium with a lining of cytotrophoblast cells and contain multiple MIB-Ki 67 positive cells and a loose embryonic mesenchymal stroma that lacks vessels. The stromal cells exclusively express vimentin. Longitudinal growth is assumed to occur via a similar process to the trophoblast cell columns (2). Intermediate villi of the immature type are, for the first time, seen in gestational week 5–6 and are clearly visible until gestational week 20.
- *Intermediate villi of the mature peripheral type* are elongated villi with a loose, reticular and moderately collagenous stroma that contains vimentin and desmin positive cells. They contain many capillaries, some of which show actin positive cells in the vessel wall. The capillaries may show sinusoidal dilatation and be tightly connected to the epithelial surface, forming vasculosyncytial membranes. The syncytiotrophoblast is discontinuously seen with varying numbers of nuclei, cytotrophoblast cells and nuclear sprouts visible on the villous surface.

- *Function:* The mature peripheral intermediate villi take part in the regulation of the microcirculation and also have an endocrine and metabolic function.
- *Terminal villi* normally originate from the peripheral type intermediate villi but some arise directly from stem villi or the central type intermediate villi; this especially occurs in the subchorionic region. They contain capillaries and venous sinusoids, both of which are in contact with the epithelial surface. The sinusoids fuse with the epithelial cytoplasm and form nuclear free epithelial areas, known as vasculosyncytial membranes. At term, and in normal maturation, vasculosyncytial membranes are found in ca. 40 % of the terminal villous surface and the mean feto-maternal diffusion distance is 4.8 nm. The membranes are interrupted by syncytial nuclear buds/ knots and cytotrophoblast cells are rare. The stroma of the terminal villi is reduced to narrow bridges between the capillaries and sinusoids.

Function: The terminal villi are the main feto-maternal unit for gas exchange and simple diffusion processes. Together with the peripheral intermediate villi they take part in metabolic activity and hormone incretion. The detailed mechanisms of the formation and growth of the terminal villi are still unknown.

One mechanistic theory of terminal villus development suggests formation begins with the passive dilatation and protrusion of vessels with secondary membrane-like narrowing of the syncytiotrophoblast. Another dynamic theory proposes development occurs by capillary proliferation and vascularization of a transient precursor tissue "Platzhaltergewebe" [14] in the peripheral villi, with subsequent regional differentiation of the chorionic epithelium into nuclear free and nuclear containing parts and vasculosyncytial membranes.

1.2 Placental circulatory system

Feto-maternal circulatory unit

The intervillous space is filled by maternal blood, and both fetal and maternal blood is conducted to the functional units of the placenta, the *placentons*. Each fetal cotyledon is served by one spiral artery [5,15,16], and the inflow of maternal blood is reported to be predominantly to the central part of each unit [16,17]. A vessel connection, on the fetal aspect, between adjacent feto-maternal units does not exist; in contrast, maternal units are not anatomically separated from each other. Feto-maternal units show a lower villous density centrally compared to the periphery and the relative proportion of intermediate villi of the immature type is greater centrally than in the periphery [15,18]. These regional differences become more pronounced in placentas at gestational week 28. (Fig. 1.7).

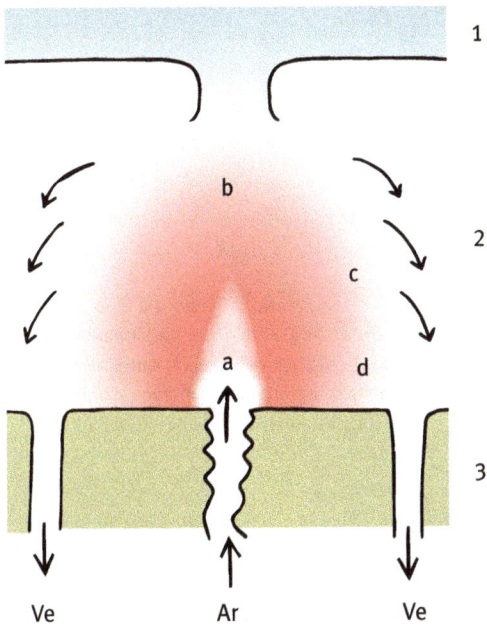

Fig. 1.7: Illustration. Feto-maternal circulatory unit: (1) Chorionic plate, (2) intervillous space, (3) basal plate. (a) Spiral artery (Ar) inflow to the cotyledon centre with (b) decreased villous density from (3) basal to (1) chorionic, (c) central to lateral and (d) central to peripheral, venous outflow (Ve) from the basal plate (modified after Moll 1981) [19].

1.3 Villous development

1.3.1 Early development

The early development of the human placenta, according gestational age, is well documented. The following stages may be differentiated:

- Pre-implantation, until day 5/6 p. c.
- Implantation, day 6–12 p. c.
- Villous development, day 13–21 p. c.

Pre-implantation

Pre-implantation starts with the formation of a zygote. Multicellular stages originate in the ovarian tube via cell division, and the first differentiated cell line is the trophoblast. The morula stage (32-cell stage, 3rd to 4th day p. c.) shows an outer trophoblast cell layer and an inner cell group. In the blastocyst stage (64-cell stage) the single-layered trophoblast differentiates from the inner embryoblast (Fig. 1.8). Trophoblasts differentiate into the syncytio- and cytotrophoblasts of the definitive placenta, and the inner cell mass differentiates into an epiblast and hypoblast at this time. The embryo, amnion and extra embryonic mesenchyme (villous stroma) develop from the epiblast and the yolk sac from the hypoblast.

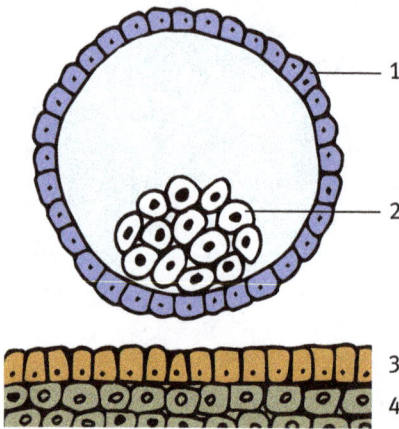

Fig. 1.8: Illustration. Blastocyst at four days p. c. Outer single-cell-layer and inner cell group: (1) trophoblast, the first differentiated cell line; (2) inner cell group with embryonic pole; (3) superficial endometrial cell line; (4) decidua.

Implantation

The blastocyst reaches the uterine cavity at day 4 p. c. and implantation occurs at day 5/6 p. c., when the embryonic pole of the blastocyst first attaches to the endometrium. At this implantation site (pole) the trophoblasts in contact with the endometrium rapidly proliferate and the cells infiltrate the maternal mucosa. This infiltrative process is facilitated by lytic secretions which are detectable in embryonic and maternal cells [20–23]. In the following days, trophoblast cells infiltrate the decidual epithelial layer and at this point two trophoblast cell types can be differentiated; syncytio- and cytotrophoblasts. Syncytiotrophoblast cells are in direct contact with maternal tissue; these cells merge and develop into solid cell formations. Cytotrophoblasts are internally attached to the extraembryonic mesenchyme (chorionic mesoderm), they possess a high mitotic activity and are considered to be the trophoblast reserve pool. The expanding implantation syncytiotrophoblast infiltrates by proteolytic and fibrinolytic activity into the decidua and the maternal vessels. Between the solid trabecular cellular networks the hollow spaces are filled with maternal blood and these spaces define

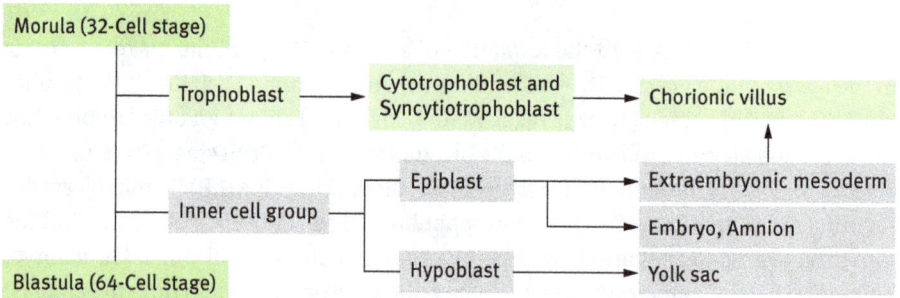

Fig. 1.9: Illustration. Chorionic villi originating from the trophoblast and extraembryonic mesoderm; embryo and amnion originating from the inner cell group.

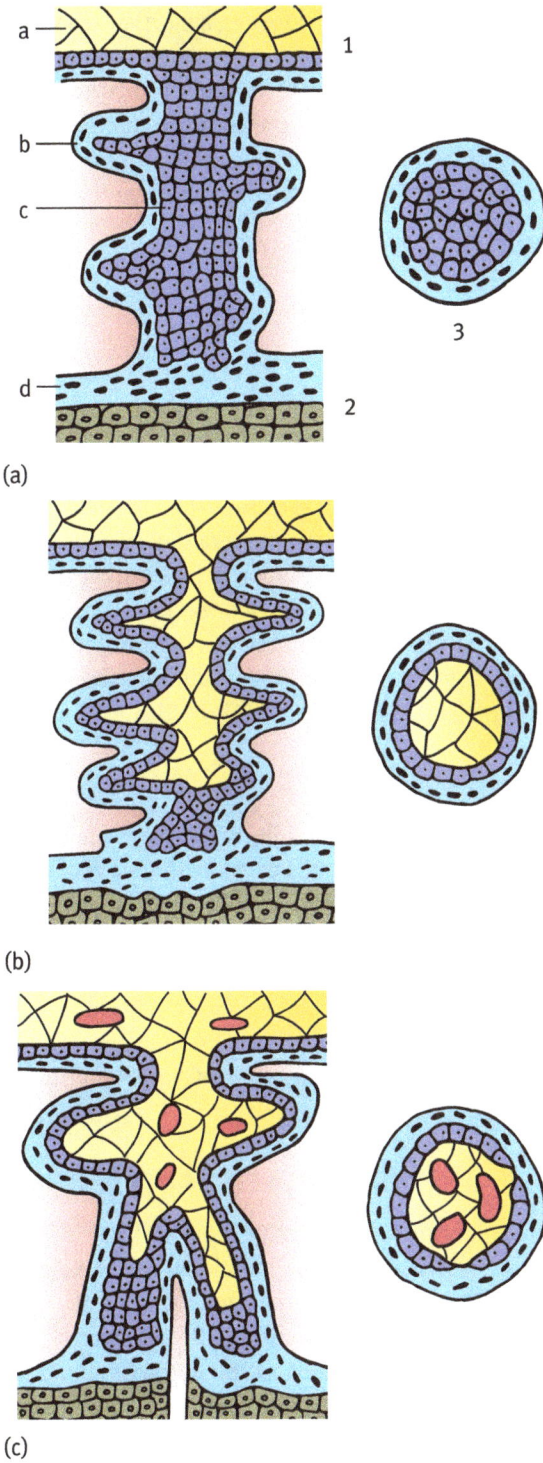

Fig. 1.10: Illustration. (a) *Primary* villus day 13–15 p. c.: (1) primary chorionic plate with (a) mesenchymal stroma (extraembryonic mesoderm), (b) lateral trabeculae with syncytiotrophoblast cells, (c) cytotrophoblast cells, (d) preliminary basal plate, (2) endometrial cells, (3) cross section. (b) Illustration. (b) *Secondary* villus day 15/16 p. c.: characteristic mesenchymal infiltration. (c) Illustration. (c) *Tertiary* villus day 17/18 p. c.: characteristic vasculogenesis.

the lacunae. The lacunae merge and are coated by the growing syncytial trabeculae. At the end of this early trabecular stage, day 9–12 p. c. [4], the blastocyst is completely enveloped by endometrium. In the later trabecular stage, day 12/13 p. c., cytotrophoblast cells infiltrate from the chorionic mesoderm of the presumptive chorionic plate into the axes of the trabeculae. The trabeculae, consisting of an inner cytotrophoblast and outer syncytiotrophoblast, function as a barrier between the maternal and fetal circulations. (Figs. 1.9, 1.10)

1.3.2 Villous morphogenesis day 13–21 p. c.

Primary villi

Villous development starts with the formation of primary villi, day 13 to day 15 p. c. The central trabecular axes are enriched by abundant and highly mitotically active cytotrophoblasts. They develop laterally and form new trabeculae that extend towards the maternal lacunae. Solid trophoblastic columns develop from the basal syncytial trophoblasts and connect to the trophoblast plate. The cellular network of the trophoblast lining gets progressively infiltrated and loosened by cytotrophoblast cells and, as soon as the trophoblast cells lose their connection to the basal membrane, their mitotic activity decreases. This allows migration, with further infiltration and expansion, in the implantation bed to occur.

Secondary villi

Transformation from primary villi into the secondary villi, which form the central stromal axis, begins from day 15 to 16 p. c. Mesenchymal cells migrate from the chorionic mesoderm into the central axes of the primary villi and transform the solid, cellular axes into mesenchymal stroma. The continued development of primary and secondary villi causes the conversion of the lacunar system into an intervillous space.

The embryo is suspended on its connecting stalk in the chorionic space, and the connecting stalk and its vessels develop in the extraembryonic mesoderm. The vessels become connected to the intraembryonic vascular system and extend centrally to reach the primitive chorionic plate at day 17 to 18 p. c.

Tertiary villi

Tertiary villous development begins with the appearance of capillary vessels in the villous stroma from day 17/18 p. c. Mesenchymal invasion into the secondary villi precedes autochthonic intravillous capillary development. The merging of the chorionic plate vessels with the villous capillaries, and the development of the embryonic-, and later feto-placental circulation is assumed to be influenced by haemodynamic factors, such as the start of rhythmic foetal heart activity and intravascular pulsation.

Histologically, the primitive walled chorionic plate/umbilical cord vessels and the villous capillaries closely attached to the chorionic plate can be seen.

1.3.3 Histology of the embryonic period (Gestational Week 6–12)

The formation of tertiary villi and an established embryonic-placental circulation concludes early placental development; subsequent growth and maturation defines the fetal period.

Development of placental villi is accomplished by growth, both longitudinal and branching, and maturation. Villous growth results in an increased number of functional trophoblast groups, increased villous tissue volume and increased villous surface area.

Villous maturation enables expansion of the fetal capillary system, differentiation of the chorionic epithelium, enlargement of the feto-maternal exchange surface

Table 1.1: Histological characteristics and changes in the chorionic plate, stem villi and peripheral villi in Gestational Weeks 5 to 12 (GW).

GW	Structure		
	chorionic plate	stem villi	peripheral villi
5–6	embryonic stroma, few Hofbauer cells, connecting stalk/UC vessels, suprachorionic capillaries, embryonic blood cells	embryonic stroma, primitive vessel branches, solid trophoblast columns, basal connecting villi	embryonic stroma, capillaries, double-layered villous epithelium, villous columns, mesenchymal stroma without vessels, villous sprouts
7–8	chorionic plate with sub-amniotic and paravascular connective tissue fibers in a loose stroma, thin walled fetal vessels	central villous vessels, paravascular loose fibers, apical villous columns, mesenchymal stroma without vessels	embryonic stroma, capillaries close to the epithelium, few syncytial columns, solid trophoblast islands
9–10	cell rich and well orientated reticular connective tissue, small vessels with tunica media that extend into the UC branches	tunica media in larger vessels, paravascular fibers	embryonic stroma, double-layered epithelium, few gaps in the cytotrophoblast, increased syncytial columns
11–12	fibrous stroma, large vessels containing tunica media	medium sized vessels contain a tunica media, subepithelial embryonic reticular stroma	one/few capillaries per villus, few gaps in the cytotrophoblast

and the minimisation of diffusion distance between the maternal and fetal circulations.

Villous growth and maturation are prerequisites for the architecture and structure of the intervillous space which facilitates fetal and maternal placental blood flow.

The placenta of the embryonic period is defined by the morphological characteristics of villous and chorionic plate development [24].

Placenta in Gestational Week 5/6

The chorionic plate consists of embryonic tissue with a junctional layer between the amniotic and chorionic portions. Primitive walled umbilical cord vessel branches are seen in the chorionic stroma and single capillaries can be found in the suprachorionic stroma.

Stem villi develop from the chorionic plate and draw chorionic plate vessels and autochthonic capillaries away from the chorionic plate.

The villi have a large and relatively evenly distributed villous diameter with a loose network of embryonic stroma containing fine cytoplasmic filaments and star-like mesenchymal cells. In the stroma, a few Hofbauer cells may be seen with eccentric nuclei and a homogeneous and eosinophilic, or finely vacuolated, cytoplasm. A few, incidental, autochthonic capillaries are distributed in the stroma and nucleated embryonic erythrocytes may be seen in the lumen.

The chorionic epithelium is continuously double-layered and has large nuclei. The mesenchymal villi show trophoblast columns. Rudimentary trophoblast coats are visible, in addition to deposits of Rohr-fibrinoid, close to the basal plate [25].

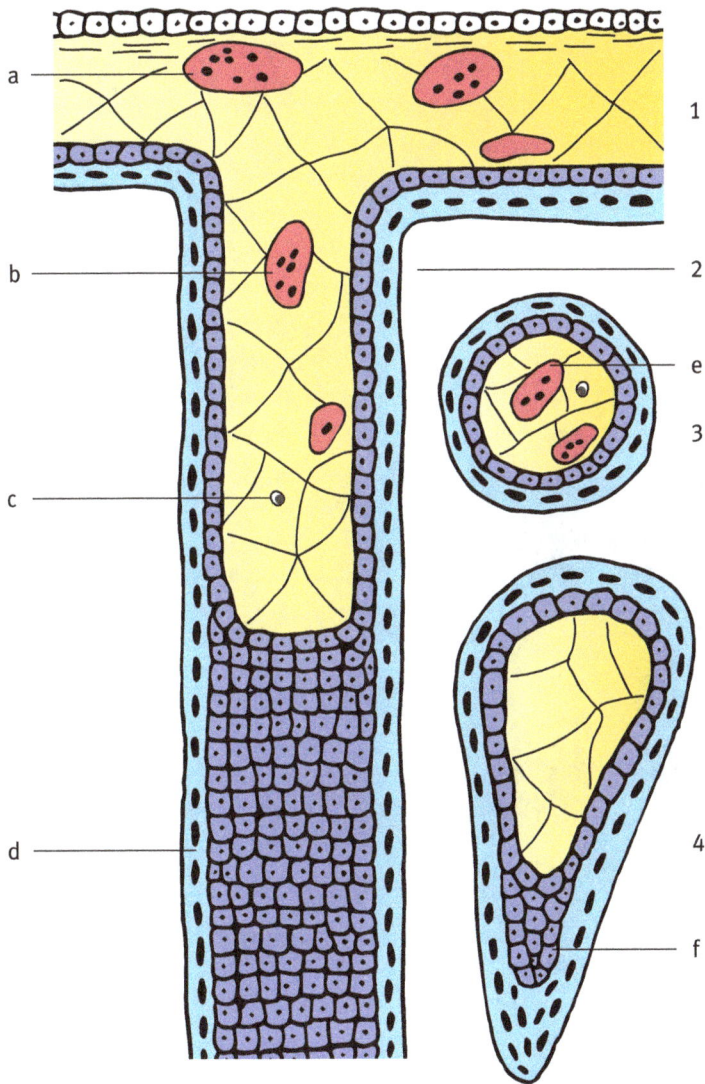

Fig. 1.11: Illustration. Histological characteristics in Gestational Week 5/6: (1) chorionic plate, (2) stem villus with trophoblast column. Cross sections: (3) peripheral villus, (4) mesenchymal villus with villous sprout. (a) Primitive walled branches of fetal (umbilical cord) vessels, (b) thin walled fetal vessels in the axis of the stem villus (if located close to the chorionic plate), (c) single Hofbauer cells in a loose embryonic stroma, (d) syncytium, (e) thin walled capillaries, (f) villous sprout.

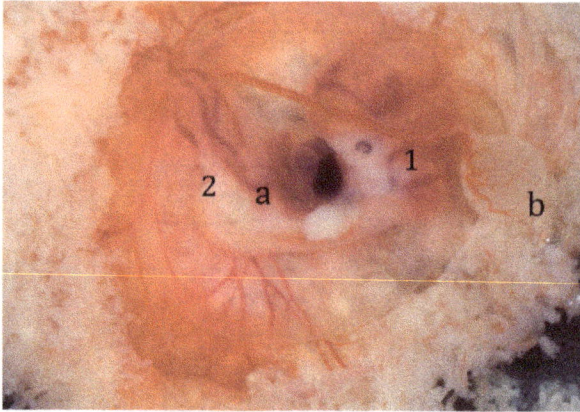

Fig. 1.12: Gestational sac in Gestational Week 6: sac diameter measured to be ca. 15 mm, embryo ca. 6 mm (Crown-Rump-Length). (1) Embryonic cranial pole; (2) embryonic caudal pole. (a) Umbilical cord, (b) yolk sac (by courtesy of Dr. N Sarioglu, Department of Pediatric Pathology and Placentology, Charité Berlin, Germany).

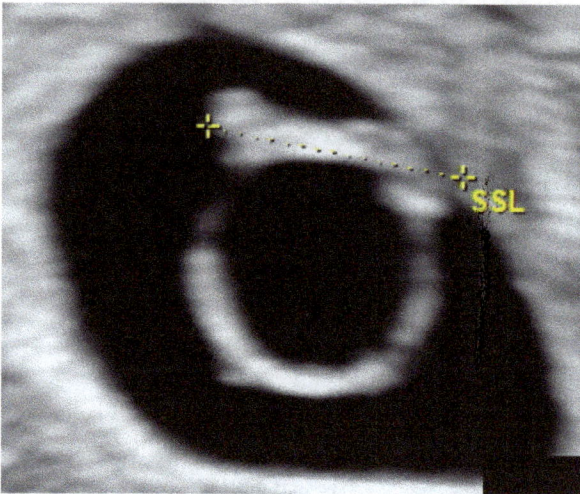

Fig. 1.13: 2D Ultrasound. Embryo in Gestational Week 6: sac diameter marked as SSL (German for Crown Rump Length) (by courtesy of Dr. Brückmann, Office for Prenatal diagnostic, Erfurt, Germany).

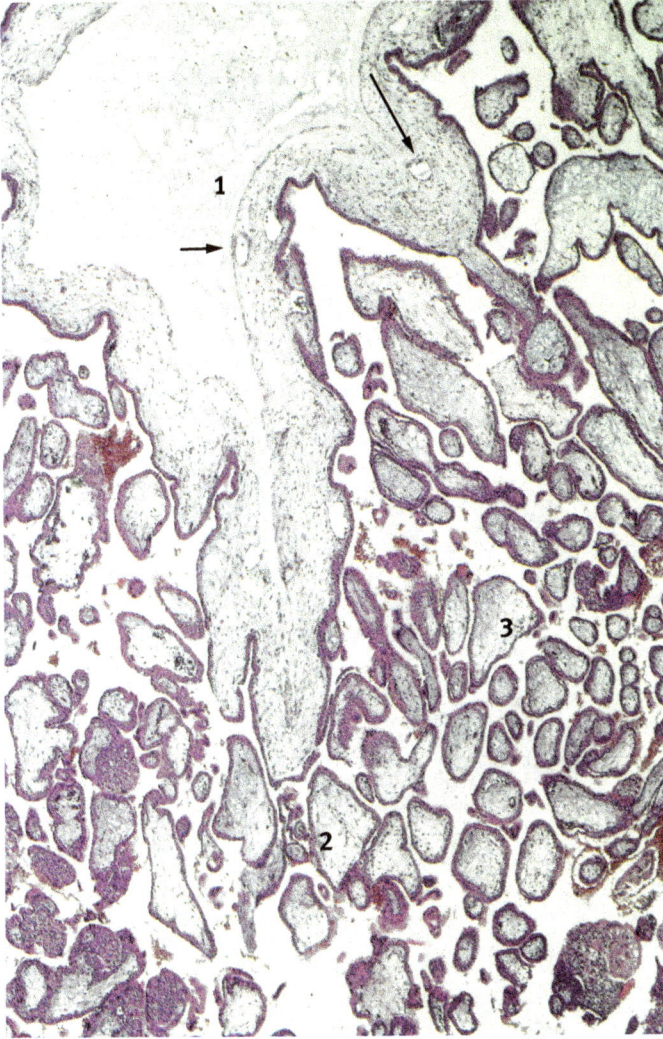

Fig. 1.14: Histology in Gestational Week 6. (1) Chorionic plate with thin walled fetal vessels (arrows), (2) stem villus, (3) mesenchymal villi without capillaries.

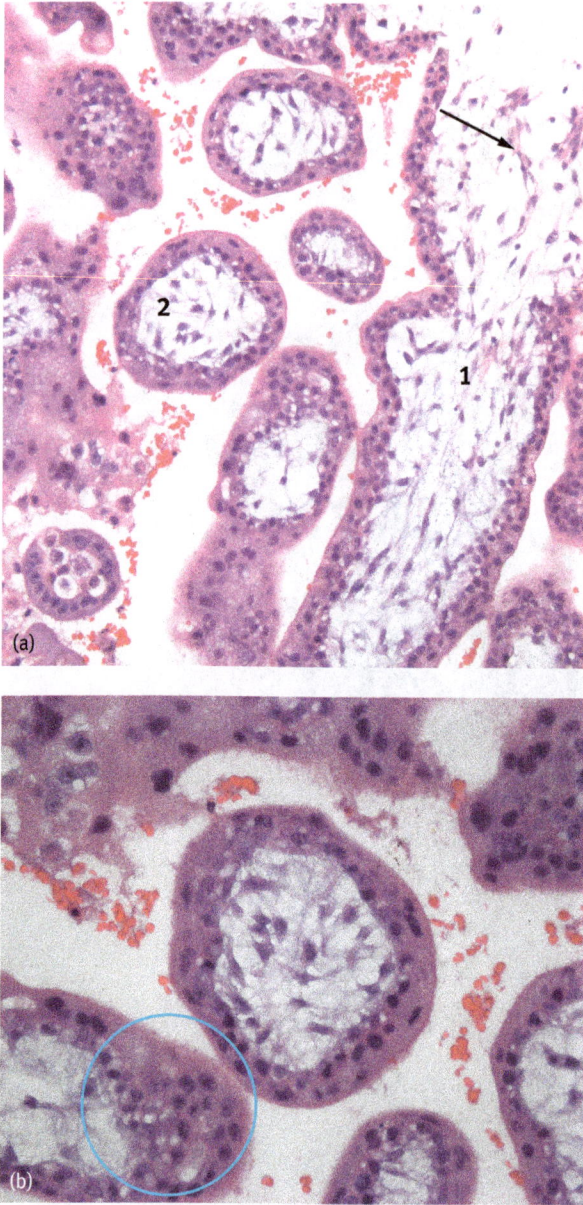

Fig. 1.15: (a) Histology in Gestational Week 6. (1) Stem villus with a large diameter and thin walled fetal vessels (arrow), (2) mesenchymal villus without capillaries. (b) Basal villous sprout, (encircled).

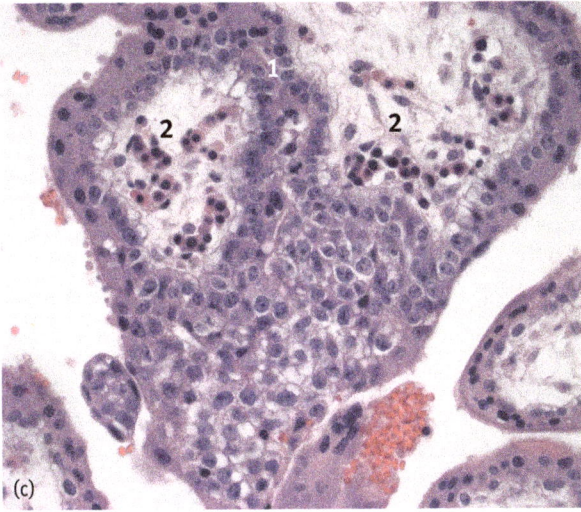

Fig. 1.15: (continued) (c) (1) Short portions of the villous trophoblastic columns, (2) villous vessels containing nucleated erythrocytes.

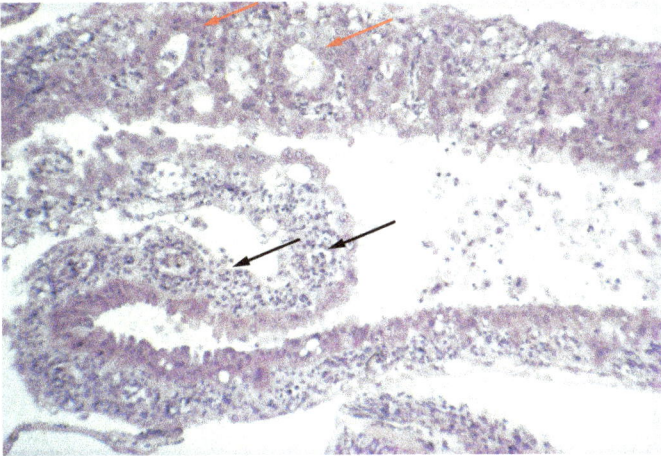

Fig. 1.16: Yolk sac: microcystic structure (red arrows), (2) blood islands (black arrows). Abortion in Gestational Week 5.

Placenta in Gestational Week 7/8

Fine collagenous tissue fibers are visible in the chorionic plate, subamniotically and along the primitive walled branches of the umbilical cord vessels. Amniotic and chorionic stroma may merge and be difficult to distinguish. The villous tree consists of 7–8 villous cross sections in each medium power field (MPF) and the villi have an embryonic stroma containing Hofbauer cells. Stem villi adjacent to the chorionic plate contain branches of the chorionic plate vessels in the villous axes and small tracts of collagen tissue fibers. Autochthonic capillaries are located subepithelially. The chorionic epithelium is double-layered and some syncytiotrophoblast proliferations are visible.

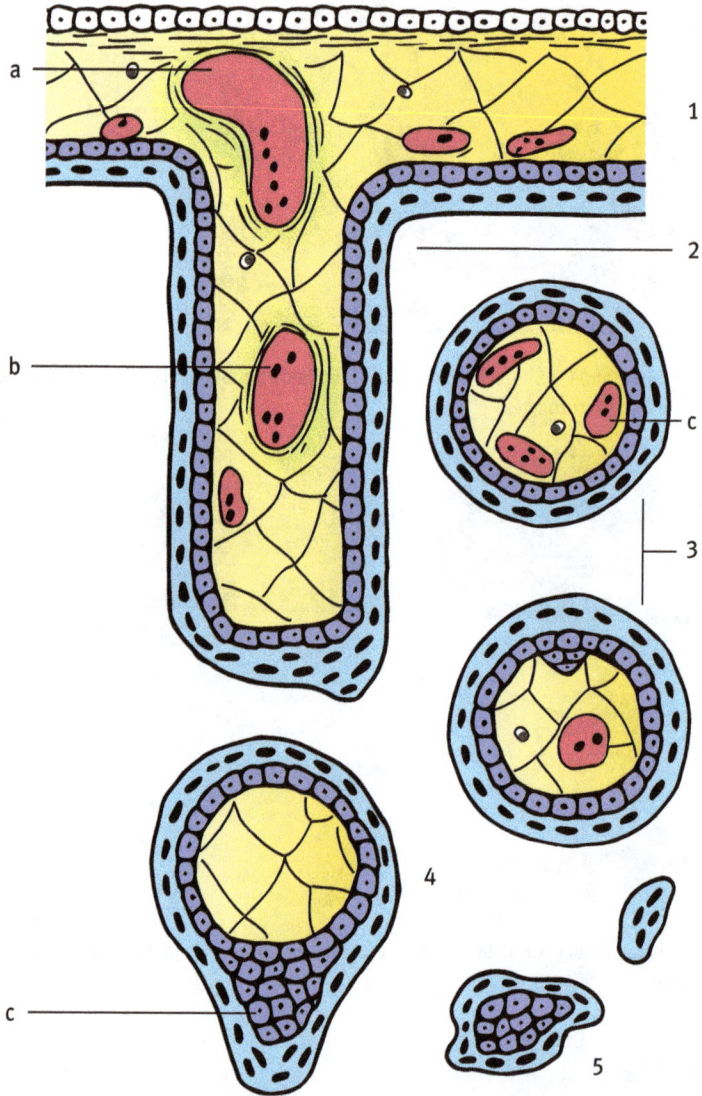

Fig. 1.17: Illustration. Histological characteristics in Gestational Week 7/8: (1) chorionic plate, (2) stem villus with trophoblast column, (3) peripheral villi (cross sections), (4) mesenchymal villus with trophoblast sprout, (5) solid intervillous trophoblast islands. (a) Primitive walled branches of fetal (umbilical cord) vessels, (b) thin walled fetal vessels in the axis of the stem villus (if located close to the chorionic plate), (c) villous sprout.

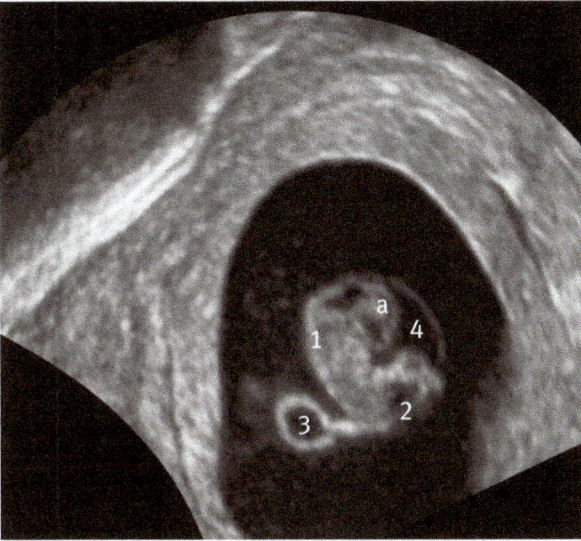

Fig. 1.18: 2D Ultrasound. (1) Embryo in Gestational Week 7 + 3: (a) head flexure, (2) developing umbilical cord as ductus omphaloentericus towards (3) the yolk sac. (4) Surrounding amniotic membrane (by courtesy of Prof. Dr. Chaoui, Prenatal diagnostic center, Berlin, Germany).

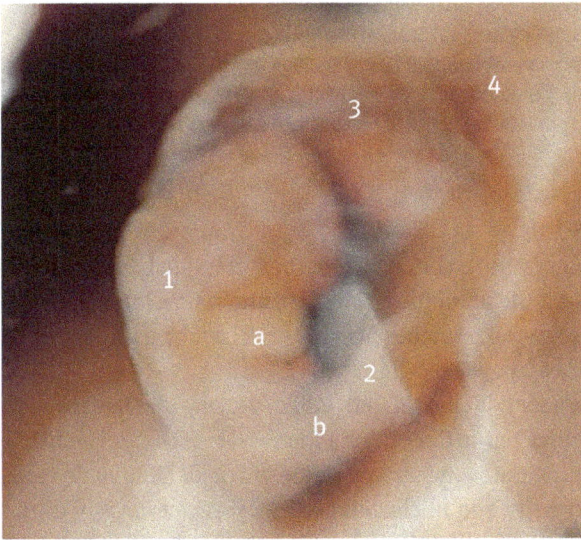

Fig. 1.19: 3 D Ultrasound. (1) Embryo in Gestational Week 8: (a) buds of the arms and (b) legs, (2) ductus omphaloentericus towards the (3) yolk sac and enveloped by the (4) amniotic membrane. The surrounding fluid is the extra-embryonic coelom (by courtesy of Prof. Dr. Chaoui, Prenatal diagnostic center, Berlin, Germany).

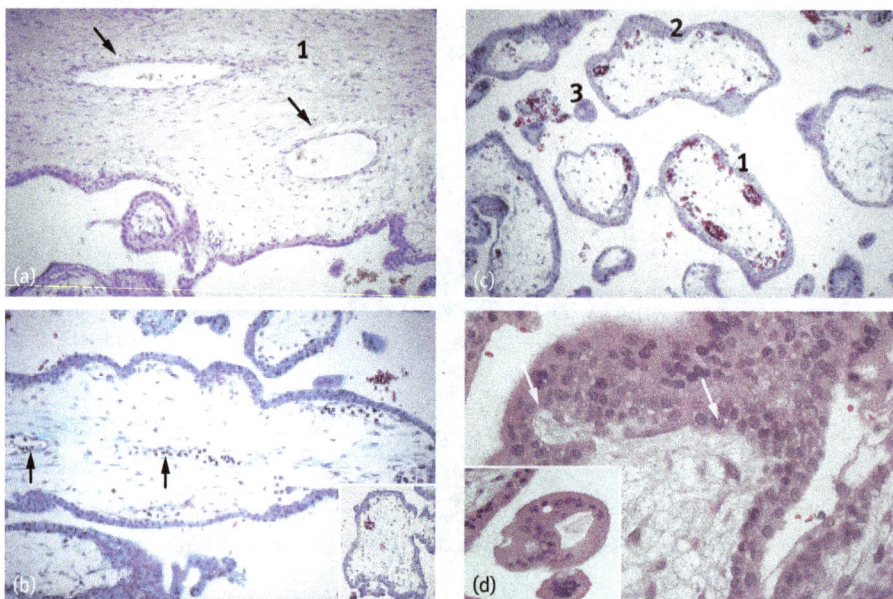

Fig. 1.20: (a) Gestational Week 8. (1) Chorionic plate with subamniotic and paravascular loosely meshed fibers, thin walled fetal vessels (arrows). (b) Stem villus with centrally located vessels and a loose and incomplete paravascular fiber network (inlet) (arrows). (c) Peripheral villi with embryonic stroma. (1) Capillaries subepithelially, (2) double-layered villous trophoblast, (3) syncytial sprouts in the intervillous space. (d) Villous sprout (arrows) with a mesenchymal stroma without capillaries, syncytial sprout (inlet).

Placenta in Gestational Week 9/10

The chorionic plate shows an increase in connective tissue, orientated in parallel fibers, and dense collagen beneath the amniotic epithelium and alongside the umbilical cord vessel branches. These vessel branches are characterized by a thin, smooth muscle layer with desmin and actin positive cells.

The villous tree shows, cross sectionally, ca. 9–10 villi of varying diameter in each MPF. Loosely arranged collagenous tissue fibers along the vessels of the stem villi are visible in the basal periphery. Generally, the stroma of the villi is of embryonic type, it shows variation in nuclear density and nucleated erythrocytes can be seen in the fetal vessel lumen. The chorionic epithelium is mainly flat, double-layered and gaps in the trophoblast cell layer are only partially visible. Nuclear sprouts develop on the villous surface and free syncytiotrophoblast cell groups can be found in the intervillous space.

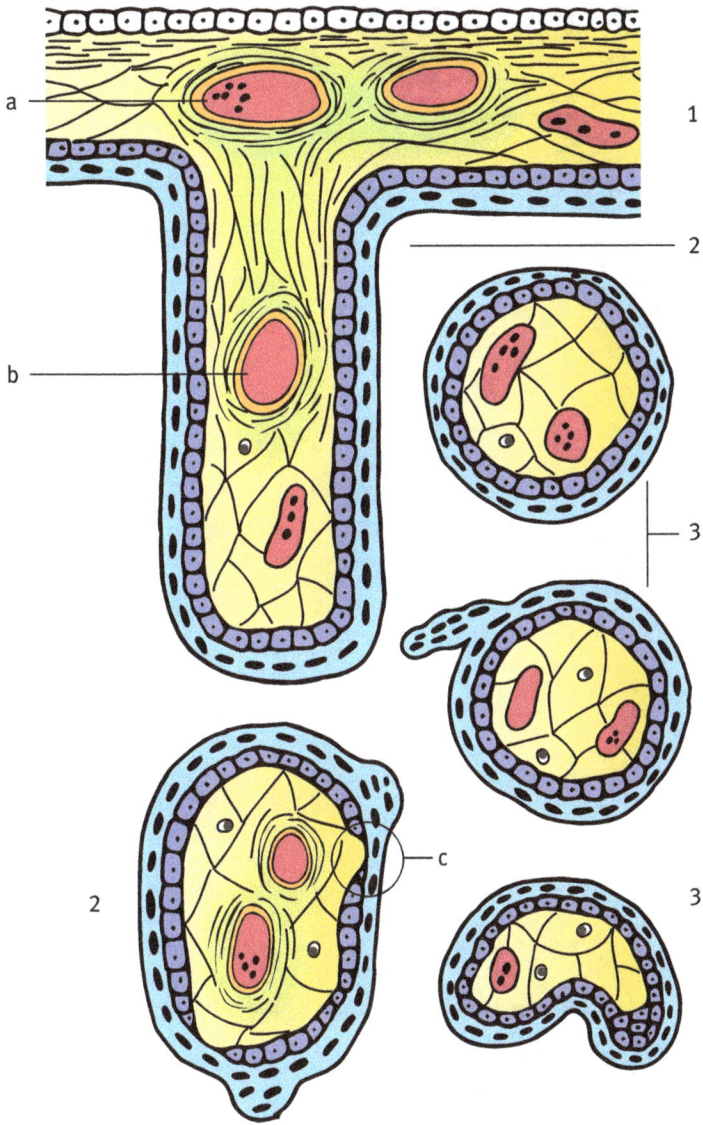

Fig. 1.21: Illustration. Histological characteristics in Gestational Week 9/10: (1) chorionic plate, (2) proximal portion of a stem villus proliferating from the chorionic plate, (3) peripheral villi with terminal ramifications and an increased number of peripheral villi (cross section), (a) fetal vessel with slender tunica media and nucleated red blood cells in the vessel lumen, (b) fetal vessel with paravascular collagenous fibers in the proximal part of the stem villus, (c) few gaps in the cytotrophoblast.

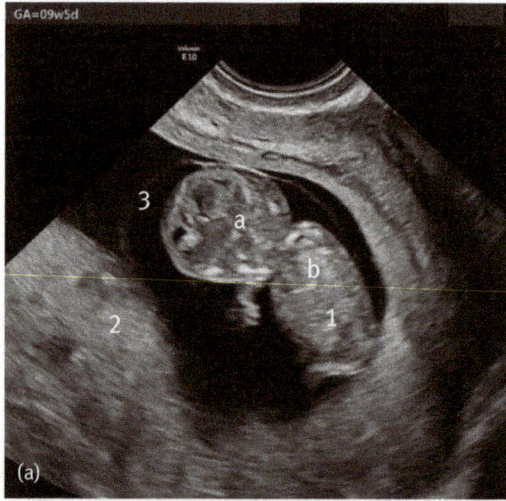

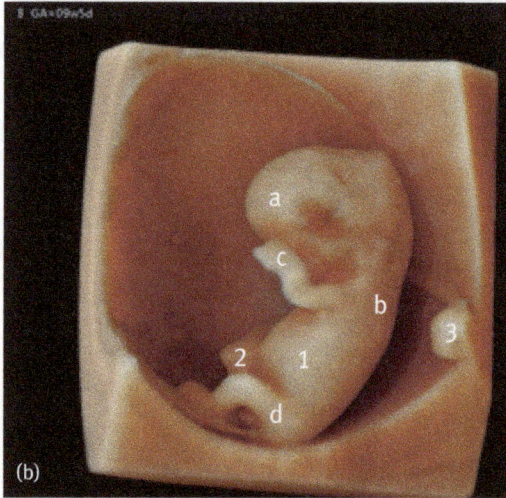

Fig. 1.22: (a) 2D Ultrasound. (1) Fetus in Gestational Week 9 + 5: (a) head, (b) body, (2) developing placenta, (3) amniotic membrane around the fetus (by courtesy of Prof. Chaoui, Prenatal diagnostic center, Berlin, Germany). (b) 3D Ultrasound. (1) Fetus in Gestational Week 9 + 5: (a) head, (b) body, (c) hand, (d) leg. The umbilical cord (2) becomes thinner and the yolk sac (3) behind the fetus is regressing (by courtesy of Prof. Dr. Chaoui, Prenatal diagnostic center, Berlin, Germany).

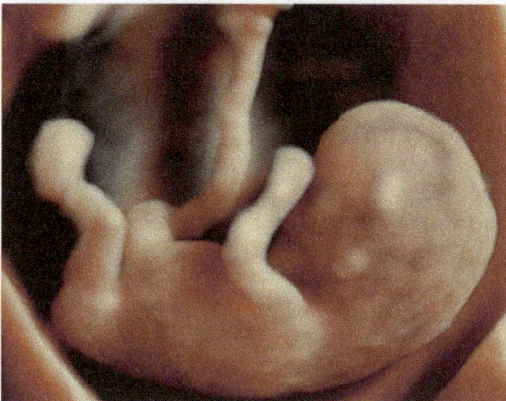

Fig. 1.23: 3D Ultrasound in Gestational Week 9: (by courtesy of Dr. Brückmann, Office Prenatal diagnostic, Erfurt, Germany).

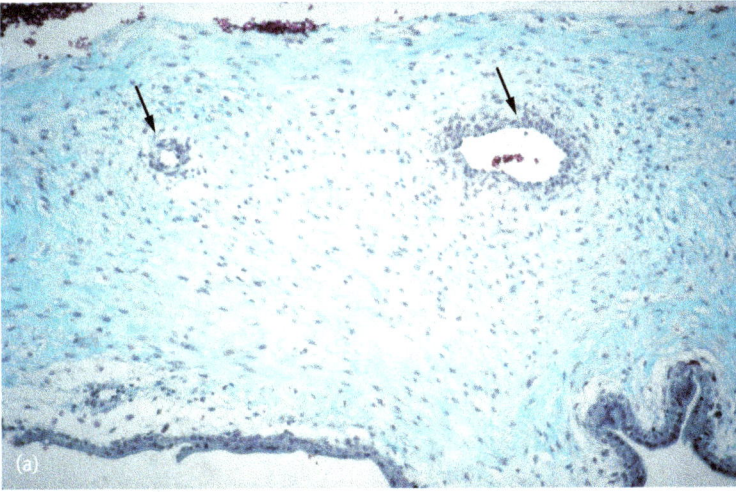

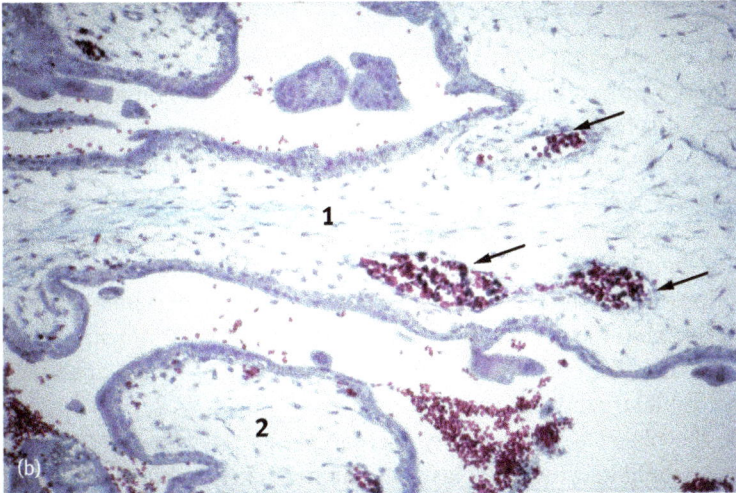

Fig. 1.24: (a) Histology in Gestational Week 10: chorionic plate with cell rich and stream like connective tissue, fetal vessel branches with tunica media (arrows). (b) (1) Stem villus with stream like collagenous fibers, (arrows) fetal vessels containing nucleated red blood cells, (2) peripheral villi.

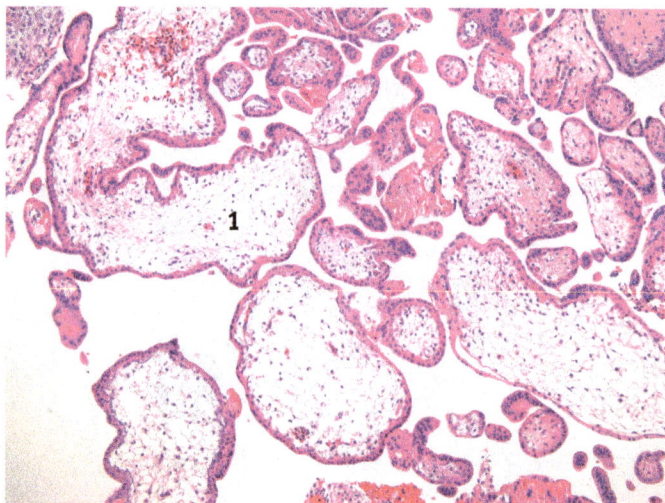

Fig. 1.25: (1) Peripheral villi of varying diameter with a nuclearrich epithelial layer (by courtesy of PD Dr. C. Tennstedt-Schenk, Mühlhausen, Germany).

Placenta in Gestational Week 11/12

The chorionic plate shows a collagenous stroma. The central vessels contain a tunica media, and in the suprachorionic stroma a few capillaries can be found.

The villous tree shows a gradual transition from larger to smaller diameter villi. The stem villi adjacent to the chorionic plate contain paravascular collagenous tissue fibers, and even vessel branches in the periphery can demonstrate a tunica media. The stroma of the stem villi is more tightly organized than the loose embryonic stroma of the peripheral villi and each villus contains one, or more, capillaries. Primarily non-nucleated erythrocytes can be seen in the vessel lumina. The syncytiotrophoblast is flat and the cytotrophoblast shows multiple gaps. The intervillous space shows multiple syncytial trophoblast sprouts.

Additionally, the placenta in the embryonic period shows trophoblast islands consisting of the basophilic cytotrophoblast, the intermediate trophoblast and the syncytiotrophoblast.

Small fibrin deposits on the villous surface, and later in the intervillous space, are regularly visible from gestational week 8 onwards.

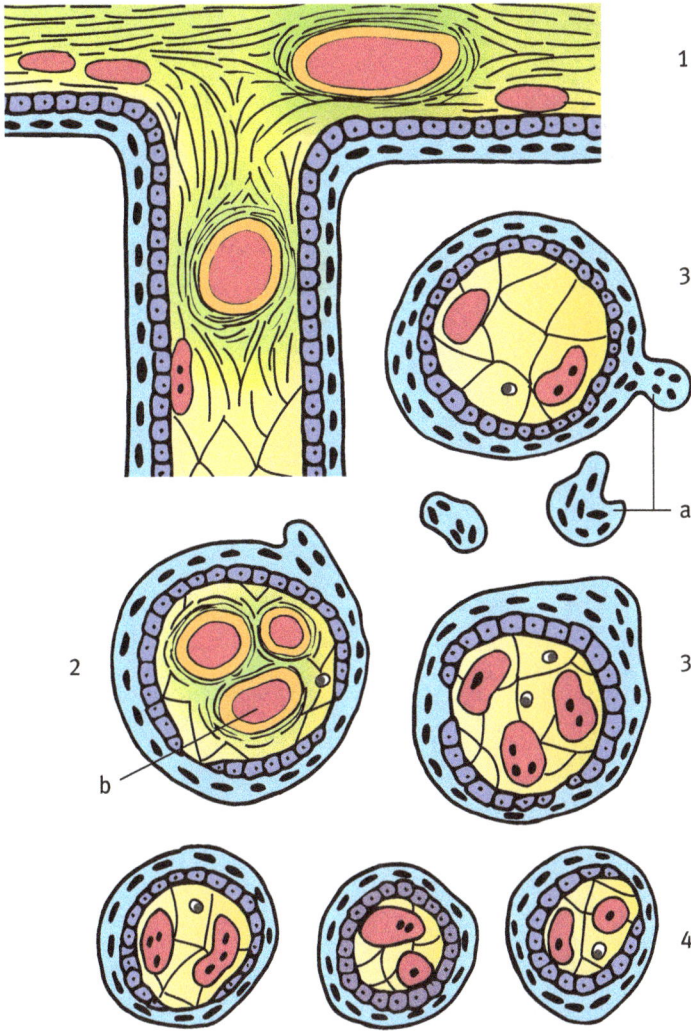

Fig. 1.26: Illustration. Histological characteristics in Gestational Week 11/12: (1) chorionic plate, (2) stem villus (cross section), (3, 4) increased number of peripheral villi (cross section), (a) trophoblast sprouts, (b) relatively thick tunica media within vessels in a distal stem villus.

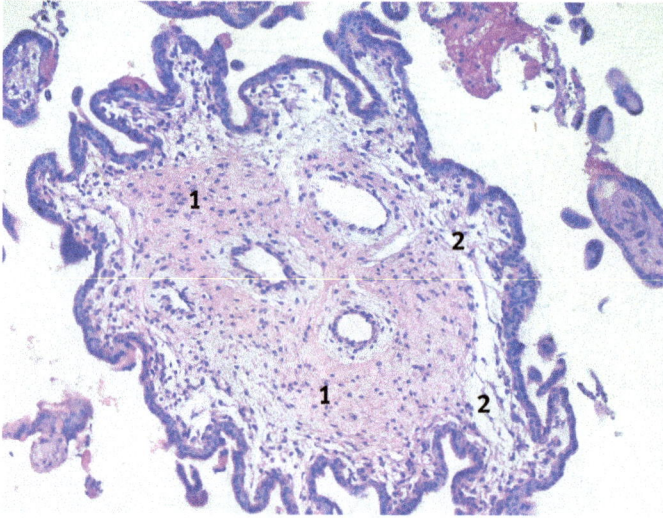

Fig. 1.27: Histology in Gestational Week 11. Subchorionic stem villus: (1) thick paravascular fiber ring, (2) loose and immature stroma in the subepithelial periphery (by courtesy of PD Dr. C. Tennstedt-Schenk, Mühlhausen, Germany).

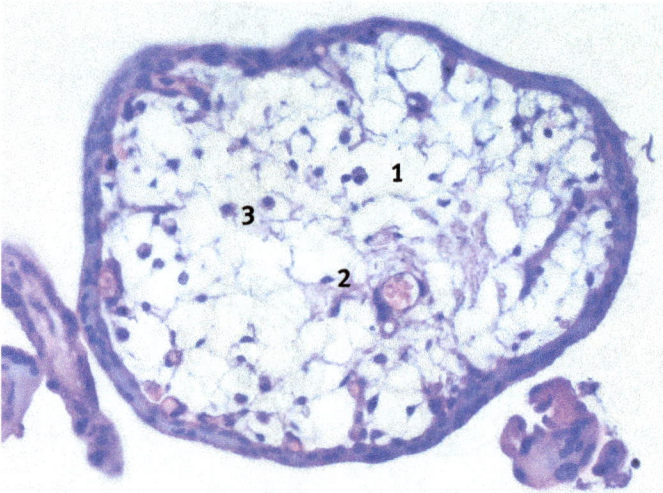

Fig. 1.28: Histology in Gestational Week 11. Peripheral chorionic villus: (1) loose embryonic stroma, (2) central and subepithelial fetal capillaries, (3) Hofbauer cells (by courtesy of PD Dr. C. Tennstedt-Schenk, Mühlhausen, Germany).

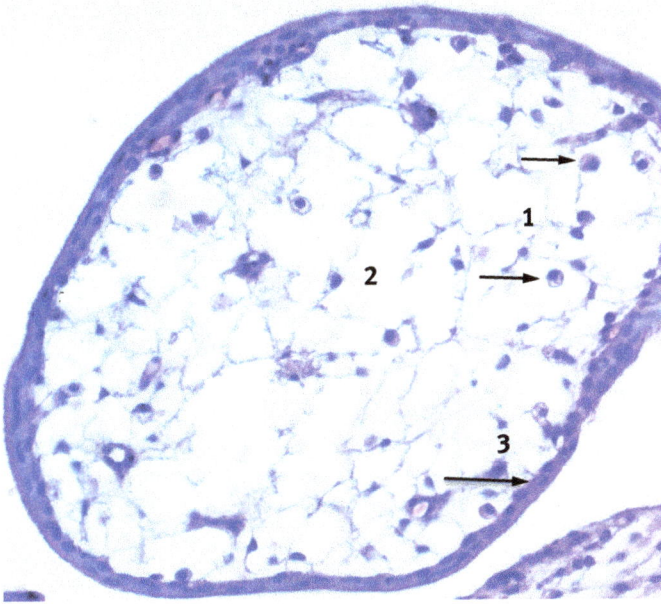

Fig. 1.29: Peripheral villus. (1) Loosely packed stroma, (2) Hofbauer cells (black arrows), (3) few cytotrophoblast gaps (by courtesy of PD Dr. C. Tennstedt-Schenk).

1.3.4 Histology from middle to late pregnancy (Gestational Week 16–40)

In the fetal period, villous maturation to term is characterized by:
- numeric and longitudinal growth of the villi with branching (seen in cross sections as increasing villous density per unit area),
- intravillus vessel and capillary growth,
- stromal differentiation,
- villous trophoblast differentiation.

Table 1.2: Percentage distribution in a MPF of the different types of villi from Gestational Week 16 to 40 (modified after M. Vogel) [26].

GW	Distribution of villous types	Villous types in %	Villous types
16		= 20	stem villi
		> 50	intermediate villi, central type
		30	intermediate villi, peripheral type
20		> 10	stem villi
		50	intermediate villi, central type
		< 40	intermediate villi, peripheral type
24		10	stem villi
		> 30	intermediate villi, central type
		50	intermediate villi, peripheral type
		< 10	terminal villi

Table 1.2: (continued) Percentage distribution in a MPF of the different types of villi from Gestational Week 16 to 40 (modified after M. Vogel) [26].

GW	Distribution of villous types	Villous types in %	Villous types
28		10	stem villi
		< 20	intermediate villi, central type
		> 50	intermediate villi, peripheral type
		20	terminal villi
32		10	stem villi
		10	intermediate villi, central type
		50	intermediate villi, peripheral type
		= 30	terminal villi
36		= 10	stem villi
		= 5	intermediate villi, central type
		> 40	intermediate villi, peripheral type
		< 40	terminal villi
40		10	stem villi
		> 30	intermediate villi, peripheral type
		< 60	terminal villi

dark green = stem villi; yellow = intermediate villi, central type; light green = intermediate villi, peripheral type; red = terminal villi (see Fig. 1.48)

Placenta in Gestational Week 16

In the early fetal period, the chorionic plate has reached its definitive form and subsequent alterations of the structure are considered to be caused by secondary changes, such as inflammatory, diffusion or metabolic disturbances and vascular malperfusion.

The villous tree is characterized by uniformly distributed medium sized villi, predominantly of the intermediate type (greater than 50 % are of the central immature type and 30 % of the peripheral mature type). They are characterized by a loose reticular stroma with stromal canaliculi. The syncytial trophoblast is flat with uniform nuclei and the cytotrophoblast shows gaps and epithelial knots, as well as epithelial invaginations, at the surface. Capillaries are, in low numbers, attached to the basal membrane of the syncytiotrophoblast and this arrangement is a precursor to the vasculosyncytial membranes. The medium diffusion distance at this stage is measured to be ca. 40 nm [25].

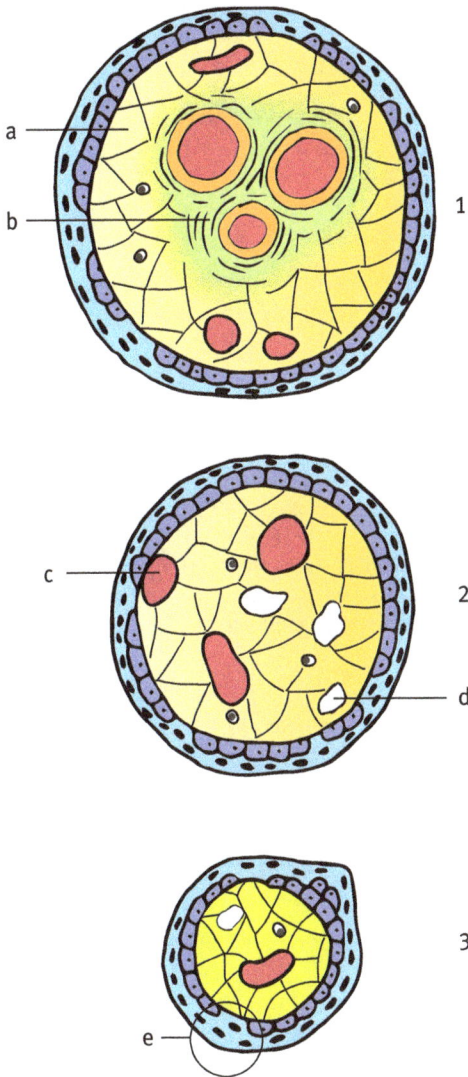

Fig. 1.30: Illustration. Histological characteristics in Gestational Week 16: (1) stem villus, (2) intermediate villus of the central immature type, (3) intermediate villus of the peripheral mature type, (a) subepithelial embryonic / loose reticular stroma, (b) fetal vessel surrounded by circumferential connective tissue fibers, (c) subepithelial fetal capillaries, (d) stromal canaliculi, (e) cytotrophoblast with gaps and syncytial sprouts.

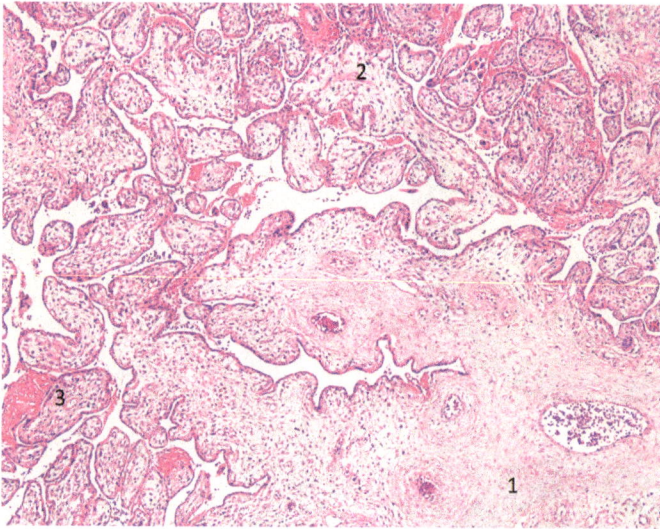

Fig. 1.31: Histology in Gestational Week 16 MPF (Medium Power Field): (1) stem villi with embryonic stroma and central fetal vessels with a tunica media, (2) intermediate villi of the central immature type, (3) intermediate villi of the peripheral type with a smaller diameter and greater cellular density.

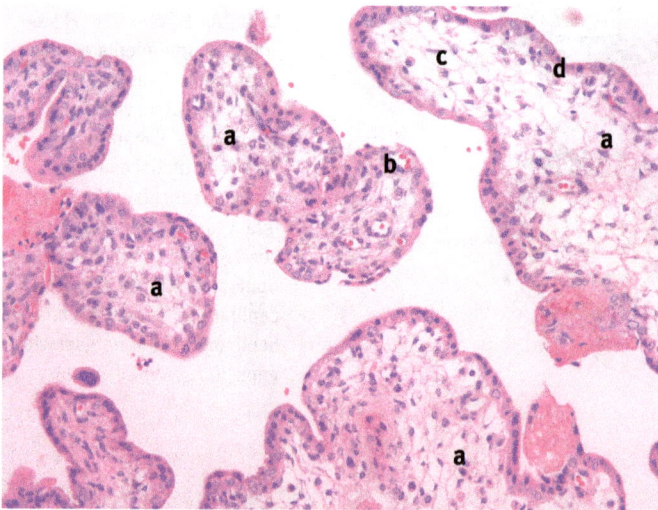

Fig. 1.32: Histology in Gestational Week 16 (HPF): (a) intermediate villi of the central immature type, with reticular and embryonic stroma; (b) subepithelial fetal capillaries; (c) stromal canaliculi; (d) cytotrophoblast gaps.

Placenta in Gestational Week 20
Differentiation into three villous subtypes occurs at this time:
1. stem villi
2. intermediate villi
3. terminal villi

Each subtype has a distinct function and these subtypes represent 2% of the villous surface. At this stage of gestation the medium diffusion distance is 27.7 nm [25].

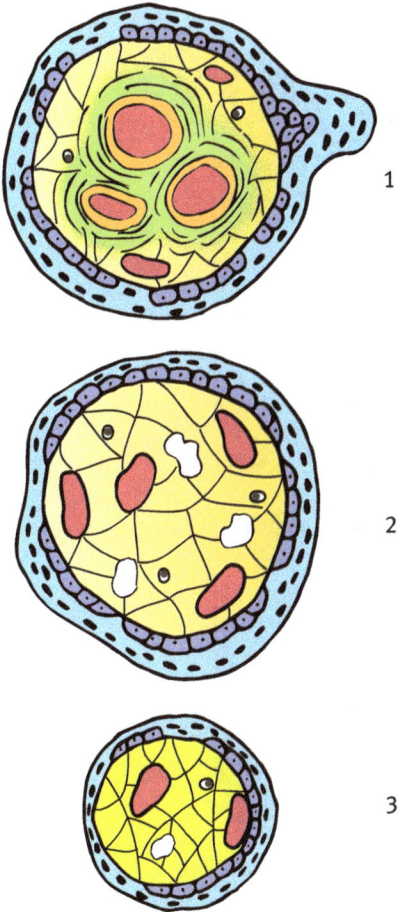

Fig. 1.33: Illustration. Histological characteristics in Gestational Week 20: (1) stem villus; (2) intermediate villus of the central immature type with embryonic stroma, Hofbauer cells and canaliculi (empty spaces); (3) intermediate villus of the peripheral type with a small diameter, loose reticular stroma and capillaries that are sometimes tightly related to the cell rich villous epithelium.

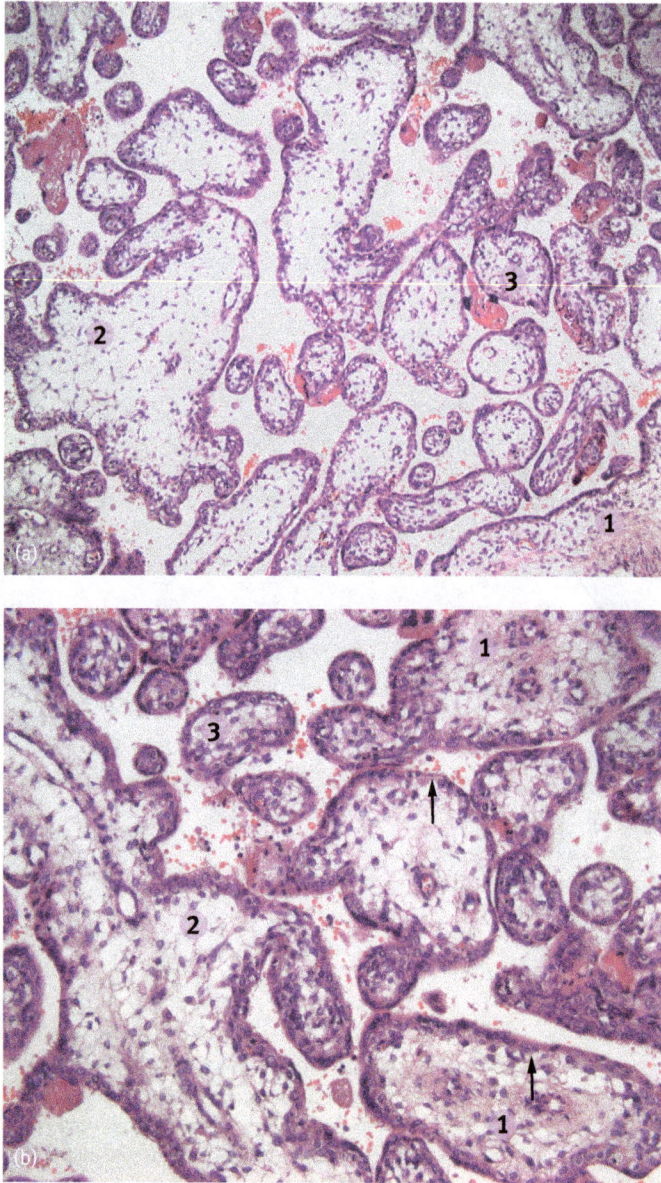

Fig. 1.34: Villous histology and distribution in Gestational Week 20: (a) (1) stem villus with a central vessel, containing a tunica media, and subepithelially an immature stroma; (2) intermediate villi of the central type with a embryonic stroma; (3) intermediate villi of the peripheral mature type with a reticular stroma and a higher cellular density. (b) Stem villus with reticular and embryonic stroma; (2) Intermediate villi of the peripheral type with a reticular stroma, a higher cellular density, villous trophoblast with cytotrophoblast gaps (arrows).

Placenta in Gestational Week 24

Uniform branching of the villous tree is seen and ca. 80 % of the villous cross sections are of intermediate villi.

The intermediate villi are of the central type and are characterized by a loose and immature stroma with Hofbauer cells, whereas the stroma of the intermediate villi of the peripheral mature type (accounting for 50 % of villi in a MPF at this stage of

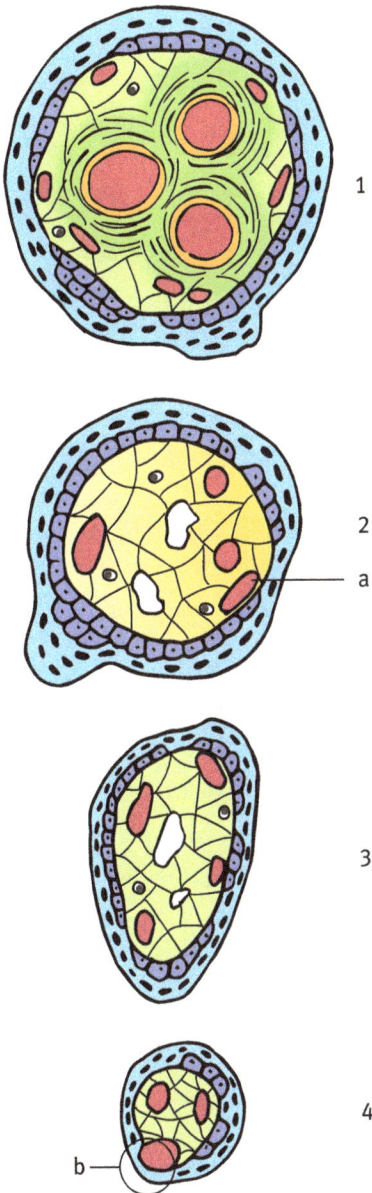

Fig. 1.35: Illustration. Histological characteristics in Gestational Week 24: (1) stem villus with dense and fiber rich paravascular stroma;(2) intermediate villus of the central immature type; (3) intermediate villus of the peripheral mature type; (4) terminal villus; (a) fetal capillaries close to, and beneath, the gaps of the nuclear rich syncytiotrophoblast and irregular cytotrophoblast; (b) vasculosyncytial membranes.

gestation) (Table 1.2) is more nuclear rich but contains less Hofbauer cells. Both types of intermediate villi show a nuclear rich syncytiotrophoblast and irregular cytotrophoblast gaps.

The terminal villi are characterized by a condensed stroma and few vasculosyncytial membranes. The medium maternal-fetal diffusion distance is more than 20 nm [27].

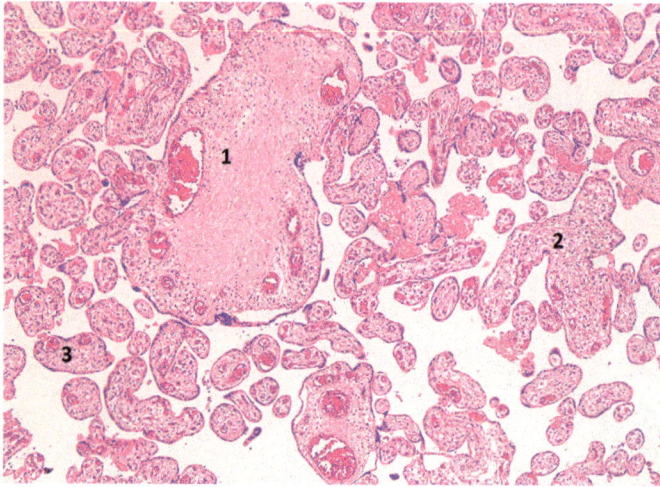

Fig. 1.36: Villous histology and distribution in Gestational Week 24: (1) stem villus, (2) intermediate villi with immature and mature stroma, (3) terminal villus with vasculosyncytial membranes.

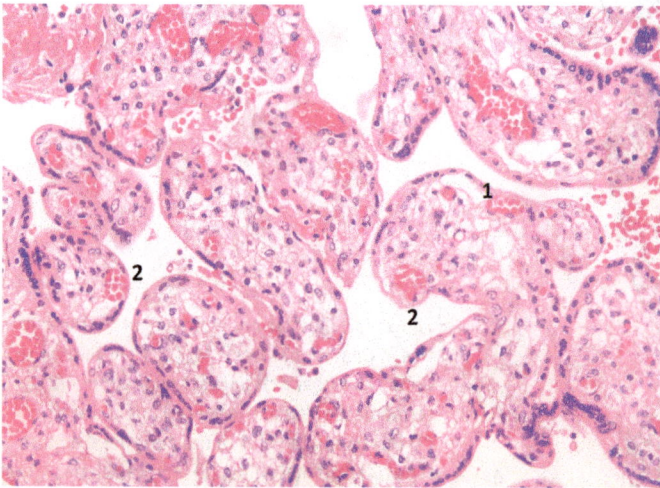

Fig. 1.37: Histology in Gestational Week 24: (1) fetal capillaries beneath the trophoblasts, (2) vasculosyncytial membranes in a terminal villus.

Placenta in Gestational Week 28

The fundamental differences in comparison to GW 24 are an increased villous density and an increased number of small diameter villi. 70 % of the villi are of the intermediate peripheral type, which have stromal canaliculi. Intermediate villi with a loose stroma and Hofbauer cells are rare. The chorionic epithelium of the stem and intermediate villi is double-layered with a nuclear rich syncytiotrophoblast.

The terminal villi show some sinusoidal dilatation of the capillaries and vasculosyncytial membranes.

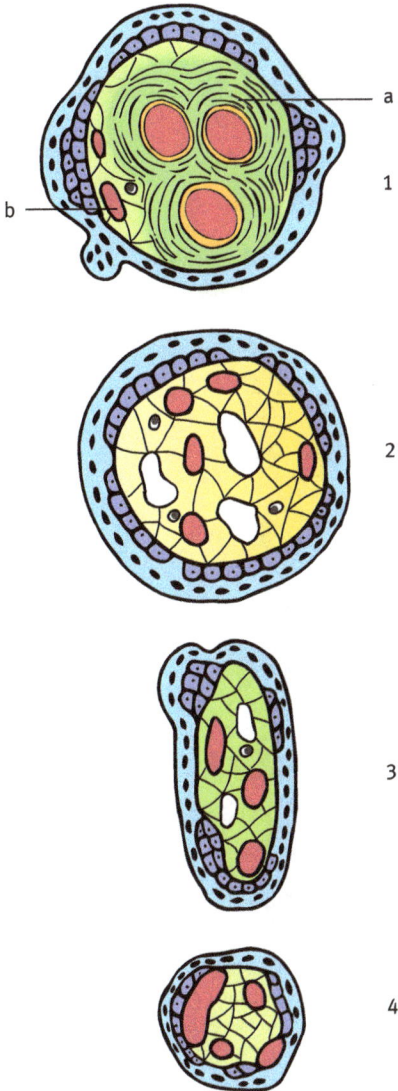

Fig. 1.38: Illustration. Histological characteristics in Gestational Week 28: (1) stem villus, (2) intermediate villus of the central immature type, (3) intermediate villus of the peripheral mature type, (4) terminal villus, (a) paravascular connective tissue ring, (b) fetal capillaries located under the epithelium with a reduced stromal rim.

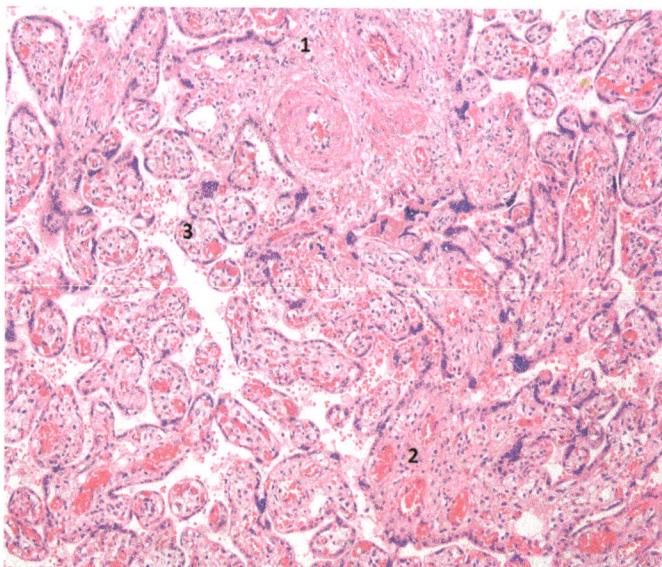

Fig. 1.39: Villous histology and distribution in Gestational Week 28: (1) stem villus, (2) intermediate villi with a loose reticular stroma and few stromal canaliculi, (3) terminal villi.

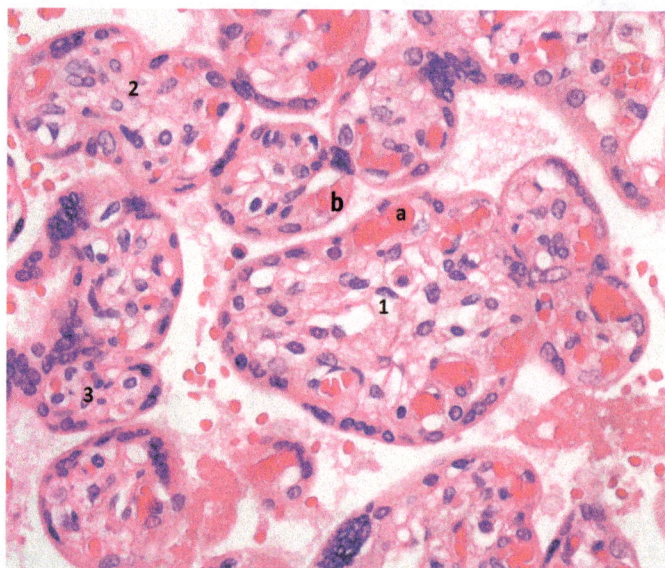

Fig. 1.40: Histology in Gestational Week 28: (1) intermediate villi with an immature reticular stroma of varying cellular density, (2) intermediate villi with a loose reticular stroma and few stromal canaliculi, (3) terminal villi, (a) subepithelial capillaries, residual nuclear in the epithelium, (b) vasculo-syncytial membranes.

Placenta in Gestational Week 32

An increased number of small diameter and uniformly branched villi, containing a loose collagenous stroma, are seen. The intermediate villi, with immature stroma and few Hofbauer cells, only represent 10 % of all villi.

Terminal villi show a cell rich, precursor tissue *"Platzhaltergewebe"* in their axes and subepithelial sinusoidal dilatation of the capillaries.

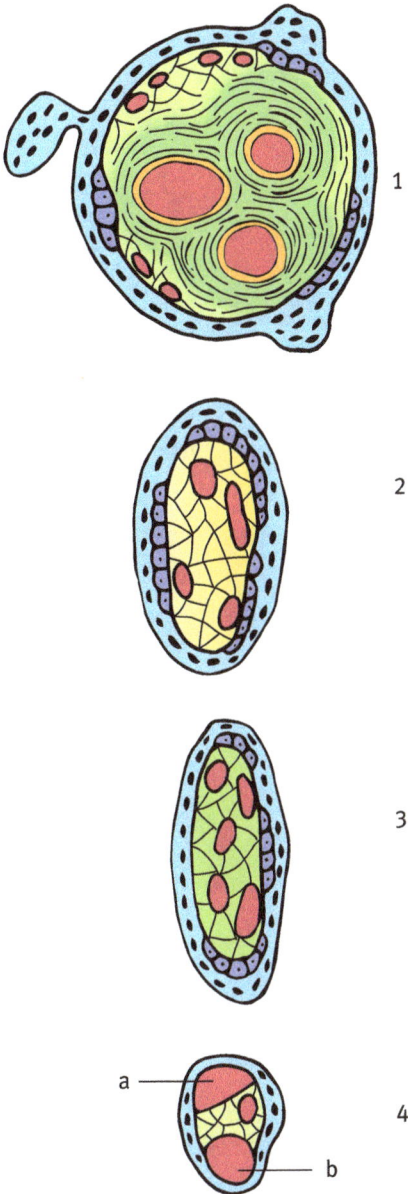

Fig. 1.41: Illustration. Histological characteristics in Gestational Week 32: (1) stem villus, (2) intermediate villus of the central immature type, (3) intermediate villus of the peripheral mature type, (4) terminal villus with (a, b) subepithelial sinusoidal dilatation of the capillaries.

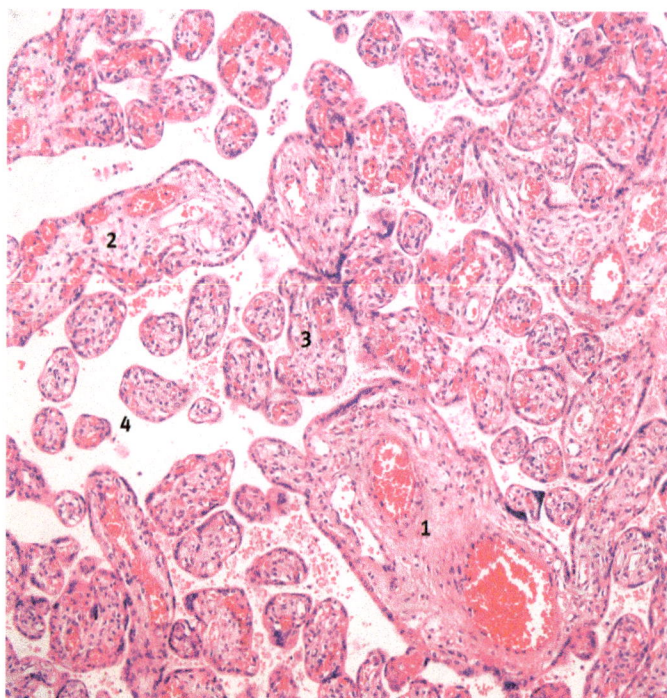

Fig. 1.42: Villous distribution in Gestational Week 32: (1) stem villus, (2) intermediate villus of the central immature type, (3) intermediate villus of the peripheral mature type, (4) terminal villi.

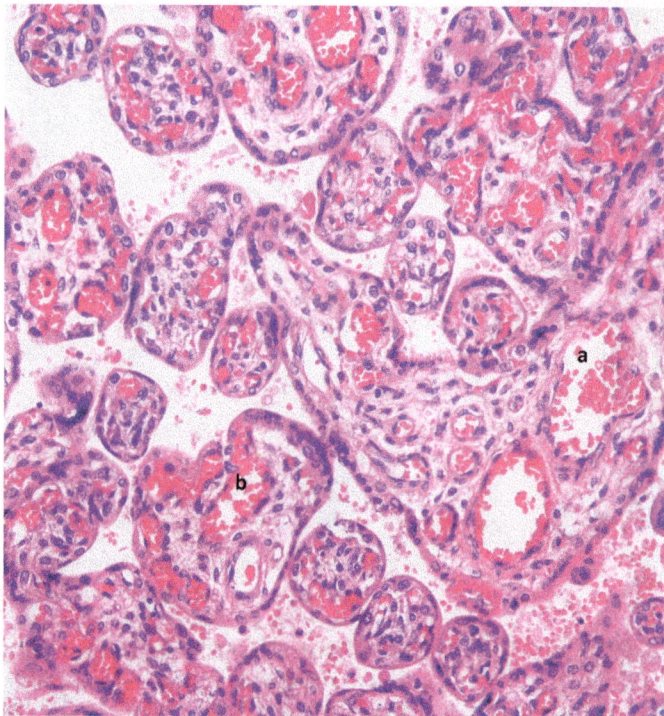

Fig. 1.43: Histology in Gestational Week 32: (a, b) subepithelial sinusoidal dilatation of the capillaries.

The villous surface measures ca. 80 % of the expected term placenta; 50 % of which contains capillaries and with vasculosyncytial membrane development in 10–15 %.

Placenta in Gestational Week 36

Intermediate villi of the peripheral type and terminal villi dominate the histological picture. The intermediate villi of the immature type are not equally represented in every MPF but are more prominent centrally in the feto-maternal circulatory unit.

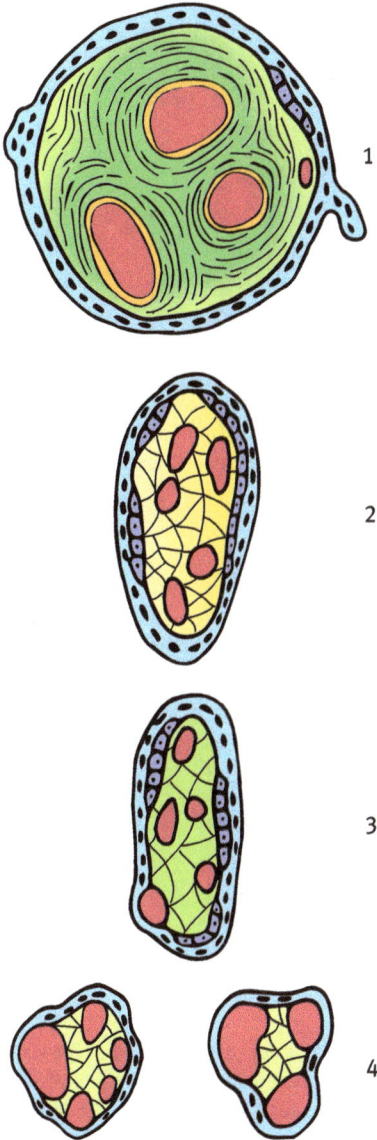

Fig. 1.44: Illustration. Histological characteristics in Gestational Week 36: (1) stem villus with small rests of subepithelial stroma; (2) intermediate villus of the central immature type with embryonic stroma and a dense nuclear villous trophoblast; (3) intermediate villus of the peripheral mature type, capillary rich and with partly developed vasculosyncytial membranes; (4) terminal villi containing capillaries and sinusoids that are in contact with the epithelium and with frequent formation of vasculosyncytial membranes.

Terminal villi contain capillaries and sinusoids which are separated by cell rich stromal bands. Each terminal villus contains several vasculosyncytial membranes and the maternal-fetal diffusion distance is decreased to 11.7 nm [25].

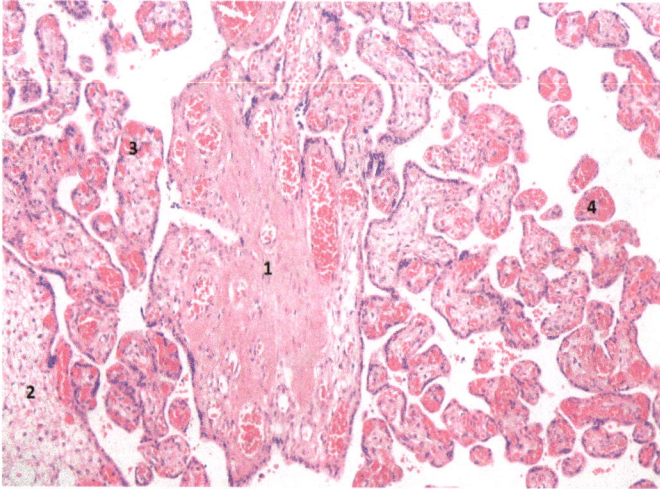

Fig. 1.45: Villous distribution in Gestational Week 36: (1) stem villus, (2) intermediate villus of the central immature type, (3) intermediate villus of the peripheral mature type, (4) terminal villi.

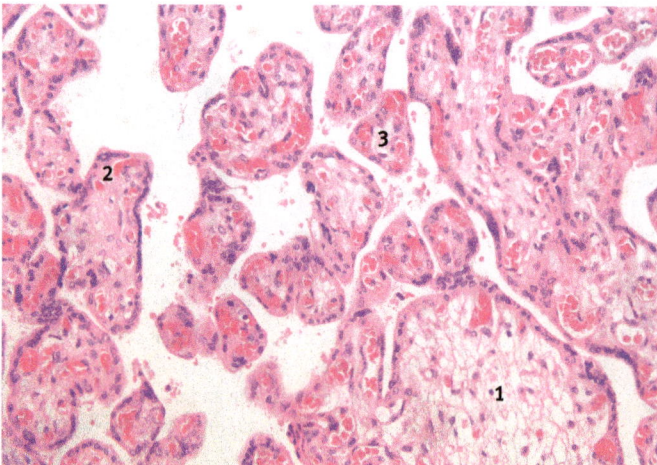

Fig. 1.46: Histology in Gestational Week 36: (1) intermediate villus of central immature type with an embryonic stroma and a nuclear rich villous trophoblast, (2) intermediate villus of peripheral mature type with several capillaries and some vasculosyncytial membranes, (3) terminal villi with fetal capillaries and sinusoids adjacent to the epithelium and frequent vasculosyncytial membranes.

Placenta in Gestational Week 40

Terminal villi dominate the mature placenta in each MPF. ⅓ of MPFs show intermediate villi, of which 1–2% are of the central immature villous type and are located
centrally in the feto-maternal circulatory unit. In contrast to maturation disorders,
branching is regular with proliferation of the peripheral intermediate villi and terminal villi. In both the mature intermediate and terminal villi, the capillaries are located
close to each other. Dilated sinusoidal capillaries in the terminal villi are reported to
belong to the venous system [28].

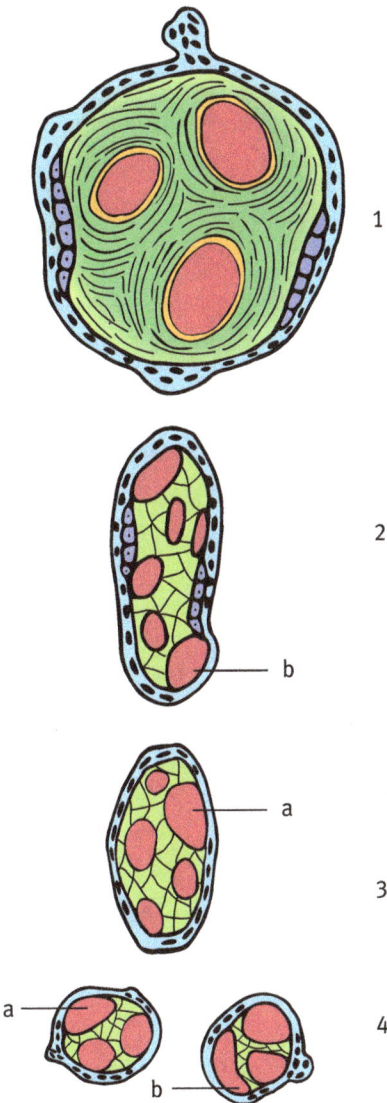

Fig. 1.47: Illustration. Histological characteristics in Gestational Week 40: (1) stem villus,
(2) intermediate villus of the central immature
type, (3) intermediate villus of the peripheral immature type, (4) terminal villi, (a) subepithelial
capillaries, (b) vasculosyncytial membranes.

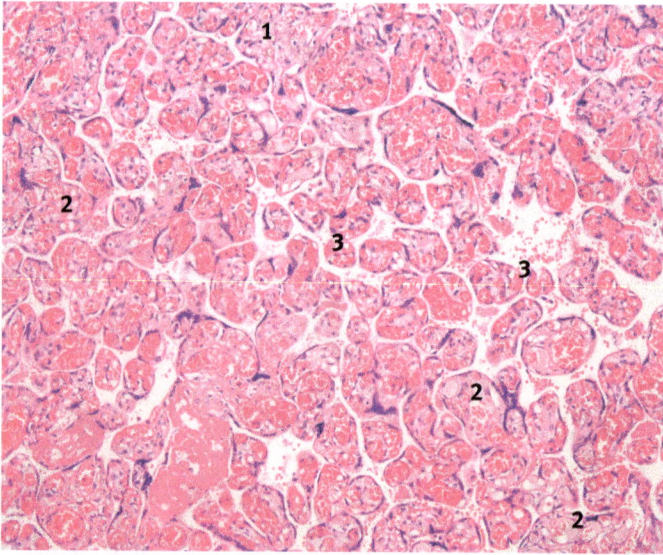

Fig. 1.48: Villous distribution, predominantly intermediate villi and terminal villi, in gestational week 40: (1) intermediate villus of the central immature type, (2) intermediate villus of the peripheral mature type, (3) terminal villi.

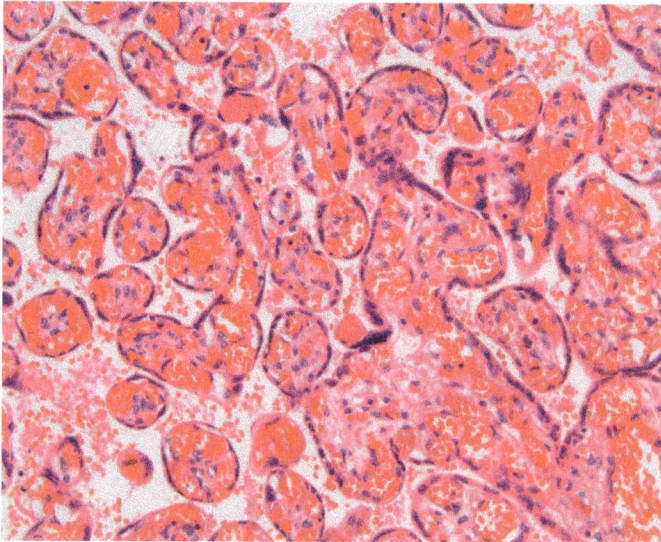

Fig. 1.49: Histology in Gestational Week 36: terminal villi with vasculosyncytial membranes and some syncytial sprouts. No subepithelial stroma is seen.

In the terminal villi each capillary and sinusoid is connected to the chorionic epithelium, in contrast to the capillaries of the peripheral intermediate villi which are close to, but not connected, to the surface and are located centrally in the villous stroma.

Approximately 40 % of the villous surface is transformed into vasculosyncytial membranes and the medium maternal-foetal diffusion distance is now 4.8 nm [25].

References

[1] Faye-Petersen OM, Heller DS, Joshi VV. Placental Pathology. NY: Taylor & Francis; 2006.
[2] Benirschke K, Burton GJ, Baergen RN. Pathology of the Human Placenta. 6 ed. Heidelberg, NY, London: Springer; 2012.
[3] Gruenwald P. The development of the placental lobular pattern in the human. Review and rein-terpretation of the material. Obstetrics and gynecology. 1977;49(6):728–732.
[4] Boyd ID, Hamilton WJ. The Human Placenta. Cambridge: Heffer; 1970. 365 p.
[5] Wilkin P. Pathologie du Placenta. Paris: Masson; 1965.
[6] Wigglesworth JS, Singer DB. Textbook of fetal and perinatal pathology. Oxford: Blackwell; 1991.
[7] Gruenwald P. Fetal deprivation and placental pathology: concepts and relationships. Perspectives in pediatric pathology. 1975;2:101–149.
[8] Gruenwald P. The placenta and its maternal supply line. Lancaster: Medicine and Technic; 1975.
[9] Kaufmann P, Sen DK. Scweikhart G. Classification of human placental villi. Cell Tissue Res (Histology): 1979;200:409–426.
[10] Graf R, Schonfelder G, Muhlberger M, Gutsmann M. The perivascular contractile sheath of human placental stem villi: its isolation and characterization. Placenta. 1995;16(1):57–66.
[11] Arts NF. Investigations on the vascular system of the placenta. I. General introduction and the fetal vascular system. American journal of obstetrics and gynecology. 1961;82:147–158.
[12] Lutz J, Backé G, Huang X, Brinckwirth B, Vogel M. Immunhistochemischer Nachweis von KP-1 positiven Makrophagen in Blasenmolen und Partialmolen – ein Beitrag zur Diskussion über die Herkunft der Hofbauerzelle. VerhDtschGesPathol. 1994;78:579.
[13] Castellucci M, Zaccheo D. The Hofbauer cells of the human placenta: morphological and immunological aspects. Prog Clin Biol Res. 1989;296:443–451.
[14] Hormann G. [Contribution on functional morphology of the human placenta]. Arch Gynakol. 1954;184(1):109–123.
[15] Crawford JM. Vascular anatomy of the human placenta. American journal of obstetrics and gynecology. 1962;84:1543–1567.
[16] Freese UE. The uteroplacental vascular relationship in the human. American journal of obstetrics and gynecology. 1968;101(1):8–16.
[17] Ramsey EM, Donner MW. Placental vasculature and circulation. Stuttgart: Thieme; 1980.
[18] Schuhmann R, Kraus H, Borst R, Geier G. [Regionally different activity of enzymes within placentones of human term-placentas. Histochemical and biochemical investigations (author's transl)]. Arch Gynakol. 1976;220(3):209–226.
[19] Bauer C, Jelkmann W, Moll W. High oxygen affinity of maternal blood reduces fetal weight in rats. Respiration physiology. 1981;43(2):169–178.
[20] Carter AM. Comparative studies of placentation and immunology in non-human primates suggest a scenario for the evolution of deep trophoblast invasion and an explanation for human pregnancy disorders. Reproduction (Cambridge, England). 2011;141(4):391–396.

[21] Carter AM, Enders AC, Pijnenborg R. The role of invasive trophoblast in implantation and placentation of primates. Philosophical transactions of the Royal Society of London Series B, Biological sciences. 2015;370(1663):20140070.

[22] Pijnenborg R. Implantation and immunology: maternal inflammatory and immune cellular responses to implantation and trophoblast invasion. Reproductive biomedicine online. 2002;4(3):14–17.

[23] Pijnenborg R, Aplin JD, Ain R, et al. Trophoblast and the endometrium--a workshop report. Placenta. 2004;25(Suppl A):42-44.

[24] Vogel M. [Histological stages of development of the chorionic villi in the embryonal and early fetal period (5th to 20th week of pregnancy)]. Pathologe. 1986;7(1):59–61.

[25] Schiebler TH, Kaufmann P. Reife Plazenta. In: Becker V, Schiebler TH, Kubli F, (Eds). Die Plazenta des Menschen. Stuttgart: Thieme; 1981. p. 51–100.

[26] Vogel M. Atlas der morphologischen Plazentadiagnostik. 1. ed. Berlin: Springer; 1992.

[27] Vogel M. Atlas der morphologischen Plazentadiagnostik. 2 ed. Berlin: Springer; 1996.

[28] Nikolov SD, Schiebler TH. [Fetal blood vessel system of the human full-term placenta]. Z Zellforsch Mikrosk Anat. 1973;139(3):333–350.

2 Pathological examination of the placenta and membranes

2.1 Preliminary remarks

The pathological examination of the placenta and its membranes should be a part of the routine investigation of all at risk pregnancies and deliveries. The utility of this examination depends on a strict compliance with a pathological examination protocol, and protocols should include guidelines detailing macroscopic handling, sampling and histological assessment of the placenta. The information acquired from such an examination should be conveyed using standardized and easily understandable terminology; essential for interdisciplinary discussion and facilitating the exchange of information, both in diagnostic and research fields, globally. A simplified international placental classification system was suggested in 2012 [1] and following the consensus meeting of international perinatal and placental pathologists in Amsterdam in 2015, the international working group discussed, and agreed upon, the placental gross findings, sampling specifications, terminology and diagnostic criteria for such a classification system. The overall goal was to unify terminology and criteria for macroscopic and histological pathological placental examination and reporting worldwide [2,3].

2.2 Indication for a pathological-anatomical placental examination

Indications for examination:
- embryonic and fetal abortion,
- pre- or post-term delivery,
- intrauterine or intrapartum fetal death,
- intrauterine or intrapartum fetal hypoxia,
- prematurity (less than gestational week 30),
- placental abruption,
- IUGR/FGR and macrosomia,
- placental macrosomia or microsomia,
- fetal malformations,
- multiple pregnancy,
- amniotic infection,
- maternal infection during pregnancy,
- fetal infection,
- maternal diseases in pregnancy (chronic hypertension, preeclampsia/eclampsia, hypotension, diabetes mellitus, etc.),

https://doi.org/10.1515/9783110452600-002

- maternal drug abuse, (nicotine, alcohol, heroin, etc.),
- maternal environmental toxin exposure during pregnancy (x- rays, chemical substances, etc.),
- maternal-fetal incompatibility reactions (Rh-incompatibility included),
- fetal hydrops,
- habitual abortion,
- pregnancy complications or genetic disorders in prior pregnancies,
- oligohydramnion, anhydramnion and polyhydramnion,
- post-partum hemorrhage.

2.3 Clinical information

Relevant clinical information is essential for a useful pathophysiological interpretation of macroscopic and histological placental findings. Clinical information hidden within prose-like descriptions is counterproductive, and it will result in a substandard pathological report, one which may be incomprehensible to anyone but the examining pathologist. Such clinically useless reports, coupled with poor communication, will discourage clinicians from requesting a pathological examination of a placenta in the future [4].

Minimum clinical information required for placental examination:
- gestational age,
- birth weight,
- APGAR score,
- perinatal complications (CTG or/and STAN pathology),
- maternal disease in pregnancy,
- maternal bleeding,
- oligohydramnion, polyhydramnion,
- genetic malformation.

Gestational age is of great importance and not only for findings of maturation disorders. Even though the criteria for the histological diagnosis of maternal vascular malperfusion are not clearly defined, findings such as intervillous fibrin depositions differ in pre-term and term placentas. Different institutions use triage examination and storage systems to stratify high and low priority placentas on the basis of predicted clinical outcome [4].

2.4 Macroscopic examination

Macroscopic examination begins with:
- inspection of the placenta; chorionic surface and basal plate (Figs. 2.1, 2.2),
- placental net weight (without the umbilical cord and membranes),
- area measurement; maximum longitudinal and transverse diameters and average thickness (Fig. 2.3),
- inspection of the umbilical cord and membranes,
- inspection of serially cut slices (5–10 mm thick) (Fig. 2.10).

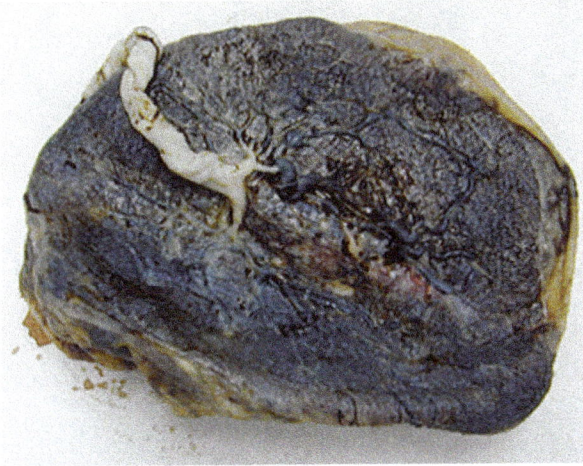

Fig. 2.1: Formalin fixed placenta. Chorionic/fetal plate with an off center umbilical cord insertion.

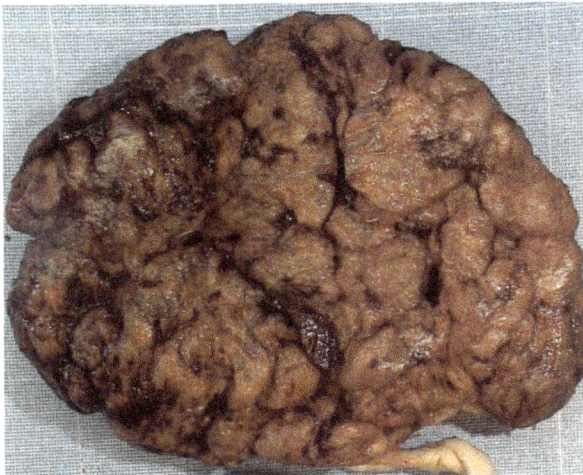

Fig. 2.2: Formalin fixed placenta. Basal/maternal plate with marked maternal basal lobes/caruncles/cotyledons.

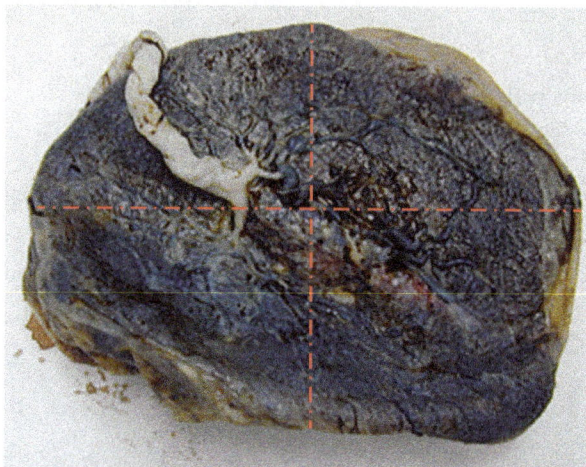

Fig. 2.3: Formalin fixed placenta at term. Red lines illustrating the measurement of the placenta in two dimensions.

2.4.1 Chorionic plate

The following changes on the chorionic plate should be documented:
– insertion of the umbilical cord (Ch. 3),
– appearance of the chorionic vessels,
– varicosis and aneurysm of the chorionic plate vessels,
– cysts and hematomas,
– fibrin plaques,
– pigment storage,
– amniotic bands,
– tumors.

The course of the vessels on the chorionic plate is determined by the umbilical cord insertion [5]. A centrally inserted umbilical cord will produce vessels that branch radially on the chorionic plate (dispersed vessel distribution, *Birch bush pattern*), while a marginally or eccentrically inserted umbilical cord will result in the chorionic vessels radiating in a rough branching pattern *(Oak tree pattern)* (Figs. 2.4a/b, 2.5, 2.6).

Almost all, more than 99 %, of the arteries on the chorionic plate cross over veins (Figs. 2.5, 2.6) [6]. The peripheral branches of the arteries dive into the chorionic plate before they reach the outer margin of the placenta *(margo externus)* (Fig. 2.7, yellow arrow). The internal margin *(margo internus)* connects the centrally located vessels to the circumferential network of vessels at the margo externus (Fig. 2.7, blue arrow). The border between the two is often defined by a whitish ring of subchorionic fibrin deposition; subchorionic fibrin and fibrinoid depositions can also be seen in the branching area of the large stem villi and here they may represent a reduced intervillous flow (subchorionic pseudoinfarct, Ch. 7).

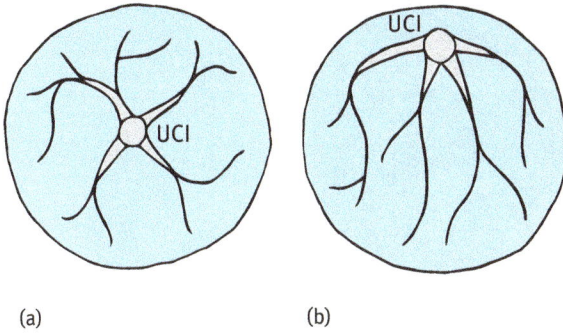

(a)   (b)

Fig. 2.4: Illustration of the umbilical cord vessels. (UCI) Umbilical cord insertion determines the course of the chorionic fetal vessels. (a) Central umbilical cord insertion with chorionic vessels running in a Birch bush pattern, (b) peripheral umbilical cord insertion with chorionic vessels arranged in an oak tree pattern (modified after Vogel) [7].

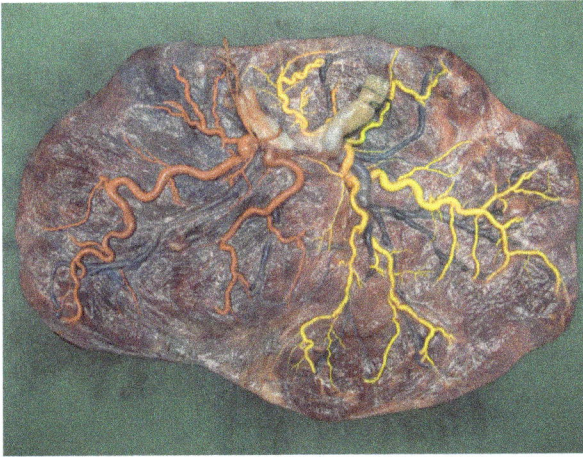

Fig. 2.5: Monochorionic-monoamniotic twin placenta with ink injected umbilical cord vessels. Centrally inserted umbilical cords with chorionic vessels running in an Oak tree pattern. Umbilical cord artery, twin 1, injected with red ink and vein, twin 1, with blue ink; artery, twin 2, injected with yellow ink and vein, twin 2, with green ink. arteries almost always cross over veins.

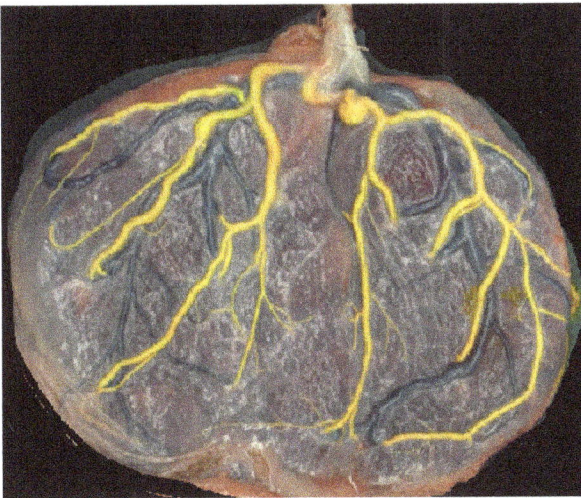

Fig. 2.6: Singleton placenta at term with a marginal umbilical cord insertion and chorionic vessels displaying an Oak tree branching pattern. Umbilical cord artery injected with yellow ink and vein injected with green ink.

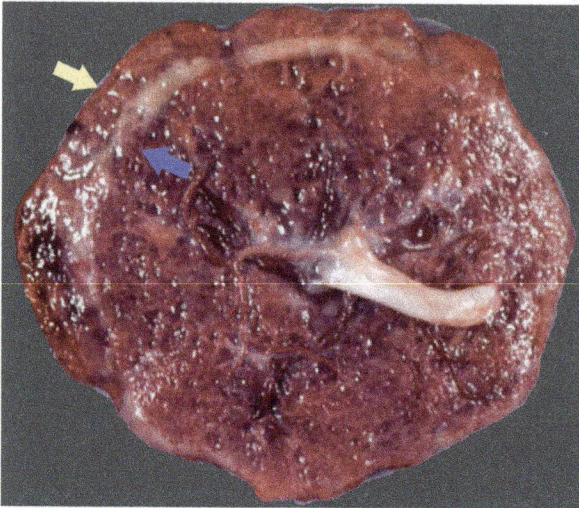

Fig. 2.7: Margo internus marked with a blue arrow and the margo externus marked with a yellow arrow at the external margin.

Discoloration of the chorionic plate may be caused by:
- ascending amniotic inflammation (Ch. 9),
- meconium release into the amniotic fluid (Ch. 4),
- rarely, hemosiderin macrophages can be found in the connective tissue of the chorionic plate and are often the result of bleeding in early and middle pregnancy.

Umbilical cord (Ch. 4)

Examination of the umbilical cord should be documented with particular attention to the following:
- length,
- number of the umbilical cord vessels,
- true and false knots,
- edema and cysts,
- hematoma and thrombosis,
- hypercoiling and strictures,
- nodules on the amniotic surface.

The umbilical cord, at term, has an average length of ca. 50–65 cm and an average diameter of 1.2 to 1.5 cm; both length and diameter are independent of placental and fetal weight [3,6].

The number and distribution of the umbilical cord vessels should be examined on several cross sections. Normally, the umbilical cord has two arteries, one vein and is surrounded by Whartons' Jelly. A physiological Hyrtl anastomosis is evidence against a diagnosis of (SUA) single umbilical artery.

Membranes (Ch. 9)

The amniotic membrane lines the gestational sac and is thin, transparent and easy to separate from the chorionic plate. It lies close to the extraplacental gestational sac and the amniotic membrane continues directly into the fetal skin at the fetal umbilical port.

Macroscopic color changes and focal nodules are readily identifiable on the membrane and can be caused by:
- amniotic inflammation,
- amniotic pigmentation,
- amnion nodosum,
- epithelial metaplasia,
- amniotic polyps (Ch. 9).

2.4.2 Basal plate of the placenta

The basal plate is divided into ca. 20 placental lobes measuring 1–3 cm in diameter. They may show (Fig. 2.8):
- coagulated blood on the basal plate and organized retroplacental hematomas,
- defects of the basal plate surface,
- calcification (see below, and Ch. 7).

Blood clots originating from placental detachment are often attached to the basal plate. Fresh blood is easy removable and the decidua below is unharmed, without any indentation from the hemorrhage. This must be differentiated from retroplacental

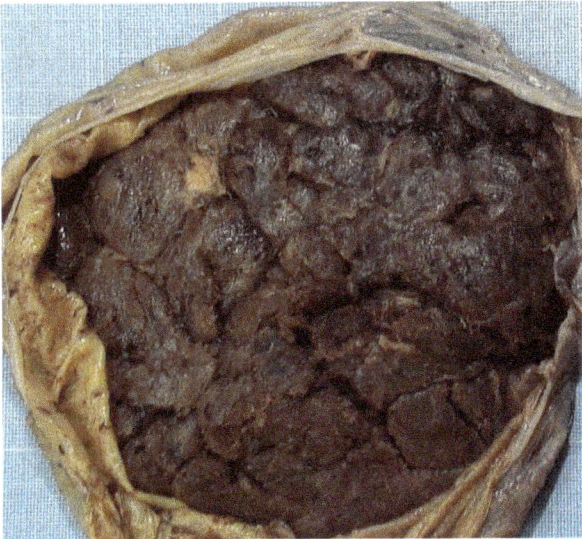

Fig. 2.8: Placenta at term. Lobes of the basal / maternal placental area with normal depositions of blood after delivery.

hematomas, due to premature placental abruption, and marginal hematomas, both of which affect the underlying decidua.

Identification of a basal plate defect is part of the routine macroscopic placental examination in the delivery room. The grey-glassy decidua shows irregular interruptions on the basal surface and portions of the placenta may even be missing. Evaluation of the completeness of the basal plate may be challenging in some cases.

Calculation of the basal plate area

The area, in cm², of the basal plate is calculated analogous to an idealized circle:

$$a \, \tfrac{1}{2} \times b \, \tfrac{1}{2} \times \pi.$$

2.4.3 Organ weight

The net weight (placental disc only) must be differentiated from the gross weight (placental disc with umbilical cord, membranes, blood and amniotic fluid). The net weight is taken after the umbilical cord is removed, at ca. 5 cm from its point of insertion on the chorionic plate, and after the membranes are trimmed around the margin. It should be documented if the placenta was examined in a fresh or formalin fixed state.

2.4.4 Placental cut sections

The placental parenchyma should be inspected on serial cut sections, ca. 1 cm thick, and macroscopic findings should be documented.

Cut sections from a mature placenta show, depending on blood content, a medium to dark red color. Organization of the parenchyma into feto-maternal circulatory units is obvious in term placentas; the central portions appearing as small, collapsed blood filled spaces. This structure is missing in placentas from fetal abortions and immature placentas from prematurely born children prior to gestational week 32. This also corresponds to ultrasound measurements estimating placental maturity. A diffuse or focal pallor of the cut sections, without any additional macroscopic changes, may be due to:
- villous immaturity
- anemia in the villi and/or in the intervillous space

Pallor, with an increased density or greater granularity of the cut sections is seen in:
1. increased fibrin deposition in the intervillous space,
2. villous stromal fibrosis, endangiopathia obliterans,

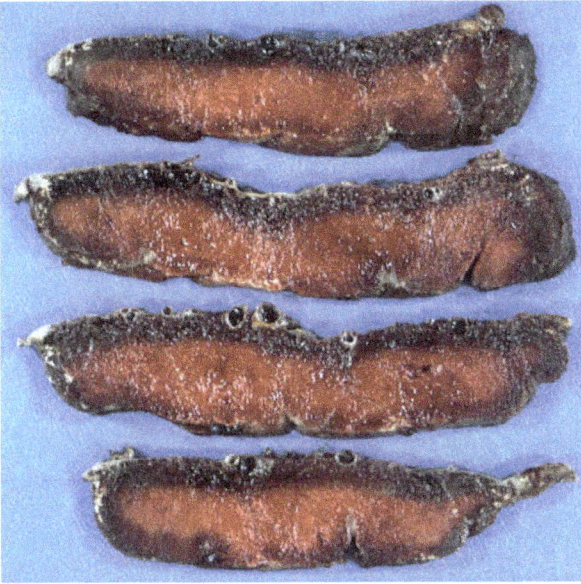

Fig. 2.9: Macroscopic examination of 5 to 10 mm thick placental slices for the documentation of parenchymal color, density, bleeding, infarcts, thrombosis, etc.

3. increased number of placental islands (these placentas are usually large with an increased weight, the cause is unknown).

Focal changes must be documented, especially if related to vascular disturbances.

Placental thickness: The minimum and maximum placental thickness should be documented; a thickness less than 5 mm is suggestive of placenta membranacea.

Calcification of the placenta: Macroscopic calcification is often seen as mm sized granular changes in the mature placenta at term. It should be documented and the percentage of the placenta involved estimated [8].

Depositions are most often located near the basal plate, but they can also be seen nearby the septa, islands, stem villi and in the subchorionic intervillous space, in the first $\frac{1}{3}$ of the total parenchymal thickness. Stromal microcalcifications in the peripheral villi may be seen histologically. Abortion material and placentas from IUFD and vascular disturbances may show fine granular or laminar calcification near the epithelial and vascular basal membranes, as well as along stromal fibers.

Pathogenesis: Calcification is seen in tissue undergoing fluctuations in pH. Necrobiotic tissue is locally acidotic and becomes more alkaline when completely necrotic. This pH change causes precipitation of calcium salts and these calcium depositions are frequently associated with:
– maternal serum calcium concentration,
– trophoblast transport capacity,
– the regulatory function of serum estrogen concentration [8].

Correlation with systemic maternal diseases is unknown and there is no known effect on the nutrition of the fetus.

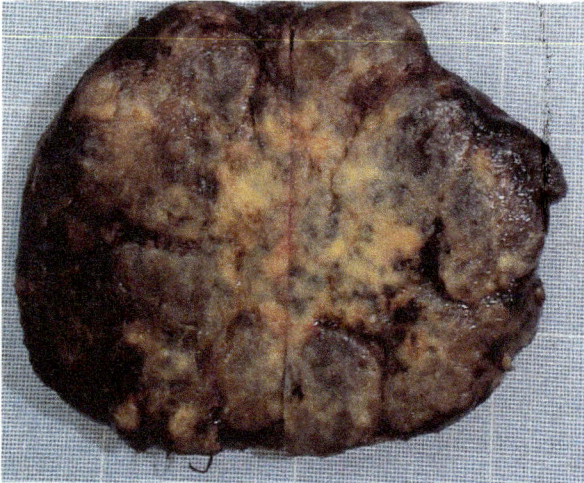

Fig. 2.10: Term placenta with yellow, firm lesions on the basal plate.

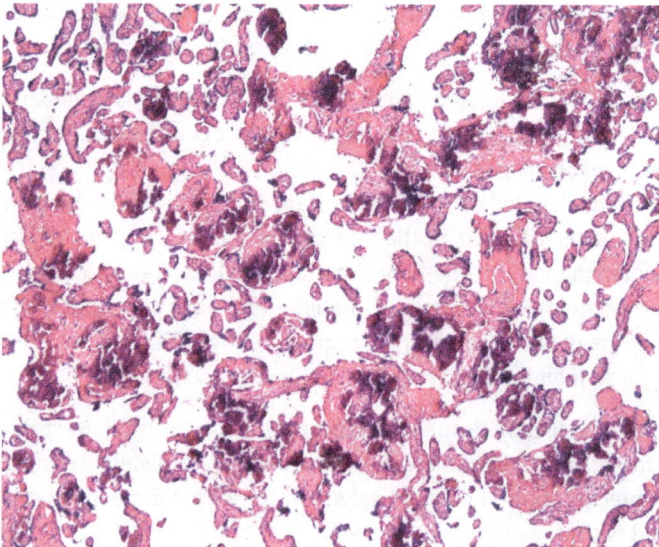

Fig. 2.11: Term placenta histology (Fig. 2.10) with calcification in the intervillous space and of the villous stroma.

2.5 Methodology

As a consequence of the Amsterdam placental workshop group consensus meeting, the following 4 block, minimum, placental sampling protocol is recommended:
- one roll of the extraplacental membranes, from the rupture edge to the placental margin, and a part of the marginal parenchyma,
- cross sections of the umbilical cord, one from the fetal end and another approximately 5 cm from the placental insertion,
- full thickness sections from macroscopically normal parenchyma.

Full thickness samples should be taken in the central two-thirds of the disc and include the area adjacent to the insertion site. If the transmural thickness is greater than the length of the cassette, the upper third (chorionic plate and underlying tissue) and lower third (basal aspect) of the parenchyma can be submitted in one cassette, or the gross slice can be divided into two and submitted in two cassettes.

A full thickness sample should be taken close to the umbilical cord insertion site, to allow for documentation of fetal vascular ectasia and a fetal and/or maternal inflammatory response.

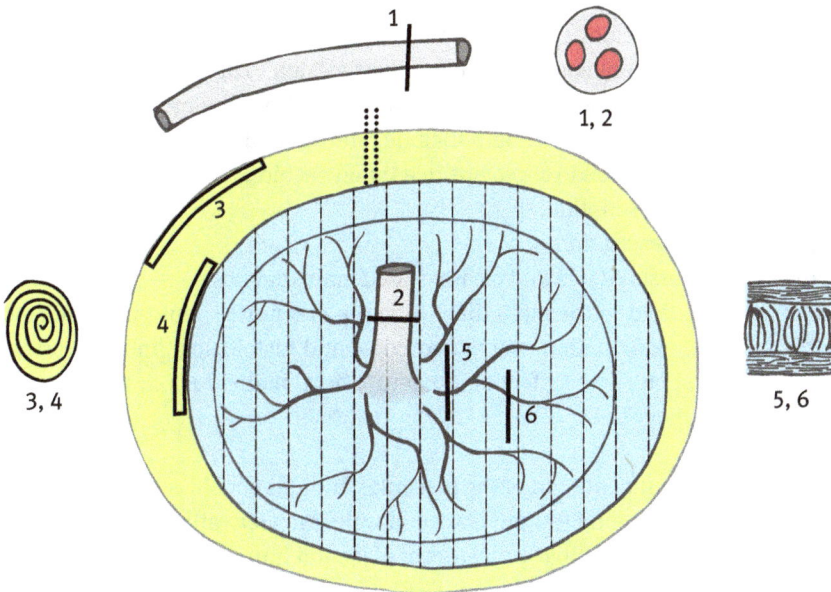

Fig. 2.12: Illustration. Recommended placental sampling for microscopic examination: (1) Cross section from the umbilical cord close to the child; (2) cross section from the umbilical cord, 5 cm from chorionic insertion; (3, 4) membrane roll from the circumferential margin; (5, 6) macroscopically normal placental parenchyma. Additional sampling of any macroscopic changes is recommended.

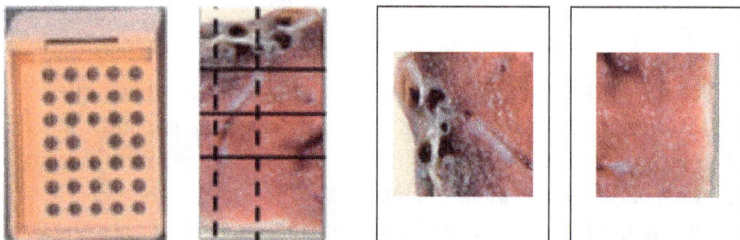

Fig. 2.13: Tissue samples distributed into standardized cassettes [3].

A consensus number of 3 parenchymal blocks was selected based on discussions on the sampling of placental lesions and evidence indicating that 62 % of villitis, a prime example of a (multi-) focal lesion, would be identified.

2.6 Pathological placental report

Previous placental pathology reports comprised of long, prose-like descriptions without a clear diagnosis. They used varying terminology and lacked therapeutic and/or prognostic information.

A unified and international placental classification and reporting system, with the primary focus of relating the main diagnostic finding to pathophysiological processes, stimulated prolonged international discussion. The Amsterdam placental workshop group consensus statement recommended a standardized pathological placental report. Such reports should include relevant and clinically useful information and be communicated to clinicians in a timely fashion. The report must include:
1. a macroscopic description,
2. a histological description,
3. an easily understandable and clearly stated main diagnosis,
4. in a separate field to the main diagnosis, the diagnosis should be correlated to the placental examination (the macroscopic and histological findings) and also to the clinical outcome (infection, maternal/fetal malperfusion, maturation defects, hemorrhage).

Description and documentation of the placental findings should include:
– Net and gross placental weight; placental weight to area ratio and fetal to placental weight ratio, as possible indicators of placental function and placental reserve capacity in fetal growth restriction (FGR) (Ch. 3). Contemporary placental weight standards should be used. (Appendix, Tables A1–A4).
– Fresh or formalin fixed placental examination; fixation will increase weight by 3 to 6 %.

- The documentation of any prior sampling of the placental parenchyma causing disruption of the basal plate.
- Placental measurement in three dimensions; placental shape and size may be associated with pregnancy complications (Ch. 5).
- Grossly identifiable lesions should be described with either an estimate of the percentage of the total parenchymal volume affected or a measurement of the two maximal dimensions of each lesion. The number and location of lesions should be counted and stated as being either single or multiple, central/paracentral or peripheral.
- Umbilical cord: diameter, length, site of insertion, hypocoiled (1 coil per 10 cm) or hypercoiled (3 coils per 10 cm). Segmental or localized areas of hypercoiling, as well as the direction of coiling, should be recorded (Ch. 3). Fixation of the cord will affect the length and therefore the coiling index, underscoring the importance of stating whether the placenta was fresh or fixed when pathologic examination was performed.
- The description of the membranes should include: color/opacity and completeness, the shortest distance between the rupture site and the placental edge, circumvallate or circummarginate membranes and the percentage of the circumference involved (Ch. 5).

References

[1] Turowski G, Berge LN, Helgadottir LB, Jacobsen EM, Roald B. A new, clinically oriented, unifying and simple placental classification system. Placenta. 2012;33(12):1026–1035.
[2] Turowski G, Parks TW, Arbuckle S, Flem Jacobsen A, Heazell A. The structure and utility of the placental pathology report. APMIS. 2018;126(7):638–646.
[3] Khong TY, Mooney EE, Ariel I, et al. Sampling and Definitions of Placental Lesions: Amsterdam Placental Workshop Group Consensus Statement. Arch Pathol Lab Med. 2016;140(7):698–713.
[4] Pathologists TRCo. Tissue pathway for histopathological examination of the placenta. In: Cox P EC, editor. London 2017.
[5] Hörmann G, Lemtis H. Die menschliche Plazenta. Klinik der Frauenheilkunde und Geburtshilfe. III. München: Urban & Schwarzenberg; 1967. p. 425–636.
[6] Smart PJ. Some observations on the vascular morphology of the foetal side of the human placenta. J Obstet Gynaecol Br Emp. 1962;69:929–933.
[7] Vogel M. Atlas der morphologischen Plazentadiagnostik. 2 ed. Berlin: Springer; 1996.
[8] Becker V, Schiebler TH, Kubli F. Allgemeine und spezielle Pathologie der Plazenta. Die Plazenta des Menschen. Stuttgart: Thieme; 1981. p. 251–393.

3 Pathology of the umbilical cord

The umbilical cord normally contains two arteries and one vein which are protected by Wharton's Jelly. In early fetal development the arterial media is divided into two equal layers, whereas the vein contains an inner muscle layer that is smaller than the outer layer. Within the vessels the endothelial and myoepithelial cells are intertwined, similar to those in the chorionic and stem villous vessels [1]. The surface of the umbilical cord is lined by amniotic epithelium and the vessels are contained within Wharton's Jelly; a gelatinous substance containing polyglycans, large fibroblasts, collagen fibers, free connective tissue cells, mast cells and desmin and actin positive muscle cells.

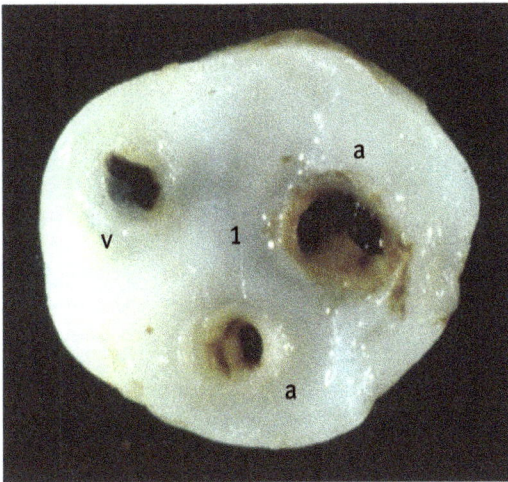

Fig. 3.1: Transverse section of the umbilical cord with three fetal vessels. Two arteries (a) and one vein (v) enclosed in Wharton's Jelly [1].

3.1 Umbilical cord length

The length of the umbilical cord, according gestational age, should be compared with that of the actual specimen (Appendix, Table A5) [2]. Longitudinal growth of the umbilical cord is assumed to be stimulated by tension during fetal growth [3]; a short umbilical cord may be due to deficient fetal movement in the 1st half of pregnancy, and in the 2nd half of pregnancy the umbilical cord length is interpreted as:
- short if less than 40 cm at term,
- overlong if more than 90 cm.

Long and short umbilical cords can be associated with adverse perinatal outcomes [2,4,5]. A short umbilical cord is found in less than 0.3 % of unselected deliveries and an overlong umbilical cord in less than 1 %.

https://doi.org/10.1515/9783110452600-003

Risks of a short umbilical cord
– *preterm placental rupture,* if the child is located in the lower uterine segment,
– vessel spasm and circulatory disorders in cases of umbilical cord overtension [6],
– *short umbilical cord complex:* complete umbilical cord absence (*achordie*) and insertion of the placenta directly on the fetal belly (limb-body wall complex or body stalk anomaly) with blood supply occurring through vasa aberrantia.

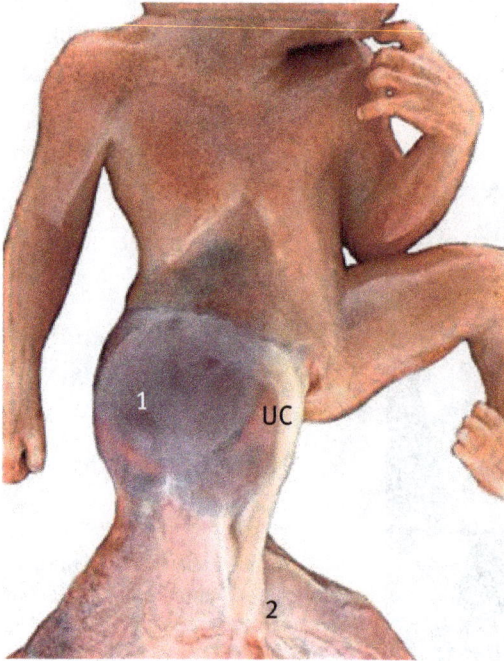

Fig. 3.2: Fetus with "body stalk anomaly". (UC) Umbilical cord; (1) lateral omphalocele; (2) umbilical cord insertion on the fetal placental plate.

Risks of an overlong umbilical cord
– fetal entanglement, with or without restriction of fetal movement (Fig. 3.3),
– true umbilical knots,
– umbilical cord prolapse following pre-term membrane rupture,
– often associated with clinical polyhydramnion.

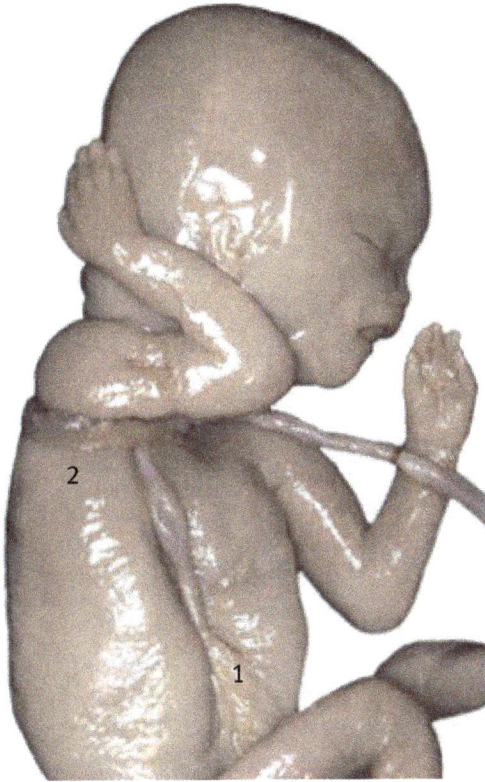

Fig. 3.3: Multiple entanglements of the (UC) umbilical cord. (1) Fetal umbilicus with umbilical cord; (2) umbilical cord entangling the fetal neck and right axilla. Fetal death in gestational week 20. Overlong umbilical cord, measuring 45 cm (normal: 23–40 cm) (2).

3.2 Umbilical cord coiling

Umbilical cord coiling describes a diffuse, or segmental, spiral like vessel configuration around the longitudinal axis of the umbilical cord; coiling is irregular, but often associated with focal deficiencies of Wharton's Jelly.

A left twist, diagonal twisting around the longitudinal axis from upper left to lower right, is most common. The clinical significance of a left versus a right twist remains unclear.

3.2.1 Hypercoiling

Hypercoiling (more than 3 coils per 10 cm) may be associated with adverse outcomes in some cases [7–10]. Hypercoiling is often localized to the periumbilical area or close to the umbilical cord insertion on the placenta. Hypercoiling may cause hypoxia or fetal demise, if there is associated edema, congestion, bleeding and/or thrombi. Deep grooves between the coils in hypercoiled cords have been associated with stillbirth.

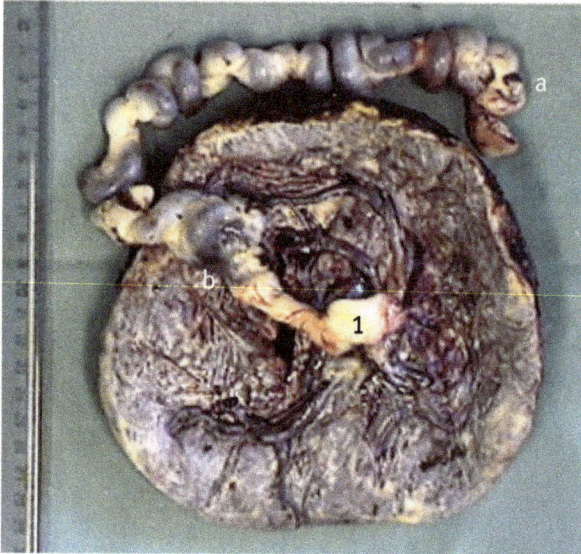

Fig. 3.4: Hypercoiling of the umbilical cord. Congestion in the middle portion between (a) and (b). (a) Fetal end of the umbilical cord; (b) congestion next to the placental insertion; (1) hypercoiling close to placental insertion.

3.2.2 Hypocoiling

Hypocoiling (less than 1 coil per 10 cm) may be associated with adverse fetal outcomes [11–13]. A hypocoiled or uncoiled umbilical cord may correlate with fetal stress and may also be associated with chromosomal anomalies.

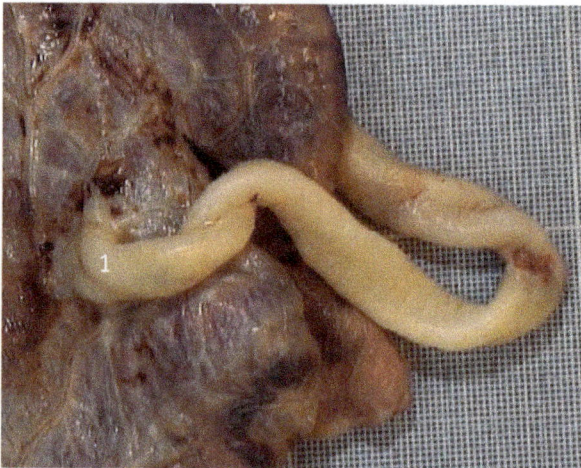

Fig. 3.5: Formalin fixed placenta with a pale and hypocoiled umbilical cord. (1) Umbilical cord insertion.

3.3 Umbilical cord knots

The umbilical cord may show true knots and false knots.

3.3.1 True knots

True knots are reported in 0.3–0.5 % of all deliveries, but in more recent prospective studies the incidence varies from 0.04–1.5 % [14].

Recent and tight (difficult to loosen) knots of the umbilical cord may be macroscopically seen next to placental insertion; with or without acute venous constriction, with or without edema and sometimes in combination with hemorrhage in Wharton's Jelly. All tight knots are characterized by deep impressions in the umbilical cord with compression of the vessel lumina and a reduction in the surrounding Wharton's Jelly. The deep impressions in the cord persist after opening the knot.

Placental changes due to true knots:
– acute collapse of vessel lumina in stem villi,
– vacuolization of the endothelial cells of the tunica intima and the muscle cells of the tunica media,
– fresh fibrin depositions of varying cellularity,
– reactive connective tissue proliferation with septation in the vessel lumen and/or intramural bleeding with long standing perfusion disorders.

Associated findings with true umbilical knots and fetal entanglement:
1. villous maturation disorders with absent fetal vessels,
2. signs (meconium phagocytosis) of pre-term meconium passage.

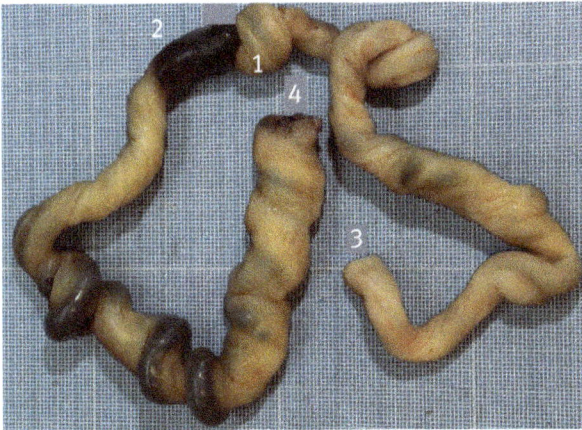

Fig. 3.6: Formalin fixed umbilical cord, 45 cm length. (1) True knot; (2) acute thrombosis; (3) placental insertion at umbilical cord end; (4) fetal end of the umbilical cord with post stenotic hypercoiling. Acute cesarean section at term due to fetal distress. Weight 3,545 g, APGAR score 7-9-9.

Predisposing factors
- overlong umbilical cord,
- polyhydramnion,
- monochorionic-monoamniotic twins,
- delayed villous maturation with a structurally restricted perfusion capacity (Ch. 8).

Structural circulatory disorders may lead to fetal hypoxia and hypermotility and this can result in true knot formation or fetal entanglement.

Consequences for the fetus
- Functional shortening of the umbilical cord and the risk of a loose knot tightening during delivery. While the majority of knots are loose and without any fetal consequences, perfusion resistance increases in tightened knots. In-vitro studies have shown that 100–110 mmHg is necessary to vascularize vessels in a knot which was tightened by a 100 g weight [15].
- Fetal hypoxic risk increases with tightening of a knot (CTG changes, pre-term meconium passage).
- Perinatal mortality increases by ca. 10 % [16].

3.3.2 False knots

False knots are:
- circumscribed accumulations and pseudocystic degeneration of Wharton's Jelly,
- summation of vessel loops with varicose dilatation.

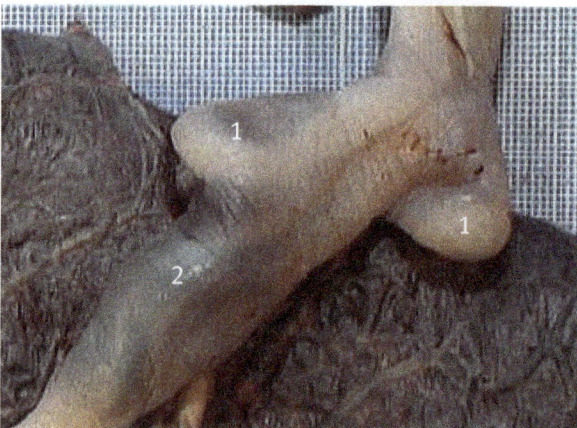

Fig. 3.7: False umbilical cord knot. (1) Prominent vessel loops; (2) thickened and congested Wharton's Jelly.

3.4 Umbilical cord stricture

The umbilical cord is extremely coiled and has a total, or subtotal, deficiency of Wharton's Jelly in a stricture. A high grade periumbilical cord stricture is found in ca. 3 % of fetal miscarriages.

Histological examination of placentas with umbilical cord strictures shows villous stromal fibrosis, endangiopathia obliterans and secondary collapse sclerosis of the stem villi.

The etiology of umbilical cord coiling/overcoiling/torsion, stricture formation and deficiencies of Wharton's Jelly remains unknown.

3.5 Thin-Cord-complex

Thin umbilical cords are associated with FGR, whereas thick cords are often associated with maternal diabetes and fetal hydrops.

A thin-cord-complex is characterized by a segmental and very thin umbilical cord with a deficiency, or complete absence, of Wharton's Jelly. It is a rare finding in late pregnancy and may be a cause of umbilical cord torsion and stricture formation.

A slim and condensed brim of Wharton's Jelly may be seen, sometimes with diffuse microcalcifications, histologically.

Risks associated with a thin-cord-complex:
– fetal abortion,
– easy mechanical irritability of the vessels (compression, cord torsion and stricture),
– rupture of the umbilical cord vessels with bleeding into the amniotic sac.

3.6 Single umbilical artery (SUA)

A SUA is an umbilical cord with a single artery. The diagnosis is made by sampling the cord at 1–2 cm intervals to confirm the absence of one of the two arteries.

Frequency
In a retrospective study of 56,919 children, 159 cases with a single artery in the umbilical cord were seen; an incidence of 0.28 % [17]. Unpublished material (Department of Pediatric Pathology and Placentology, Charité, Berlin, Germany) identified a single umbilical artery (SUA) in:
– 0.5 % of unselected deliveries,
– 1.7 % of at risk pregnancies,
– 2.4 % of multiple pregnancies,
– 3.1 % of perinatal deaths.

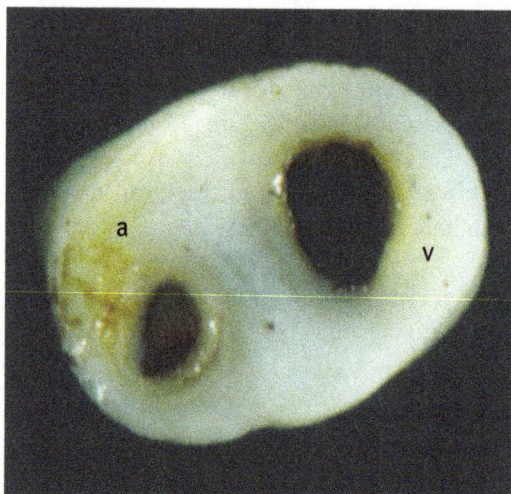

Fig. 3.8: Umbilical cord cut section. (a) One artery and one (v) vein.

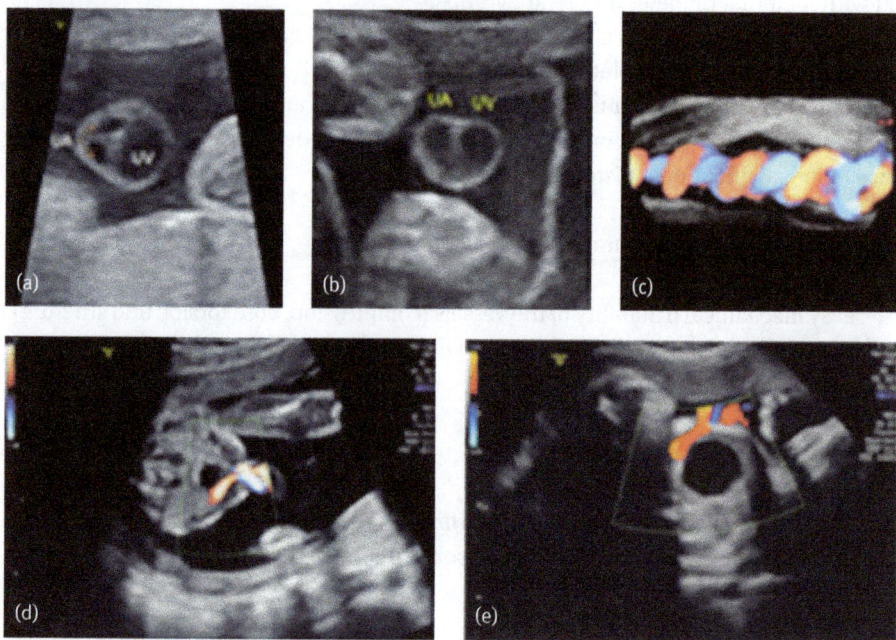

Fig. 3.9: Ultrasonographic examination of the umbilical cord should include detailed examination of both transverse (a, b) and longitudinal views (c) of a free cord loop. Due to physiological anastomoses, segments from an umbilical cord with a single artery can display more than one arterial lumen in cross section; however, color-Doppler can assist in identifying the umbilical vessels and the diagnosis can be confirmed by identifying a missing corresponding intra-abdominal portion of the umbilical artery (i. e., superior bladder) (d, e) (by courtesy of prof. B. Tutschek, Zürich, Switzerland and Prof. Dr. Th. Braun, Department of Obstetrics, Charité Berlin, Germany).

Pathogenesis

The cause of SUA is unknown. Primary agenesis, secondary atrophy or a single persisting allantois vessel have been proposed. A single umbilical artery is more common
in Caucasian fetuses (from autopsy series), in placentas with marginal or velamentous cord insertions and in fetuses with aneuploidy or other structural abnormalities.
Although it occurs more often in twins, monozygotic twin fetuses are usually discordant for SUA [18].

Consequences for the fetus

– Associated anomalies in SUA include: musculoskeletal abnormalities in 23 %,
  genitourinary abnormalities in 20 %, cardiovascular abnormalities in 19 %, gastrointestinal abnormalities in 10 % and central nervous system abnormalities
  in 8 %. SUA is also associated with aneuploidy, trisomy 13 and 18, monosomy X
  (Turner) and triploidy [18].
– Associated malformations in the surviving children are less frequently seen than
  those occurring in perinatal deaths; confirmed by pediatric follow up studies,
  children up to 4 years of age, that demonstrate no statistically significant increased incidence in fetal malformations when compared to control groups.
– Increased perinatal mortality, caused by associated malformations.
– Intrauterine fetal growth restriction in 17.5 % of cases [19].
– No functional placental dysfunction, if not associated with villous retarded maturation.

3.7 Supernumerary umbilical cord vessels

Reports of the frequency of four, or more, umbilical cord vessels are inconsistent.
More often than not careful macroscopic examination shows that these extra vessels
are small arterial, rather than venous, branches of the cord vessels. Persistence of the
v. umbilicalis dextra, two veins and two arteries on transverse sections of the umbili-

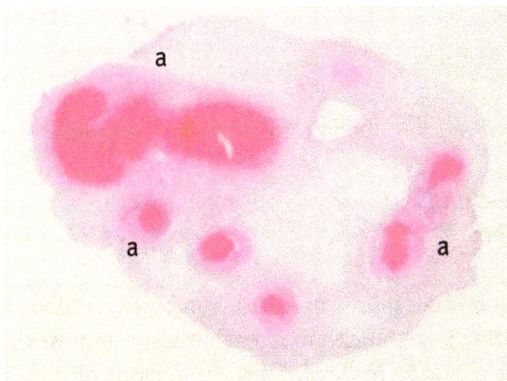

Fig. 3.10: Macroscopic view on an
embedded section sample of an umbilical cord: (a) multiple umbilical cord
vessels due to the divergence of the
two arteries

cal cord, close to the child is reported without fetal consequence. Prior to term, small arterial branches may be found in the placenta, close to the umbilical cord [20]; these vessels may represent additional yolk sac vessels [21].

3.8 Thrombosis of the umbilical cord vessels

Partial thrombosis of umbilical cord vessels was often seen in cases of inflammation.

Unpublished material from a Berlin obstetric department found thrombosis in 0.09 % of unselected placentas, and this corresponds to a prospective study in which six umbilical cord thromboses were seen in 7,738 placentas, an incidence of 0.07 % [22].

When compared to controls, thrombosis was more often associated with perinatal (0.3 %) and intrauterine (0.7 %) death. 80 % of cases with thrombosis are associated with other umbilical cord complications, such as overcoiling, strictures and hematomas, strangulation, vessel constriction, omphalovasculitis and funiculitis [22].

Case reports have documented thrombosis occurring in twin pregnancy, hydrops universalis, intrauterine fetal death in diabetic mothers and placental implantation in the lower uterine segment.

Single case reports of combined thrombosis and calcification of the vessel wall may be a result of intrauterine infection with circumscribed vessel wall necrosis, secondary calcification and tertiary partial thrombosis. A segmental vessel wall necrosis caused by hypoxia, close to old areas of torsion or cord strangulation, may also be a possibility.

Secondary changes due to thrombosis:
- intrauterine fetal death, if associated with other cord complications,
- hydrops fetalis,
- hemorrhagic infarction of the kidneys/adrenals, caused by appositional thrombosis of the vena cava and renal veins,
- origin of an intrauterine, usually paradoxical, thromboembolism.

3.9 Hematoma of the umbilical cord

A hematoma of the cord is the extravasation of blood into Wharton's Jelly and two types may be distinguished:
- hematoma without vessel compression,
- hematoma with vessel compression.

Hematomas without vessel compression occur more often in the umbilical cord next to the child and are caused by tension on the umbilical cord, mechanical compression and rupture during delivery. They are clinically irrelevant, except in cases of rhexis

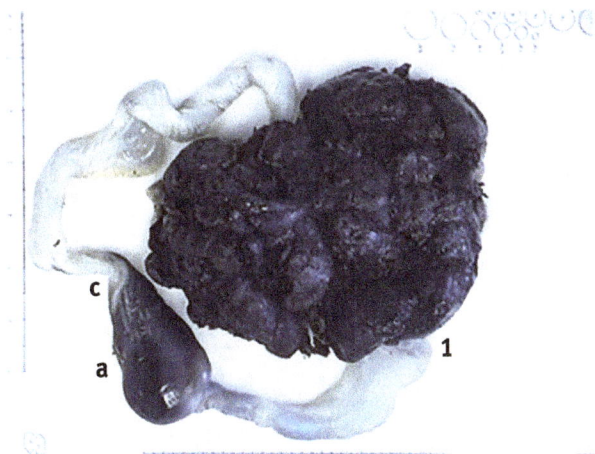

Fig. 3.11: Umbilical cord and view on the maternal plate of the placenta. Umbilical cord with (a) sac-like varicosity and acute thrombosis; (b) paravascular hematoma; (c) false knot with prominent loops. (1) Fetal end of the umbilical cord.

bleeding during delivery as this carries a risk of fatal fetal hemorrhage, and the source of the hemorrhage is frequently unknown.

Hematomas with vessel compression are very infrequent and cause a prominent and bulging black-red lesion on the surface of the umbilical cord. Abundant and partly coagulated fresh blood can be found on the cut surface and umbilical cord vessels may be difficult to visualize. The hematoma may measure several cm in length.

Pathogenesis
- hemorrhage most frequently originates from the vein, rather than the arteries of the umbilical cord,
- rupture of varix knots,
- diapedesis hemorrhage in fetal bleeding disorders with increased permeability of the vessel wall,
- bleeding from persisting omphalomesenteric vessels,
- bleeding from an umbilical cord hemangioma.

Secondary changes
- vessel compression,
- rupture of the umbilical cord surface with bleeding into the amniotic sac; risk of fatal fetal hemorrhage.

3.10 Edema and cysts

Fluid retention can increase the umbilical cord diameter by several centimeters, but the consequences of such swelling for the fetus are unknown. Fluid filled pseudocysts (cysts lacking an epithelial lining) can be seen in the swollen umbilical cord. True cysts (cysts with an epithelial lining) of the umbilical cord may be subclassified as:

- cysts representing allantois duct rests, lined by flat to cuboidal epithelium,
- cysts representing omphalomesenteric duct rests, lined by intestinal epithelium,
- inclusion cysts of the surface epithelium, lined by amniotic epithelium or squamous epithelium.

Pseudocysts are frequent, whereas true cysts are rare. Both are without any clinical relevance.

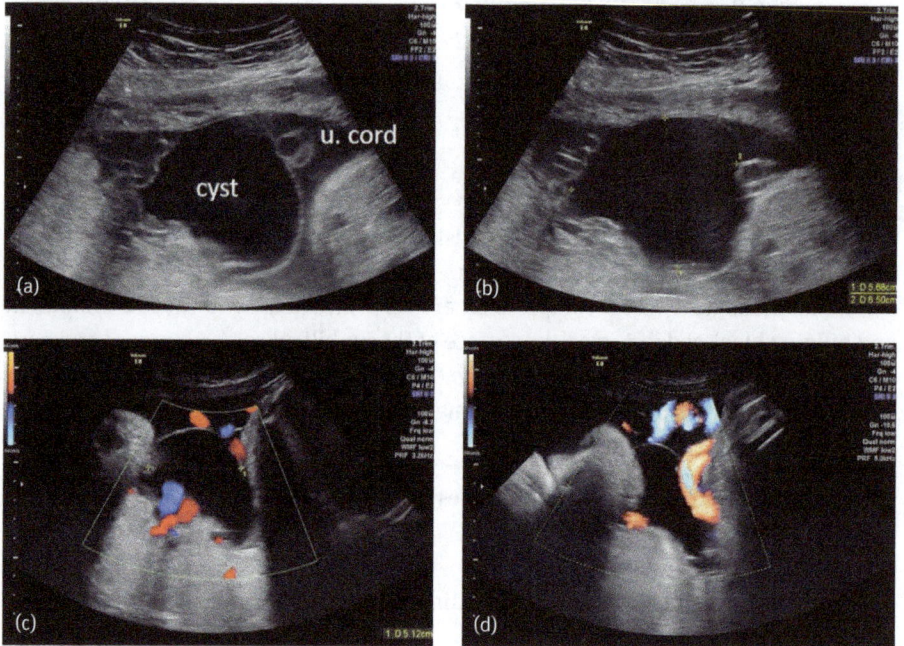

Fig. 3.12: Umbilical cord cysts. (a, b) sonographic cysts shown as fluid filled masses within the umbilical cord, usually seen near the fetal end; (c, d) detectable blood flow on color-Doppler examination (by courtesy of Prof. Dr. Th. Braun, Department of Obstetrics, Charité Berlin, Germany).

3.11 Umbilical cord polyp

Umbilical cord polyps are a rarely described benign lesion [23].

Intestinal polyps, with small bowel mucosa on histology, can be found on the umbilical cord surface, close to the fetal umbilical cord segment [24]. Secondary changes, such as mucosal defects, hemorrhage and inflammation may be seen.

Polyps are believed to develop from persisting elements of the ductus omphalomesentericus.

The ductus normally regresses by gestational week 10, but should it persist, parts of the ductus can prolapse and anomalies such as polyps, fistula and cysts of the umbilical cord and fetal bowel may develop [25].

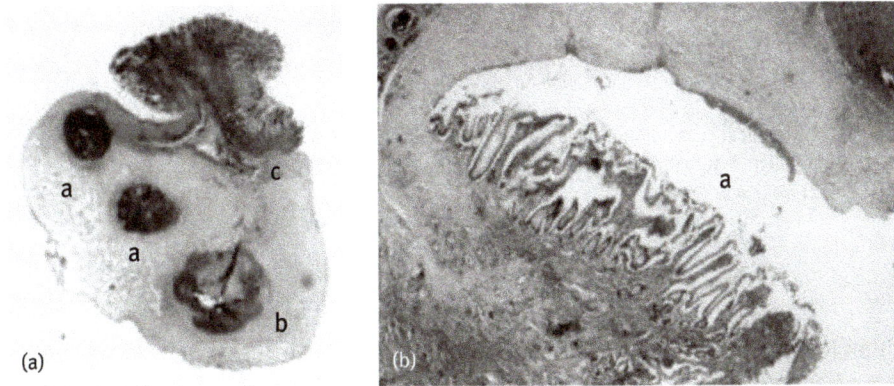

Fig. 3.13: (a) Umbilical cord with a small intestine polyp on the surface (LPF). (a) Umbilical cord arteries; (b) umbilical cord vein; (c) intestinal mucosa on the surface. (b) Umbilical cord with an intestine polyp (HPF). Small intestine mucosal fold and (a) muscularis mucosa (by courtesy of Thieme, Publisher, Stuttgart) [25].

3.12 Umbilical cord tumor

To be differentiated are hemangiomas, teratomas and angiomyxomas [26,27].

3.12.1 Hemangioma

Hemangiomas of the umbilical cord may be found in Wharton's Jelly and appear as well defined, non-encapsulated lesions. They are usually only microscopically visible (micro-hemangiomas) and are most often of the capillary type, rather than the cavernous or mixed types.

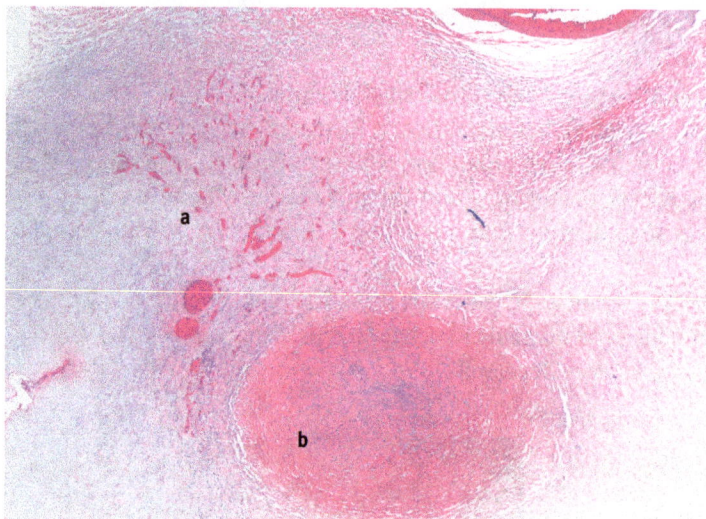

Fig. 3.14: Umbilical cord hemangioma. (a) Small capillaries with a diffuse distribution in Wharton's Jelly; (b) umbilical artery. Clinically fetal distress and umbilical cord prolapse. Forceps delivery in gestational week 41.

3.12.2 Teratoma

Umbilical cord teratomas are only documented in isolated case reports. They are always benign, only showing the histological characteristics of differentiated teratomas. They lie intrafunicularly, but in few cases on the chorial surface. This enables the differentiation of acardius amorphous in monochorionic twin pregnancies.

Their formation/origin is assumed to be due to an aberrant migration of germinal center cells in the connecting stalk (later the umbilical cord).

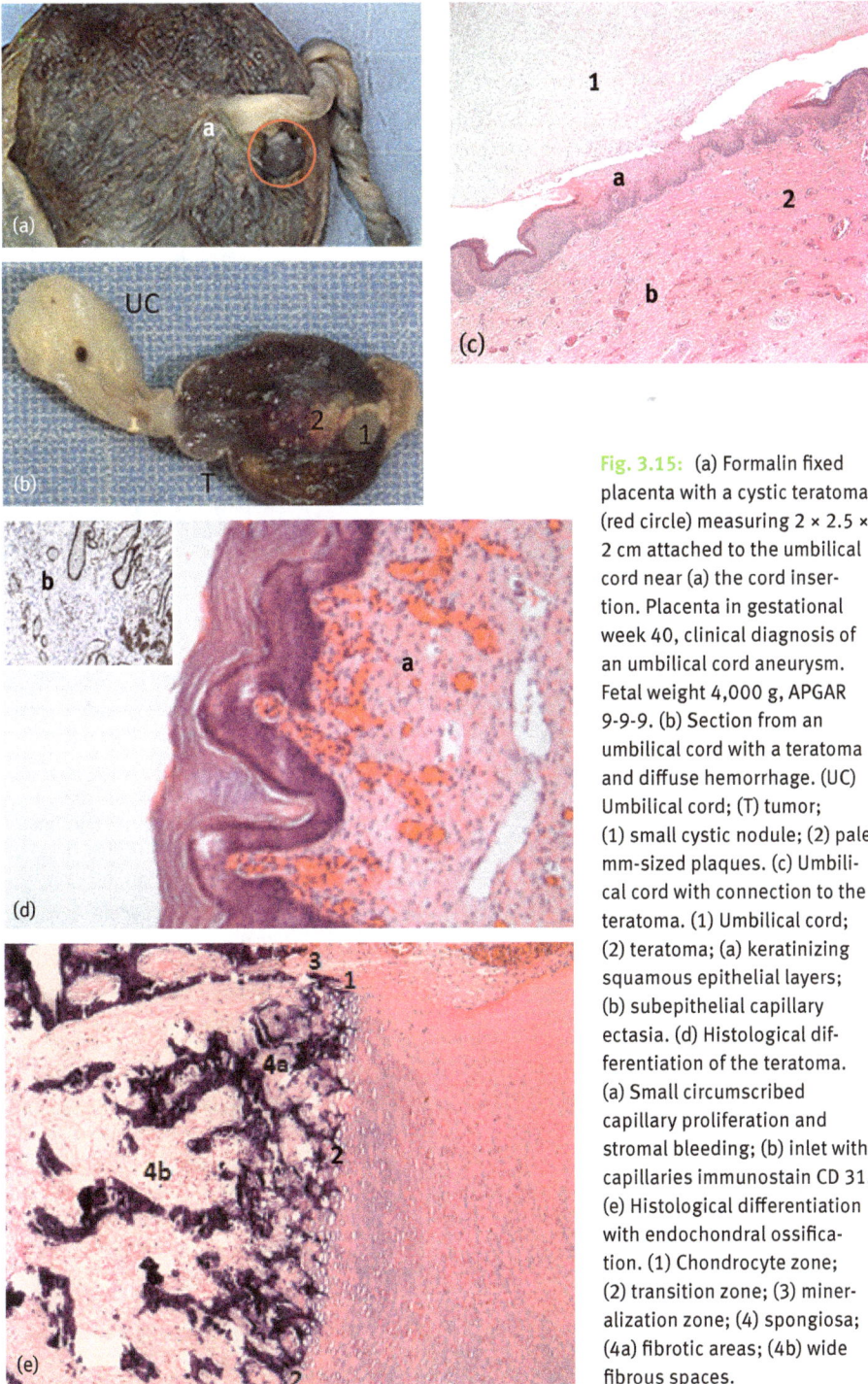

Fig. 3.15: (a) Formalin fixed placenta with a cystic teratoma (red circle) measuring 2 × 2.5 × 2 cm attached to the umbilical cord near (a) the cord insertion. Placenta in gestational week 40, clinical diagnosis of an umbilical cord aneurysm. Fetal weight 4,000 g, APGAR 9-9-9. (b) Section from an umbilical cord with a teratoma and diffuse hemorrhage. (UC) Umbilical cord; (T) tumor; (1) small cystic nodule; (2) pale mm-sized plaques. (c) Umbilical cord with connection to the teratoma. (1) Umbilical cord; (2) teratoma; (a) keratinizing squamous epithelial layers; (b) subepithelial capillary ectasia. (d) Histological differentiation of the teratoma. (a) Small circumscribed capillary proliferation and stromal bleeding; (b) inlet with capillaries immunostain CD 31. (e) Histological differentiation with endochondral ossification. (1) Chondrocyte zone; (2) transition zone; (3) mineralization zone; (4) spongiosa; (4a) fibrotic areas; (4b) wide fibrous spaces.

3.12.3 Angiomyxoma

An angiomyxoma is a benign tumor of the umbilical cord mesenchyme and capillaries that arises from pre-existing umbilical cord vessels.

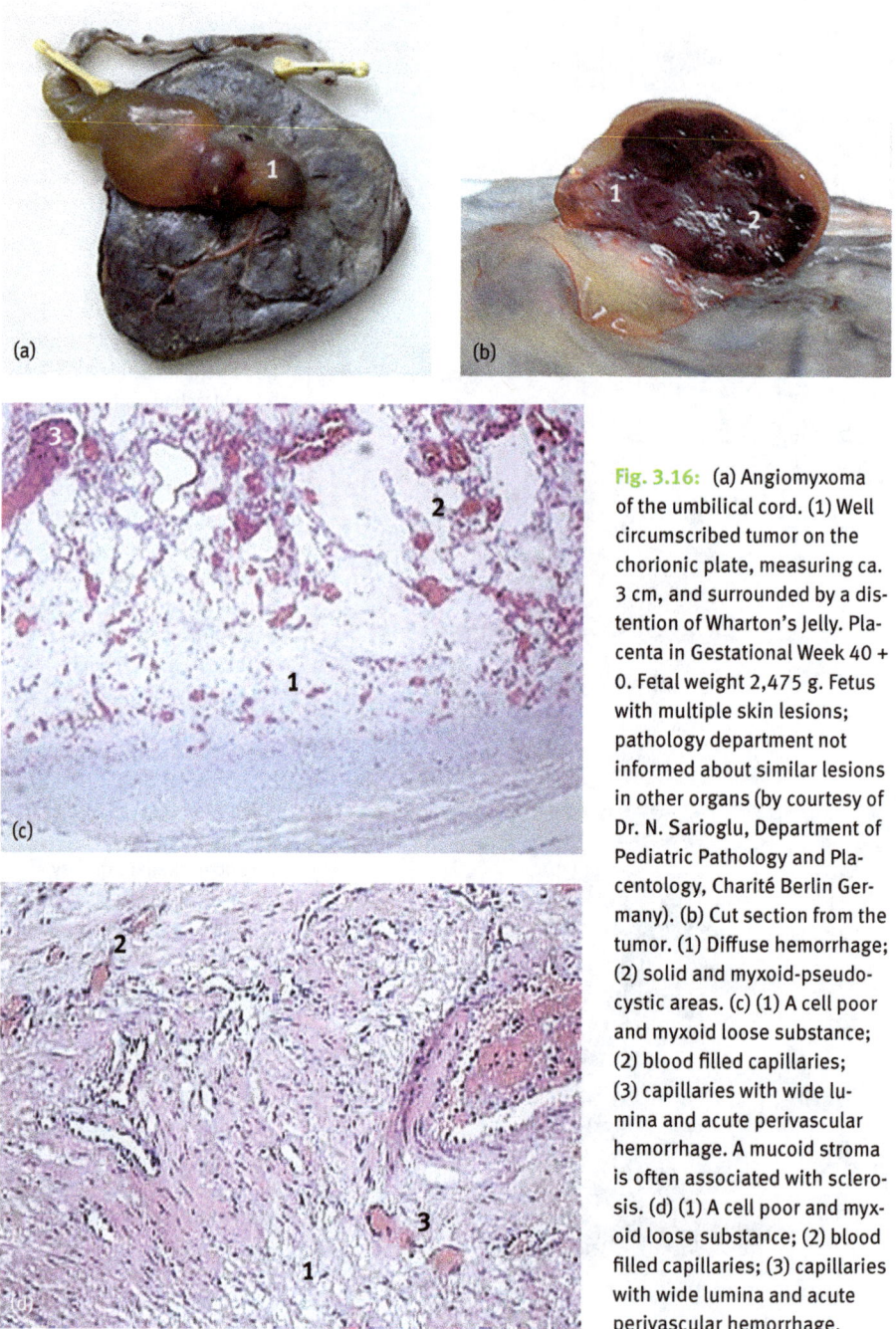

Fig. 3.16: (a) Angiomyxoma of the umbilical cord. (1) Well circumscribed tumor on the chorionic plate, measuring ca. 3 cm, and surrounded by a distention of Wharton's Jelly. Placenta in Gestational Week 40 + 0. Fetal weight 2,475 g. Fetus with multiple skin lesions; pathology department not informed about similar lesions in other organs (by courtesy of Dr. N. Sarioglu, Department of Pediatric Pathology and Placentology, Charité Berlin Germany). (b) Cut section from the tumor. (1) Diffuse hemorrhage; (2) solid and myxoid-pseudocystic areas. (c) (1) A cell poor and myxoid loose substance; (2) blood filled capillaries; (3) capillaries with wide lumina and acute perivascular hemorrhage. A mucoid stroma is often associated with sclerosis. (d) (1) A cell poor and myxoid loose substance; (2) blood filled capillaries; (3) capillaries with wide lumina and acute perivascular hemorrhage.

Pathogenesis: Unknown.

Fetal risk: The tumor is rare and there are only a few cases, associated with premature delivery, fetal growth restriction and fetal death, described in the literature. Fetal growth restriction and fetal death may be a result of a disturbed and reduced fetal blood supply due to mechanical compression of the umbilical cord.

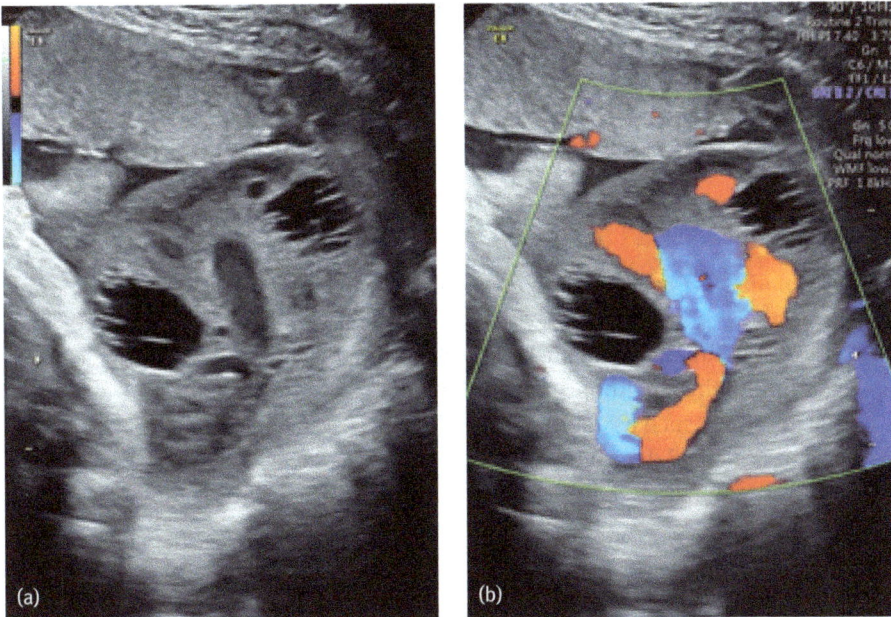

Fig. 3.17: Angiomyxoma on ultrasound. The tumor presents as a hyperechogenic mass with variably sized pseudocysts near the umbilical vessels. Color-Doppler ultrasound helps to identify low velocity blood flow in the echogenic component of the tumor. Angiomyxomas near the fetal cord insertion can mimic omphaloceles. (by courtesy of Prof. Dr. Th. Braun, Obstetric Department, Charité Berlin, Germany).

3.13 Umbilical cord rupture

Total rupture of the umbilical cord is extremely rare (ca. 1:35,000 deliveries). Partial rifts are more often found as rifts of veins in intrafunicular hematomas. If the umbilical cord surface is torn, the hemorrhage will be visible on the outside.

Incomplete ruptures of the umbilical cord are more often found towards the fetal end and close to the placental insertion, as opposed to the middle third.

Causes
–   short umbilical cord length,
–   sudden delivery,

- segmental hypoplasia of Wharton's Jelly,
- vessel wall defects,
- breech birth,
- amniocentesis,
- umbilical cord paracentesis.

Consequences for the fetus
- hemorrhagic shock in acute and large bleeds,
- anemia,
- hemorrhage into the amniotic sac and occasionally the amniotic fluid,
- aspiration of blood.

3.14 Miliar umbilical cord plaque

Flattened miliar foci can be found on the umbilical cord surface and such findings may suggest:
- Squamous epithelial metaplasia (isles of multiple-layered and partly keratinizing epithelium), this is without clinical significance.
- Infectious foci, such as Candida funiculitis, listeriosis and Staphyloccus.
- Granular calcified depositions.
- Necrotizing funiculitis.

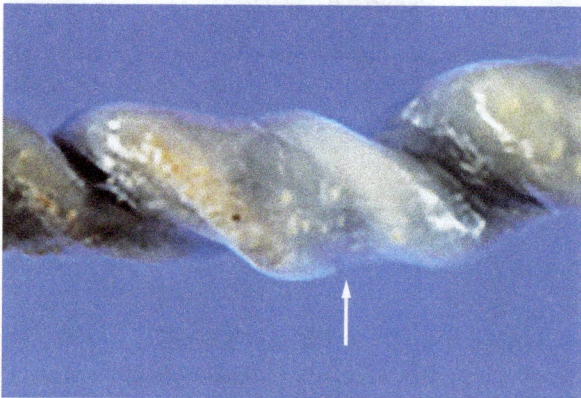

Fig. 3.18: Umbilical cord with Staphylococcus aureus depositions. Hypercoiled umbilical cord with small grey-white depositions on the surface.

References

[1]   Nikolov SD, Schiebler TH. [Fetal blood vessel system of the human full-term placenta]. Z Zell-
      forsch Mikrosk Anat. 1973;139(3):333–350.
[2]   Naeye RL. Umbilical cord length: clinical significance. The Journal of pediatrics.
      1985;107(2):278–281.
[3]   Moessinger AC, Blanc WA, Marone PA, Polsen DC. Umbilical cord length as an index of fetal
      activity: experimental study and clinical implications. Pediatr Res. 1982;16(2):109–112.
[4]   Baergen RN, Malicki D, Behling C, Benirschke K. Morbidity, mortality, and placental pathology
      in excessively long umbilical cords: retrospective study. Pediatric and developmental pa-
      thology : the official journal of the Society for Pediatric Pathology and the Paediatric Pathology
      Society. 2001;4(2):144–153.
[5]   Georgiadis L, Keski-Nisula L, Harju M, et al. Umbilical cord length in singleton gestations: a Fin-
      nish population-based retrospective register study. Placenta. 2014;35(4):275–280.
[6]   Bain C, Eliot BW. Fetal Distress in the First Stage of Labour Associated with Early Fetal Heart
      Rate Decelerations and a Short Umbilical Cord. Aust N Z J Obstet Gynaecol. 1976;16(1):51–56.
[7]   de Laat MW, Franx A, Bots ML, Visser GH, Nikkels PG. Umbilical coiling index in normal and
      complicated pregnancies. Obstetrics and gynecology. 2006;107(5):1049–1055.
[8]   Ernst LM, Minturn L, Huang MH, Curry E, Su EJ. Gross patterns of umbilical cord coiling:
      correlations with placental histology and stillbirth. Placenta. 2013;34(7):583–588.
[9]   Jessop FA, Lees CC, Pathak S, Hook CE, Sebire NJ. Umbilical cord coiling: clinical outcomes in
      an unselected population and systematic review. Virchows Archiv : an international journal of
      pathology. 2014;464(1):105–112.
[10] Khong TY. Evidence-based pathology: umbilical cord coiling. Pathology. 2010;42(7):618–622.
[11] de Laat MW, Franx A, van Alderen ED, Nikkels PG, Visser GH. The umbilical coiling index, a re-
      view of the literature. The journal of maternal-fetal & neonatal medicine : the official journal of
      the European Association of Perinatal Medicine, the Federation of Asia and Oceania Perinatal
      Societies, the International Society of Perinatal Obstet. 2005;17(2):93–100.
[12] de Laat MW, van der Meij JJ, Visser GH, Franx A, Nikkels PG. Hypercoiling of the umbilical cord
      and placental maturation defect: associated pathology? Pediatric and developmental patho-
      logy : the official journal of the Society for Pediatric Pathology and the Paediatric Pathology
      Society. 2007;10(4):293–299.
[13] Dutman AC, Nikkels PG. Umbilical hypercoiling in 2nd- and 3rd-trimester intrauterine fetal
      death. Pediatric and developmental pathology : the official journal of the Society for Pediatric
      Pathology and the Paediatric Pathology Society. 2015;18(1):10–16.
[14] Fox H, Sebire NJ. Pathology of the placenta: Saunders Elsevier; 2007.
[15] Browne FJ. On the Abnormalities of the Umbilical Cord which may cause Antenatal Death. BJOG.
      1925;32(1):17–48.
[16] Scheffel T, Langanke D. [Umbilical cord complications at the Leipzig University Gynecologic
      Clinic during 1955–1967]. Zentralbl Gynakol. 1970;92(14):429–434.
[17] Leung AK, Robson WL. Single umbilical artery. A report of 159 cases. Am J Dis Child.
      1989;143(1):108–111.
[18] Debich-Spicer EG-BD. Embryo and Fetal Pathology – color atlas with ultrasound correlation. 2nd
      ed. Cambridge: Cambridge University Press; 2006.
[19] Bryan EM, Kohler HG. The missing umbilical artery. I. Prospective study based on a maternity
      unit. Archives of disease in childhood. 1974;49(11):844–852.
[20] Wunderlich M, Sandig T. [Persistence of right umbilical vein--a rare vascular abnormality of the
      umbilical cord]. Zentralbl Gynakol. 1977;99(14):891–894.

[21] Meyer WW, Lind J, Moinian M. An accessory fourth vessel of the umbilical cord. A preliminary study. American journal of obstetrics and gynecology. 1969;105(7):1063–1068.

[22] Heifetz SA. Thrombosis of the umbilical cord: analysis of 52 cases and literature review. Pediatr Pathol. 1988;8(1):37–54.

[23] Larralde de Luna M, Cicioni V, Herrera A, Casas JG, Magnin PH. Umbilical polyps. Pediatric dermatology. 1987;4(4):341–343.

[24] Lee MC, Aterman K. An intestinal polyp of the umbilical cord. American journal of diseases of children (1960). 1968;116(3):320–323.

[25] Guschmann M, Janda J, Wenzelides K, Vogel M. [Intestinal polyp of the umbilical cord]. Zentralbl Gynakol. 2002;124(2):132–134.

[26] Vogel M. Atlas der morphologischen Plazentadiagnostik. 2 ed. Berlin: Springer; 1996.

[27] Benirschke Kurt BGJ, Baergen Rebecca N. Pathology of the Human Placenta. 6 ed. Heidelberg, NY, London: Springer; 2012.

4 Pathology of the membranes and the clinical relevance of amniotic fluid

4.1 Pathology of the membranes

The membranes are formed by layers of the amnion, chorion leve and maternal decidua (Fig. 4.1).

The amnion and chorion leve act as selective semi-permeable membrane barriers that allow:
- the transfer of nutrients, water, waste products, etc. to/from the embryo/fetus,
- the retention amniotic fluid.

Pathological changes in the membranes:
- squamous and intestinal metaplasia,
- "amniotic polyps"
- pigmentation,
- inflammation,
- amniotic band amniotic rupture sequence (ADAM-complex: Amniotic-Deformities-Adhesions-Mutilations).

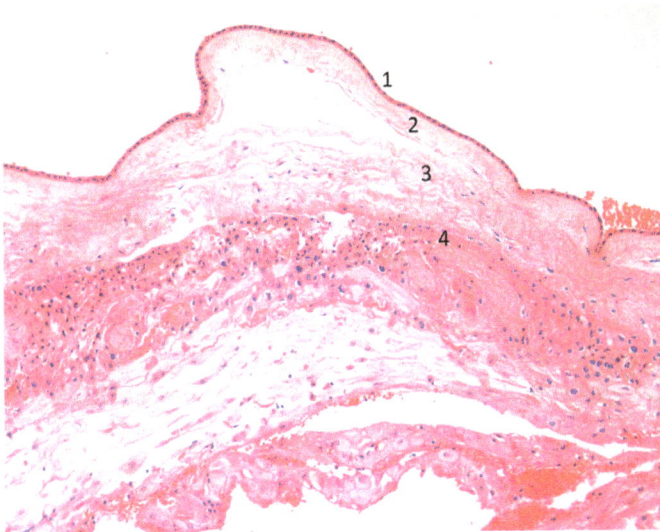

Fig. 4.1: Membrane structure. (1) Amniotic epithelium; (2) subamniotic stromal tissue; (3) loose chorionic tissue; (4) partly hypochromatic extravillous intermediate trophoblast and decidua.

https://doi.org/10.1515/9783110452600-004

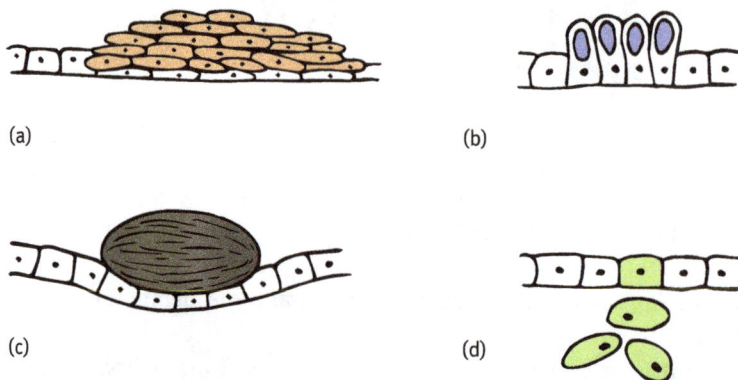

Fig. 4.2: Illustration. Most frequently seen changes in the superficial amniotic membrane. (a) Squamous metaplasia; (b) intestinal metaplasia; (c) amnion nodosum; (d) pigment deposition.

4.1.1 Metaplasia of the amniotic epithelium

Small foci of squamous epithelial metaplasia are seen in 50 % all of 3rd trimester pregnancies (Fig. 4.2). They may be found on the surface of the umbilical cord, the chorionic plate and even occasionally in the free amniotic membranes.

Intestinal metaplasia is seen less frequently and presents as foci of cylindrical epithelial cells with large cytoplasmic vacuoles and a focal positive reaction on PAS special stain.

4.1.2 Amniotic polyps

Hyperplasia of the amniotic epithelium is frequently seen as small, tree-like polyps microscopically. These polyps may be less frequent in triploidy syndrome, when compared to uncomplicated pregnancies (Fig. 4.3)

Polyps should be differentiated from amniotic folds with irregular and raised loops. These folds are projections of the subamniotic stroma and the amnion (Fig. 4.4). This is infrequently associated with a secondary loss of amniotic fluid and has a risk of recurrence.

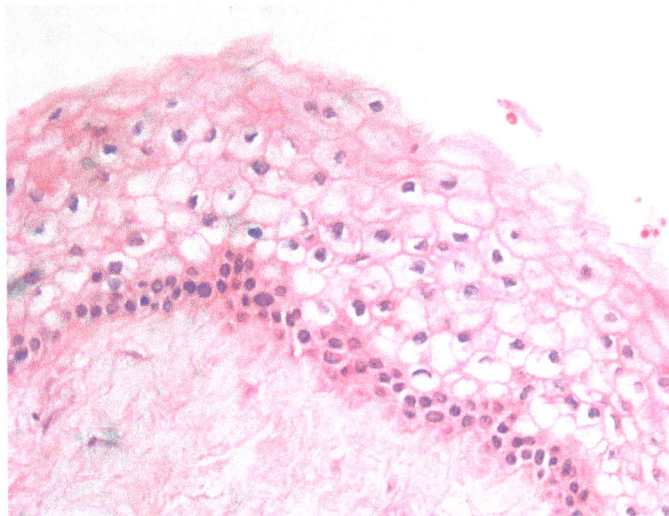

Fig. 4.3: Squamous metaplasia. Induced labor in GW 38 due to fetal growth restriction, APGAR 9-10-10.

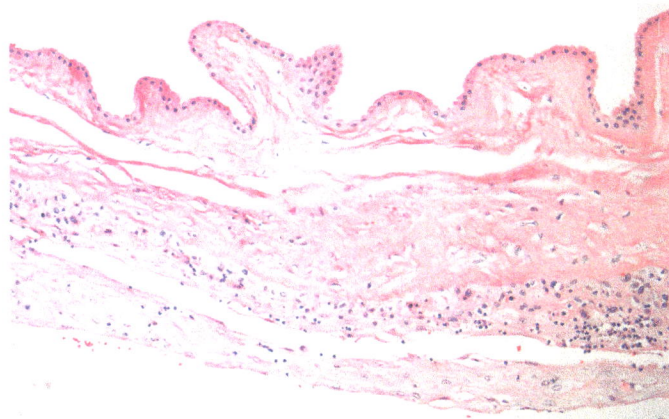

Fig. 4.4: Pseudopolypoid folds of the amniotic surface with clinical amniotic fluid loss.

4.1.3 Amnion nodosum

Nodule-like deposits of amniotic fluid on the amniotic epithelium are seen from gestational week 28. Amnion nodosum has an incidence of 1:1500 and is rarely identified in fetal abortions. It appears as small (mm sized), grey-yellow to grey-white, irreg-

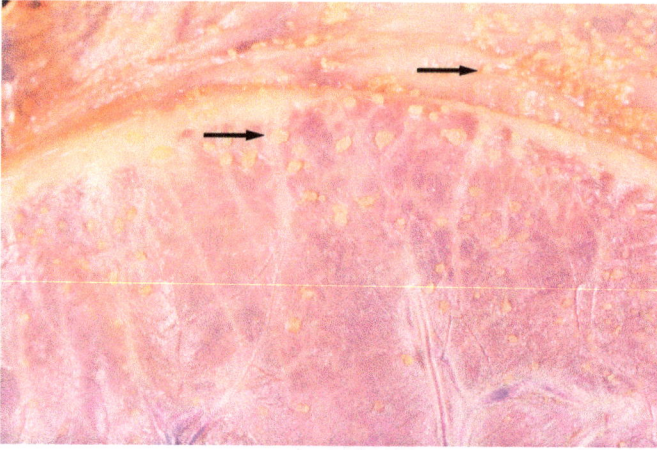

Fig. 4.5: Amnion nodosum. Chorionic surface with nodule-like spots / knots that are grey-yellow in color (occurring as part of Potter sequence). Gestational week 37.

ularly distributed nodules and may be macroscopically seen on the surface of the chorionic plate, the amnion and the umbilical cord (Fig. 4.5).

Microscopically, the nodules are sharply defined amorphic and eosinophilic deposits in a mixture of necrotic squamous epithelial cells, vernix caseosa and hair. They are compact, homogenous and are not covered by an epithelial layer. Smaller, fresher nodules react positively on PAS special stain.

Pathogenesis and causes

When the fetal skin rubs against the amniotic sac wall, cellular and amorphous particles from the skin and the wall enter the amniotic sac and attach to the placental surface along the umbilical cord.

The chronological course of amniotic nodule formation is not completely understood; however, deficient amniotic fluid (oligohydramnion), the quantity of corpuscular particles floating in the amniotic fluid and the extent of fetal contact with the dry amniotic wall are considered to play important roles.

Amnion nodosum is seen in oligohydramnion; however, plaques may attach to the amnion even if the amniotic fluid volume is normal. This may be seen if the amniotic fluid is enriched with epidermal squames and vernix caseosa; seen in cases of post-term pregnancies and fetal dystrophy (Fig. 4.6). If vernix caseosa and epithelial cells are deposited in the connective tissue of the chorionic plate and amniotic epithelium, the epithelium may split (vernix dissecans).

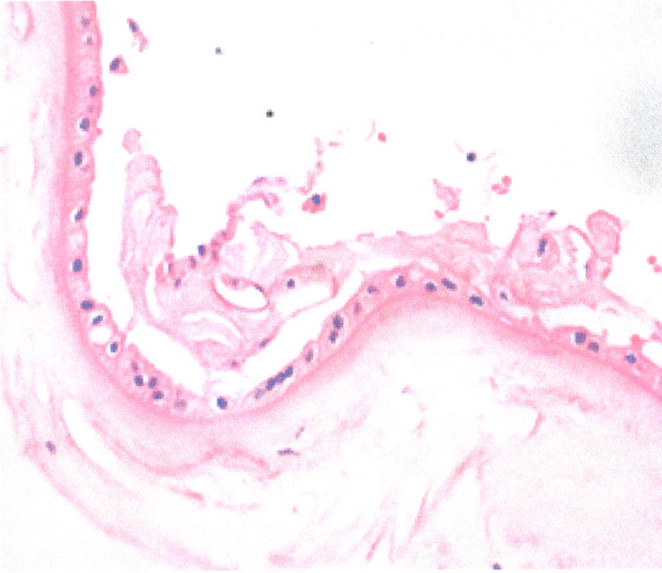

Fig. 4.6: Deposits of epidermal plaques and vernix caseosa on the outer surface of the amnion.

4.1.4 Pigmentation of the membranes

Pigmentation of the amnion may be caused by deposition of meconium pigment, lipofuscin, melanin and hemosiderin (Fig. 4.7).

Green discoloration of the amnion can be caused by fetal meconium. Meconium is green, and when diluted in amniotic fluid can appear as a green, yellow or brown discoloration. This can be the result of normal gut maturation and motilin secretion; however, a very strong green coloration of the amniotic fluid may indicate a pathological cause of meconium passage e. g. fetal hypoxia (fetal bradycardia, silent CTG, prolonged delivery). Intrauterine hypoxia can cause a temporary mesenteric vasoconstriction and intestinal ischemia; this may cause a transient increase in intestinal motility and dilatation of the anal sphincter, resulting in the pathological passage of meconium. Meconium pigment is initially found on the amniotic epithelial surface and, after two hours, phagocytosis in the amniotic epithelium causes degenerative cellular changes. It can be identified in subepithelial stromal cells after ca. 3–4 hours. The extent and intensity of phagocytosis depends on the meconium content of the amniotic fluid. Lipofuscin deposits, due to lysosomal breakdown of meconium pigment, are seen after ca. 3–4 days, even in a hyperamniotic stroma.

Meconium can cause constriction of the vessels in the umbilical cord, degeneration of myocytes, necrosis of the tunica media and even an inflammatory reaction.

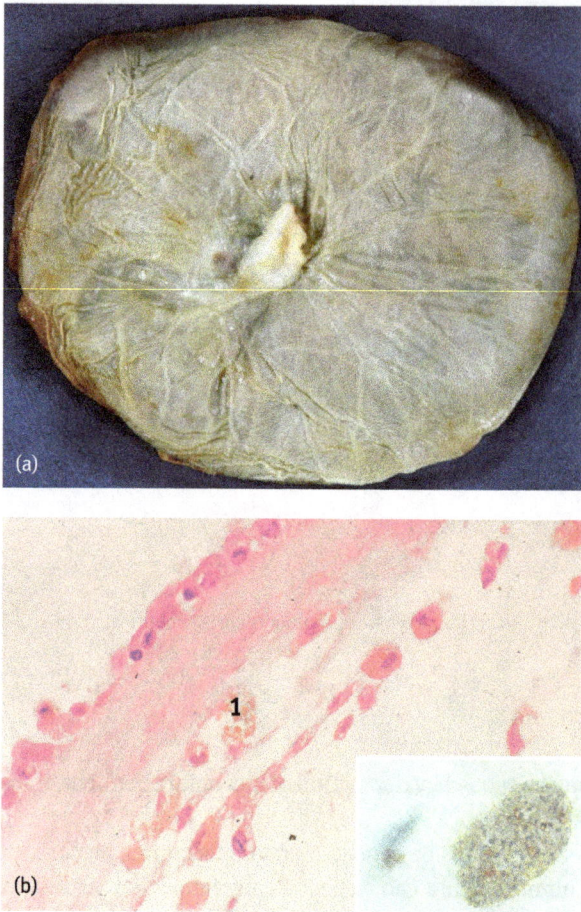

Fig. 4.7: (a) Formalin fixed placenta with green dyscoloration of the surface. (b) Histology of the chorionic plate with (1) macrophages containing meconium.

Melanin has been seen in macrophages after prolonged amniotic rupture, and in cases of dermatopathic melanosis of the placenta it is seen not only in the amniotic stroma, but also in Hofbauer cells along the villous basal membrane.

The cause and source of hemorrhage often remains unknown, but it may originate from:
- chorionic plate vessels,
- vasa aberrantia in the connective tissue of the chorionic plate and free amniotic membranes,
- decidual vessels of the extraplacental amnion,
- after puncture of the amniotic sac.

Siderophages (hemosiderin-containing macrophages) may indicate post inflammatory and fetal hemolytic diseases. Cases of amniotic siderosis, occurring in jaundice during pregnancy, are reported [1].

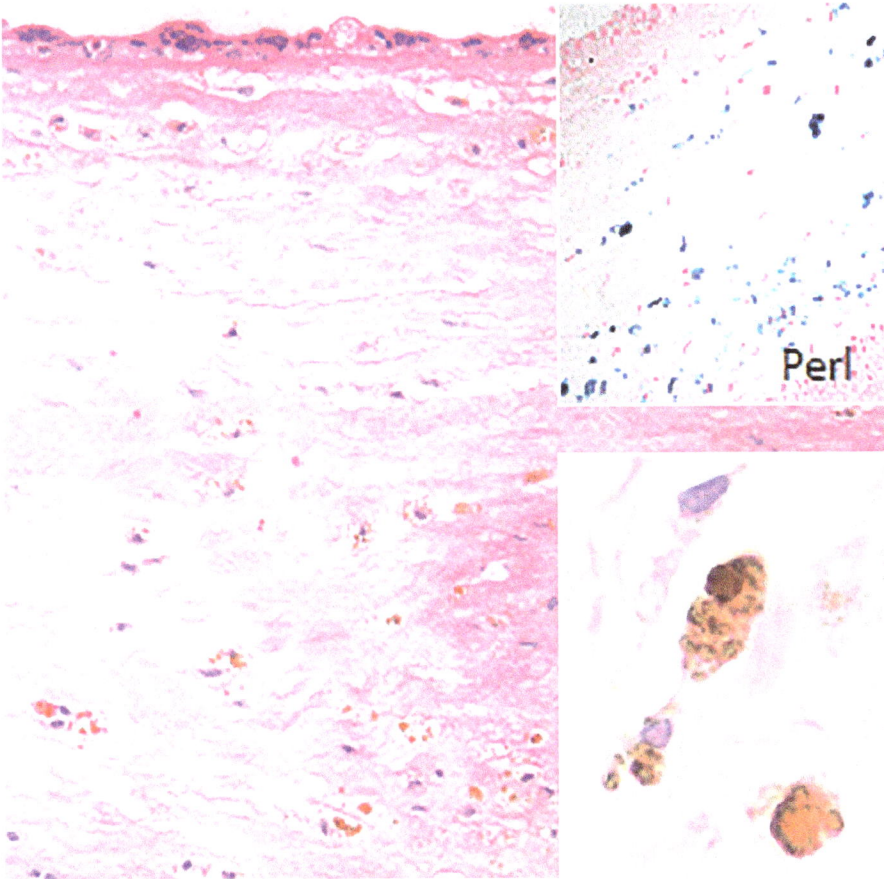

Fig. 4.8: Chorioamniotic membrane with siderophages. Perl-stain (upper inlet) and higher magnification of the granules (lower inlet). Premature spontaneous delivery in GW 23 + 4.

4.1.5 Amniotic band amniotic rupture sequence

Amniotic bands (Simonart's bands) are connective tissue strands and folds. These prolapse freely into the amniotic sac and form bridges, pouches or rings with the amniotic sac wall.

Amniotic bands are easily identifiable in fresh placentas macroscopically, but they may be difficult to find following formalin fixation (Fig. 4.9).

The most important consequence of these bands is the potential development of amniotic band amniotic rupture sequence (sequential malformations with varying degrees of entanglement, strangulation and ingrowth of the amniotic bands on the embryo/fetus). This presents as ring-like and deep impressions in the soft tissue of the fetus and may cause amputation of phalanges, or even whole extremities, and exencephaly, as well as slanting facial clefts.

Amniotic bands may entangle the umbilical cord close to the placental insertion and cause strangulation of the vessels and fetal death.

The etiology of amniotic bands remains controversial, but suggested predisposing factors include: irregular separation from the embryonic pole, irregular amniotic folding and separation of connecting stalk with formation of amniotic strands between the amnion and yolk sac [2]. This can result in constriction rings which preferentially develop in the head-neck fold or at the end of the embryonic tail and result in an ADAM complex. Amniotic rupture in early pregnancy causes separation of the amnion and chorion with the free amniotic and chorionic tissue forming folds and strands [3]. The pathogenesis of amniotic rupture due to trauma has been investigated but is not supported by evidence.

4.2 The clinical relevance of amniotic fluid

Amniotic fluid is a dynamic substance and is continuously exchanged between the mother and child. Developmental factors affecting the amniotic fluid volume are:
- fetal urine excretion from Gestational Week 10,
- fetal fluid excretion from the lung in the last trimester of pregnancy,
- the amniotic epithelium.

Amniotic fluid volume increases from ca. 5–10 ml in GW 9 to 1000 ml in gestational week 36 and subsequently decreases to ca. 800 ml in Gestational Week 40. The normal volume at term is between 300 and 1500 ml [4].

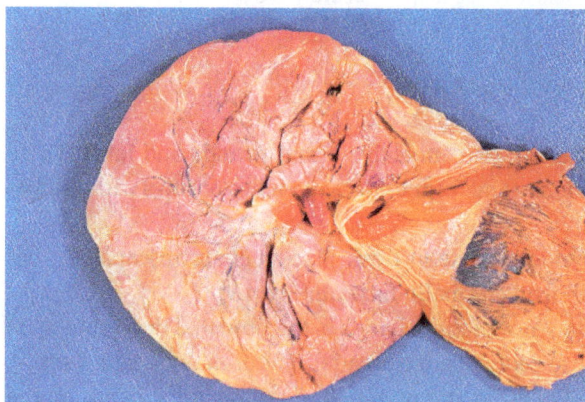

Fig. 4.9: Fetal surface of a fresh placenta. Late amniotic rupture sequence (ADAM-complex: Amniotic-Deformities-Adhesions-Mutilations) with strangulation of the umbilical cord by multiple amniotic bands. IUFD in Gestational Week 31.

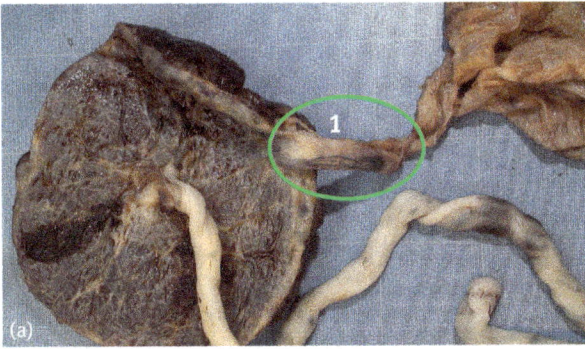

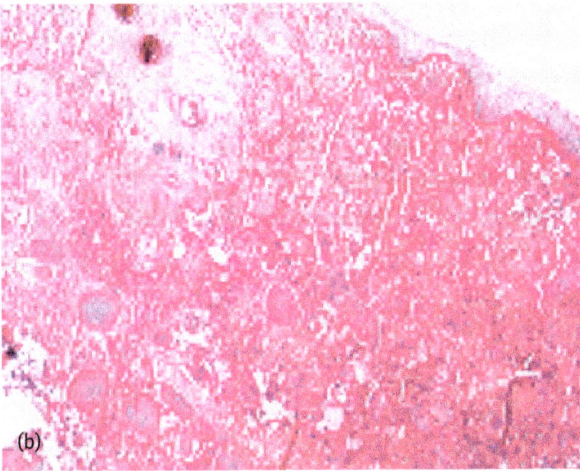

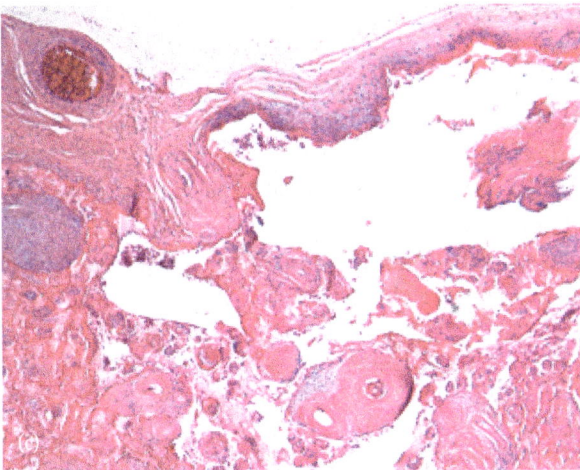

Fig. 4.10: (a) Formalin fixed placenta with an amniotic band. (1) Strand like membranes in the placental margin; umbilical cord insertion. The structure was considered to be an amniotic band on ultrasound and delivery was induced in GW 38 + 2. (b) Histology: hemorrhagic congestion of the placental parenchyma. (c) Necrotic foci in the amniotic band.

4.2.1 Polyhydramnion

Polyhydramnion is a pathological increase, up to 2 liters, of amniotic fluid and may be:
1. acute, due to an increase of amniotic fluid over a few days,
2. chronic, due to a gradual increase of amniotic fluid.

There are no characteristic changes in the amnion or amniotic epithelium, but it is often associated with villous maturation arrest.

The causes and origin of polyhydramnion may be classified as
– maternal causes: diabetes mellitus, maternal nephritis and intrauterine infection,
– fetal causes: malformations leading to disorders of swallow, anencephalus with increased fluid transudation, atresia of the gastro-intestinal tract, epignathus, etc.,
– placental causes: chorangioma (occasionally as a triad of polyhydramnion, chorangioma and pregnancy induced maternal hypertension),
– twin-twin transfusion syndrome with polyhydramnion of the recipient.

4.2.2 Oligohydramnion and anhydramnion

Oligohydramnion is a decrease of amniotic fluid to less than 100 ml and anhydramnion a complete lack of amniotic fluid.
    Associated placental changes are:
– amnion nodosum
– polypoid amniotic folding.

Causes of oligohydramnion/anhydramnion
– kidney and/or urinary tract malformations (Potter Sequence),
– chronic amniotic fluid loss due to pre-term rupture of the membranes (PROM),
– chronic amniotic fluid deficiency in chronic placental insufficiency and intrauterine fetal growth restriction,
– chronic amniotic fluid deficiency in the donor of twin-twin transfusion syndrome,
– chronic amniotic fluid loss due to intrauterine retention.

References

[1] Liebhart M, Wojcicka J. Microscopic patterns of placenta in cases of pregnancy complicated by intrahepatic cholestasis (idiopathic jaundice). Pol Med J. 1970;9(6):1589–1600.
[2] Becker V, Schiebler TH, Kubli F. Allgemeine und spezielle Pathologie der Plazenta. Die Plazenta des Menschen. Stuttgart: Thieme; 1981. p. 251–393.
[3] Torpin R. Rupture of amnion alone. Obstetrics and gynecology. 1969;33(3):450.
[4] Dudenhausen JW. Prakische Geburtshilfe. Berlin: DeGruyter; 1989.

5 Pathology of the placenta in middle and late pregnancy

5.1 Growth disorders

In a normally progressing pregnancy, the placenta increases in growth and weight according to gestational age. Placental growth is assessed against reference values from normal range percentile tables. Macrosomia and growth restriction are interpreted as a sign of growth disorder, and they are associated with villous maturation disorders and maternal metabolic and vascular disorders.

Placental growth is characterized by:
- weight
- area
- placental-fetal ratio (PF)
- fetal-placental ratio (FP)

There is some evidence to suggest that the shape and size of the placenta may be associated with pregnancy complications (FGR, reduced fetal movements) and the individual's long-term health [1–4].

5.1.1 Weight and area

The placental weight to area/size ratio is relatively constant between 1.6:1 and 2.0:1. A large placental size/area is due to implantation and perfusion, and such a placenta has a greater functional capacity than a smaller placenta of same weight. Perfusion in small, thick placentas (more than 4 cm) is reduced as the thickness is unfavorable for vascularization [5].

Macrosomic placentas are defined by a weight and/or size above the 90th percentile and may be seen in combination with:
- maternal gestational diabetes (GDM)
- early onset GDM with ineffective metabolic transport
- morbus hemolyticus neonatorum
- hydrops congenitus
- chronic intrauterine infection (congenital syphilis, hydropic toxoplasma, CMV)
- cyanotic cardiac failure
- congenital tumors (teratoma, nephroblastoma metastases, congenital leukemia)
- chorangiomatosis
- villous immaturity
- prolonged exposure to altitudes above 4000 m sea level

https://doi.org/10.1515/9783110452600-005

– genetic disorders
– mesenchymal dysplasia, Beckwith-Wiedemann

Small placentas are characterized by a weight and/or area less than the 10th percentile and may be seen in combination with:
– premature delivery
– gestational hypertonia
– essential hypertonia
– chronic kidney disease
– late stage type 2 diabetes mellitus (T2DM) with vascular changes
– collagenosis, rheumatoid vasculitis
– chronic intrauterine infection (viral) with vasculitis
– genetic disorders (trisomy)

5.1.2 Placental-fetal ratio (PF)

The placental-fetal ratio (PF) is the calculated placental net weight and fetal weight (Plw:Few). The ratio decreases in normal pregnancies as they progress (Appendix, Table A3).

An increased PF may suggest:
– increased placental weight due to villous immaturity or chorangiosis type 1
– placental hydrops
– chorangiomatosis of the placenta
– acute blood congestion (feto-placental transfusion)
– growth restricted fetuses with normal placental growth or macrosomic placental growth (triploidy)

A decreased PF may be found in:
– decreased placental growth, in combination with accelerated villous maturation or terminal villous hypoplasia, with a normal fetal weight
– macrosomic fetuses with a normal placental weight
– hydrops fetalis (without placental hydrops)
– congenital fetal tumors

A normal placental-fetal ratio does not exclude growth and maturation disorders of the placenta and/or the fetus.

5.1.3 Fetal-placental ratio (FP)

The fetal-placental weight ratio (FP) is the calculated fetal weight and the placental weight (Few:Plw). Several studies suggest this value is useful in the assessment of SGA (small for gestational age) children, who are often born with large placentas. This value may be a possible indicator of the adequacy of the placental reserve capacity in fetal growth restriction (FGR) [6–8] (Appendix, Table A4).

Consequences for the fetus

A macrosomic placenta with retarded villous maturation may favor a chronic and/or acute fetal hypoxia. A growth restricted placenta with circulatory disorders and maturation disorders may favor a chronic nutritional placental insufficiency.

Both macrosomic and growth restricted placentas should be examined, their placental weight deviations calculated and the results correlated with clinical findings.

Recurrence risk of growth disorders

The recurrence risk of growth disorders has not been examined in large studies, but in an archive of 700 placentas, the calculated recurrence risk in the subsequent pregnancy was 53 % for macrosomia and 33 % for growth restriction.

5.2 Implantation disorders

Implantation disorders have been described as macroscopic variations of form that may indicate an asymmetric distribution and growth, or extensive depth, of the trophoblasts [3]:

1. variation in the shape of the placenta
2. variation of the umbilical cord insertion
3. implantation disorders, specifically:
   - incorrect implantation location,
   - attachment disorders of the placenta.

Diagnosis may be made on ultrasound, if an increased depth of implantation is seen. Implantation disorders, umbilical cord insertion included, are seen in more than 70 % of risk pregnancies and in ca. 50 % normal pregnancies.

5.2.1 Placental appearance

The placenta is usually round and slightly oval. The shape and size of the placenta are factors that are statistically associated with complications in pregnancy (FGR, reduced fetal movements) and an individual's long-term health [1,2,4,9,10].

Deviations in shape (kidney, heart or belt-like configurations) are of minimal maternal and fetal consequence. (Figs. 5.1, 5.2)

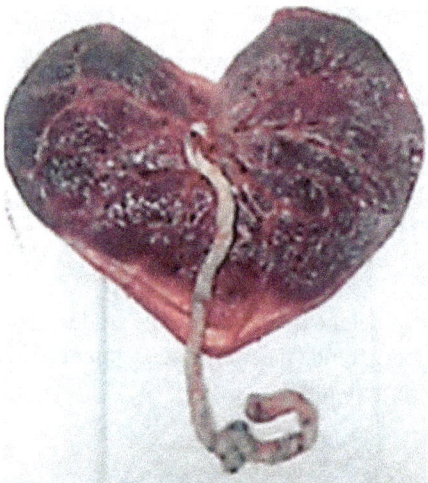

Fig. 5.1: Heart-shaped placenta (by courtesy of Prof. Dr. Anne Cathrine Staff, Division of Obstetrics and Gynecology, Oslo University Hospital, Faculty of Medicine, University of Oslo, Norway).

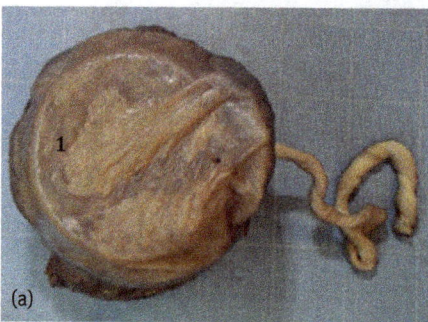

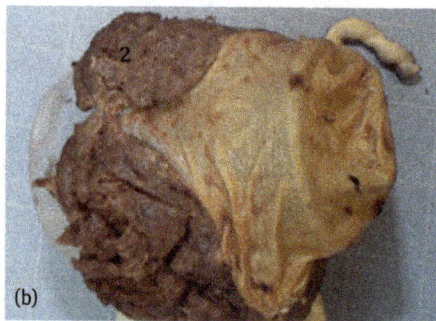

Fig. 5.2: Belt-like placenta. (a) Fetal surface; (b) maternal surface: (a) the inner part of the chorionic and basal parenchyma is replaced by membrane (1); (b) protrusion of a section of the central membrane with view in to the maternal basal surface: the external parenchyma forms like a belt around the inner membrane (2).

Placenta succenturiata is characterized by one, or more, adjacent placental lobes that are connected by membrane bridges to the main placental disc, which contains the umbilical cord insertion (Figs. 5.3a, 5.4). Vascularization of the accessory lobes

(a)

(b)

(c)

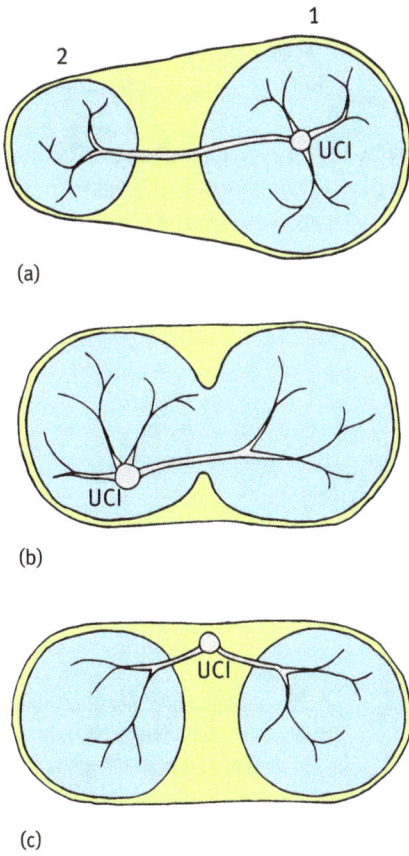

Fig. 5.3: Illustration. Variations in placental appearance with different umbilical cord insertions (UCI): (a) placenta succenturiata; UCI on the main placental disc (1); accessory lobe (2); fetal vessels running in the amniotic membrane connecting both lobes; (b) placenta bilobata: incomplete separation of the lobes; UCI on one lobe; (c) placenta bipartite: two completely separated discs; Velamentous UCI.

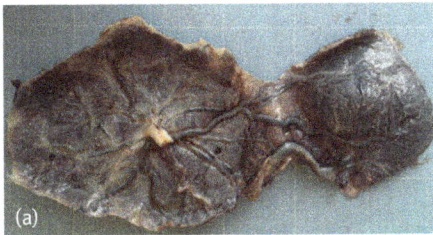

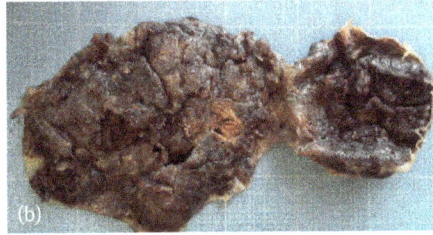

(a) (b)

Fig. 5.4: Placenta succenturiata. (a) Fetal surface with one lobe connected to the main placental disc by vessel bridges; (b) maternal surface; (UCI) umbilical cord insertion.

occurs via bridging vessels in the membrane. Diagnosis on ultrasound is important due to the risk of polyp development, which may cause:
– postpartum bleeding
– retarded uterus involution with increased hemorrhage
– endometritis puerperalis

Placenta bi/multilobata is characterized by a placental disc containing two or more placental notches in the placental margin. These notches demarcate the different lobes. The lobes may be of equal or different size. There is no associated increased fetal or maternal risk. (Figs. 5.3b, 5.5)

Placenta bi/multipartita is characterized by two or more placental discs. The discs are confined to the membranes and each has a direct connection to the velamentous umbilical cord insertion (Fig. 5.3c, 5.6). Bridging vessels between the placental discs (vasa previa) increase fetal risk and may cause:
- fetal-placental circulatory disorders
- vessel rupture, especially in premature rupture of the membranes
- incomplete placental delivery.

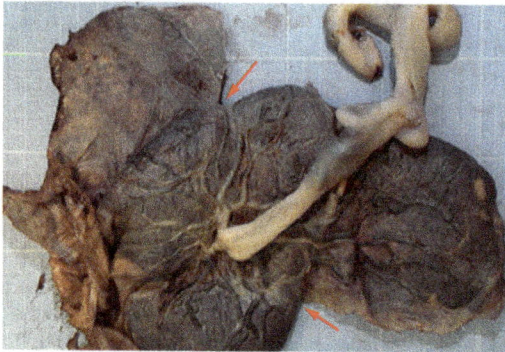

Fig. 5.5: Placenta bilobata (two lobes). The lobes are identified by two notches (arrows) in the placental margin.

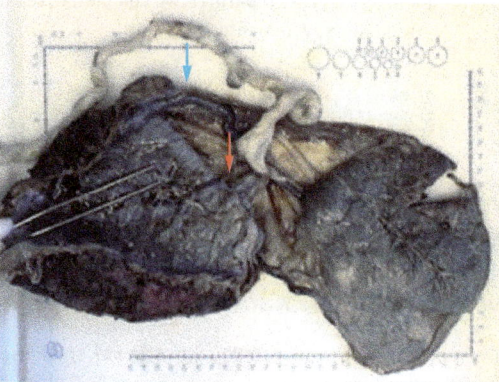

Fig. 5.6: Placenta bipartita. Velamentous umbilical cord insertion between the two placental discs: vasa previa (red arrow); vasa aberrantia (blue arrow).

Placenta extrachorialis is characterized by a disparity between the chorionic plate and placental parenchyma; this results in placental tissue lying beyond the boundaries of the chorionic plate. The distance between the margo internus and margo externus is more than 2 cm. The membranes insert in the margo internus and the transition to the chorion leve no longer occurs at the placental edge, but at varying points within the

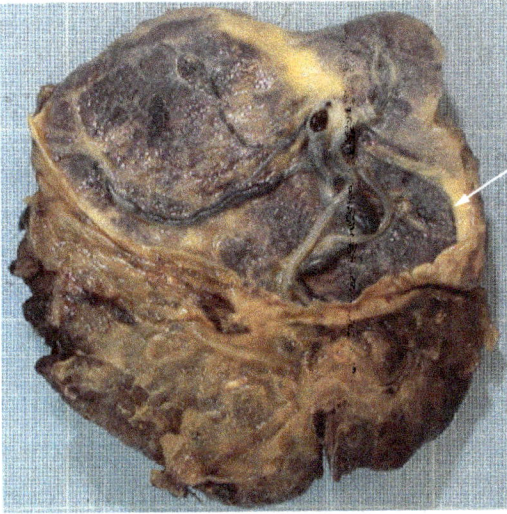

Fig. 5.7: Placenta extrachorialis marginata partialis. Eccentric UCI with chorionic vessels branching in an Oak tree pattern. Margo internus (white arrow) Placenta in GW 29.

circumference of the placenta. On ultrasound, the central part of the placental disc is depressed and surrounded, at a variable distance from the umbilical cord insertion, by a white ring. Ultrasound findings include folding of the fetal membranes back onto the fetal surface, or a brim of tissue continuous with the edge of the placenta protruding into the uterine cavity. The shape of this placental abnormality has been compared to a soup plate and has been reported in association with endometritis, retained placenta and postpartum hemorrhage [11,12]. Depending on the height of the margo internus, two different types can be differentiated [13]:

– Placenta extrachorialis marginata (less than 5 mm height).
– Placenta extrachorialis circumvallata (more than 5 mm height).

The pathogenesis of extrachorialis is not known. Deep implantation of chorion frondosum and subsequent division of the chorion frondosum and chorion laeve are considered as possible cause. During villous expansion and growth, the internal margin (margo internus) is formed centrifugally "extrachorionic" and separated from the margo externus. The space between margo externus and internus is free from vessels. Membrane insertion is pushed towards the inner margin, increasing the distance between the inner and outer margin (internus, externus). This process only affects parts of the placenta, which is why placenta extrachorialis is first seen after gestational week 14–15. It has been suggested that this placental variation develops due to recurrent venous hemorrhages, such as those in small focal and low grade placental marginal abruptions. Hemorrhages may lead to membrane folding which affects the insertion of the chorionic plate. In cases of placenta circumvallata, fibrin/fibrinoid, hemorrhage and siderophages are found in the margo internus, which may indicate

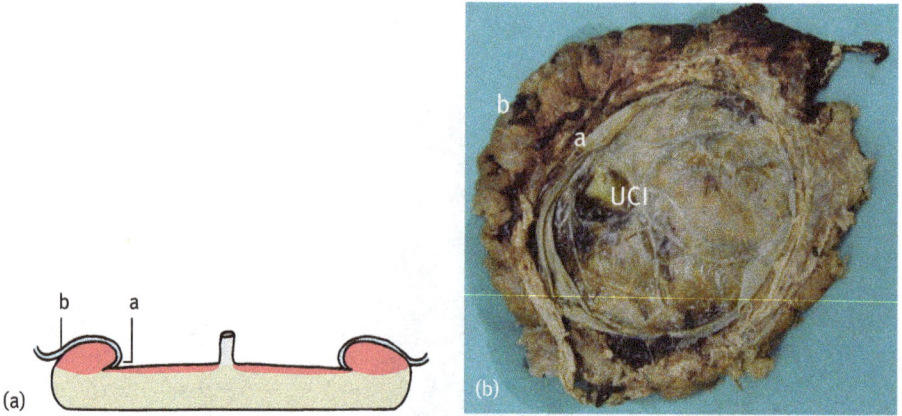

Fig. 5.8: (a) Illustration of placenta circumvallata. Fetal plate with height > 5 mm and > 2 cm distance between (a) margo internus and (b) margo externus. (b) Formalin fixed placenta circumvallata. (a) Margo internus, (b) margo externus, (UCI) umbilical cord insertion.

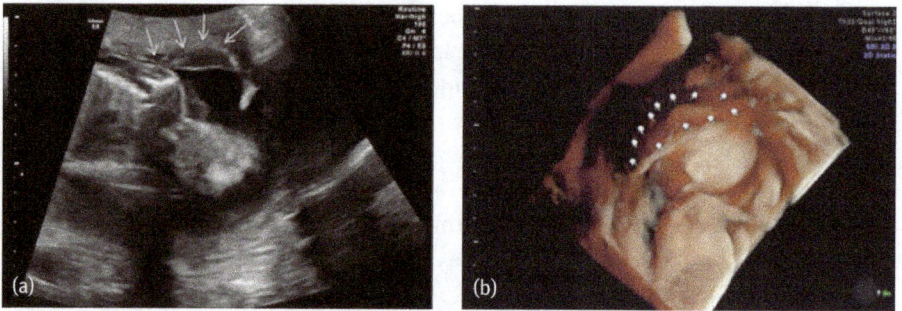

Fig. 5.9: 2D (a) and 3D (b) Ultrasound of a circumvallate placenta with a central depression and a surrounding white ring at a variable distance from the umbilical cord insertion. The white ring consists of a double-layer of amnion and chorion, necrotic villi and fibrin. The chorion and the amnion overlap to a chorio-amniotic fold or "band"; including folding of the fetal membranes back onto the fetal surface, or a brim of tissue continuous with the edge of the placenta protruding into the uterine cavity. (by courtesy of Prof. Dr. Th. Braun, Department of Obstetrics, Charité Berlin, Germany).

secondary circulatory disorders in this area. This proposed mechanism for extrachorialis marginata remains controversial.

Frequency

Placenta extrachorialis occurs in less than 10 % of non-risk pregnancies, placenta extrachorialis marginata is of 7-fold higher incidence than placenta extrachorialis circumvallata.

Perinatal risk

A circumvallate placenta may be associated with bleeding and abruption in early pregnancy. Gross examination may show a yellow-brown discoloration, and on histology iron deposition in the chorioamniotic membranes may be seen.

Both morphological variations are more frequent in multiple pregnancy, with an increased risk in circumvallata of:

- preterm delivery, 3-fold increase,
- Increased preterm marginal abruption and acute sinus bleeding [14–16].

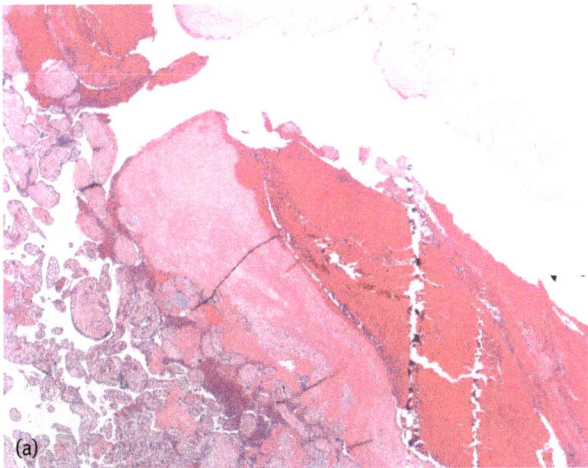

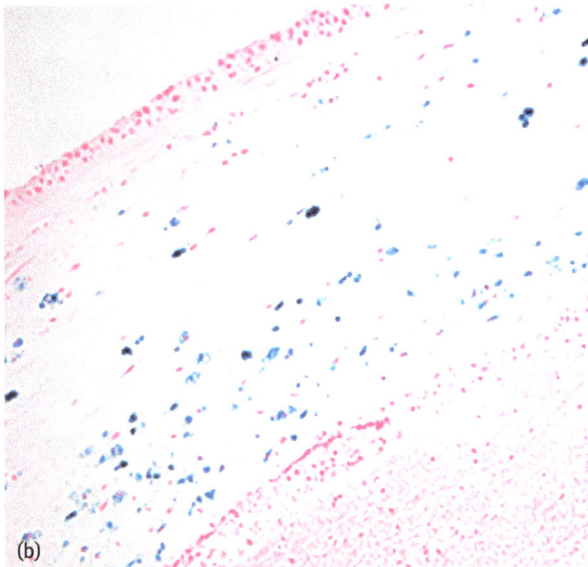

Fig. 5.10: (a) Marginal bleeding. Fibrin and blood are pushed from the margo externus into the intervillous and subchorionic space. (b) Iron deposition in the chorioamniotic membrane, Perl special stain. Placenta circumvallata in Gestational Week 36 + 4, delivered by cesarean section.

Placenta membranacea is a flattened placenta, less than 5 mm thick, and often only affects part of the placenta (placenta membranacea partialis). A diffuse placenta membranacea (placenta membranacea totalis or diffusa) is rare and usually associated with a placenta previa.

Placenta membranacea is often associated with:
– abortion,
– fetal growth restriction,
– placenta previa with subsequent hemorrhage,
– placenta accreta or increta with placenta retention.

Placenta fenestrata is an extremely rare variation of the placenta with window-like, irregular villous defects which are covered by the membrane. It is frequently seen in embryonic and early fetal abortion rather than in late pregnancy.

5.2.2 Umbilical cord insertion

Umbilical cord insertion occurs inside the inner semicircle of the chorionic plate in more than 50 % of placentas and, as a consequence, cord insertions may be:
– *Central or slightly eccentric:* insertion within the semicircle occurs in ca. 30 %.
– *Eccentric:* insertion occurs outside the inner semicircle with dichotomic branching of the fetal vessels.

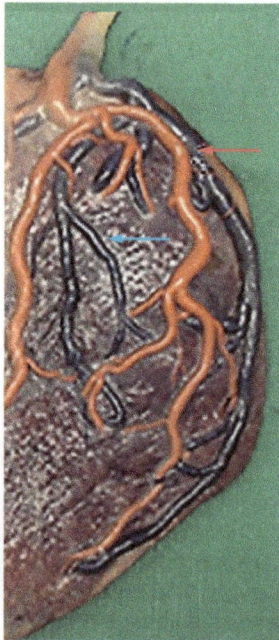

Fig. 5.11: Marginal umbilical cord insertion in a twin placenta. Vasa previa, fetal vessels running towards the central part of the placenta (blue arrow); Vasa aberrantia, fetal vessels running along the placental margin (red arrow). Dichorionic-diamniotic twin placenta in Gestational Week 36.

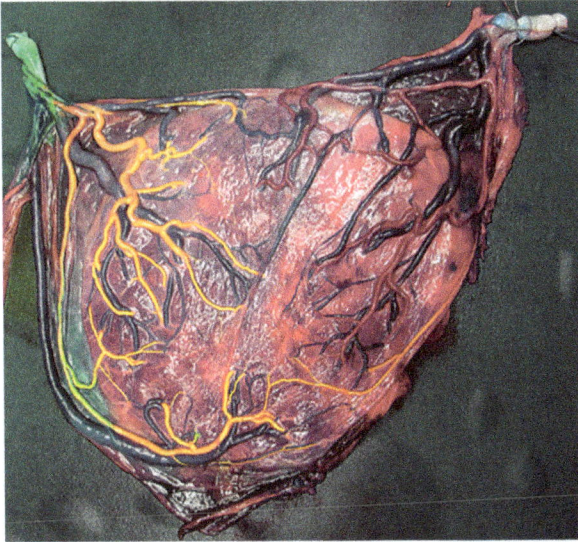

Fig. 5.12: Velamentous umbilical cord insertion in a monochorionic-diamniotic twin placenta in Gestational Week 34. Ink injection into one umbilical artery and the umbilical vein of both cords.

- *Marginal:* insertion is located in the marginal placental border.
- *Velamentous:* insertion with unprotected vessel branches running in the membranes towards the chorionic plate. The course of these vessels is either direct, the shortest way "vasa previa", or in a roundabout way, "vasa aberrantia". Ultrasound may show umbilical cord vessel branches running unprotected along the uterus wall.
- *Insertio furcuata:* characterized by a branching of the umbilical cord above the chorionic plate with fork like vessel branches running towards the chorionic plate that are unprotected by Whartons' Jelly.

Pathogenesis

Atypical umbilical cord insertions are assumed to be due to asymmetric trophoblast migration; caused by a nutritional deficiency in the maternal implantation bed [17]. The blastocyst attaches to the maternal mucosa at the embryonic pole and the location of this attachment corresponds to the connecting stalk, from which the umbilical cord develops. In structural and functional disorders, the trophoblast is not fully developed to all sides of the implantation bed and this results in a developmental asymmetry of the placenta and the umbilical cord.

Eccentric umbilical cord insertions, and morphological anomalies, are more often seen in singleton pregnancies due to in-vitro fertilization and intrauterine embryonic transfer, rather than in spontaneous pregnancies [18].

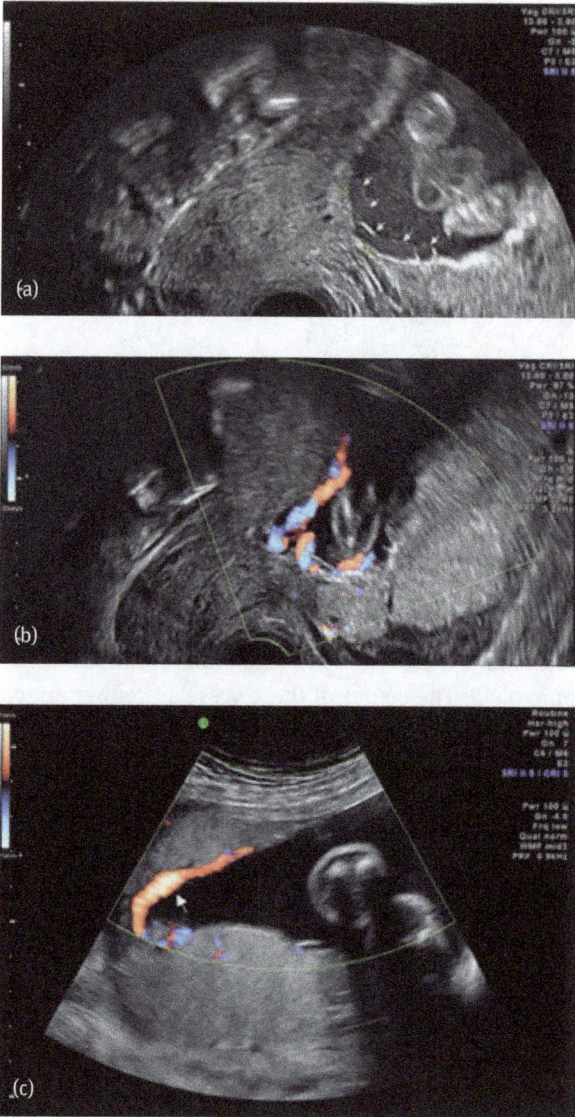

Fig. 5.13: Ultrasound of a placenta with a velamentous cord insertion. Characteristic vessels running parallel to the uterine wall, unprotected by the underlying chorion, and extending to the placental margin (c), where they connect to the chorionic vasculature. Color-Doppler (a, b) imaging aids in the identification of the vessels. A differential diagnosis may include cord loops, but a velamentous insertion remains fixed when the uterus is moved (by courtesy of Prof. Dr. Th. Braun, Department of Obstetrics, Charité Berlin, Germany).

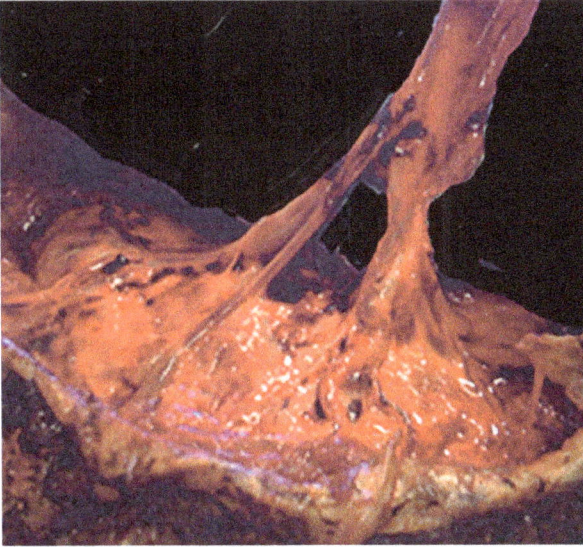

Fig. 5.14: Insertio furcuata. Velamentous umbilical cord vessels dividing within the membranes, at a distance from the chorionic surface. Caesarean section at term.

Consequences for the fetus

Increased fetal and perinatal risk is only seen in marginal, velamentous and insertio furcuata umbilical cord insertions. In a marginal insertion, vessel kinking may lead to a temporary fetal vascular malperfusion with corresponding CTG changes [19].

A velamentous umbilical cord insertion may lead to:
– Temporary circulatory disorders caused by traction; as a consequence of pressure on, or kinking of, the vessels in the membranes.
– Vessel rupture with fetal hemorrhage / anemia; especially with premature rupture of the membranes. The frequency of vessel rupture with vasa previa is reported at ca. 2 % and perinatal fetal deaths due to fetal anemia as 0.46 % [20].

5.2.3 Implantation disorders

There are two different groups of implantation disorders:
1. Placenta implanted in the wrong location:
   – placenta previa marginalis: the placenta reaches the inner cervix
   – placenta previa partialis: the placenta partly overlies the cervix
   – placenta previa totalis: the placenta completely overlies the cervix
2. Placental adhesive disorders:
   – accreta
   – increta
   – percreta

Placenta with increased implantation depth

– Placenta accreta: a partial or complete deficiency of the decidua basalis and Nitabuch's fibrinoid. Chorionic villi extend into the basal myometrium, either focally or completely [21].
– Placenta increta: villi and trophoblast islands show infiltration within the superficial or deep myometrium.
– Placenta percreta: villi penetrate through the full thickness of the myometrium to the serosa.

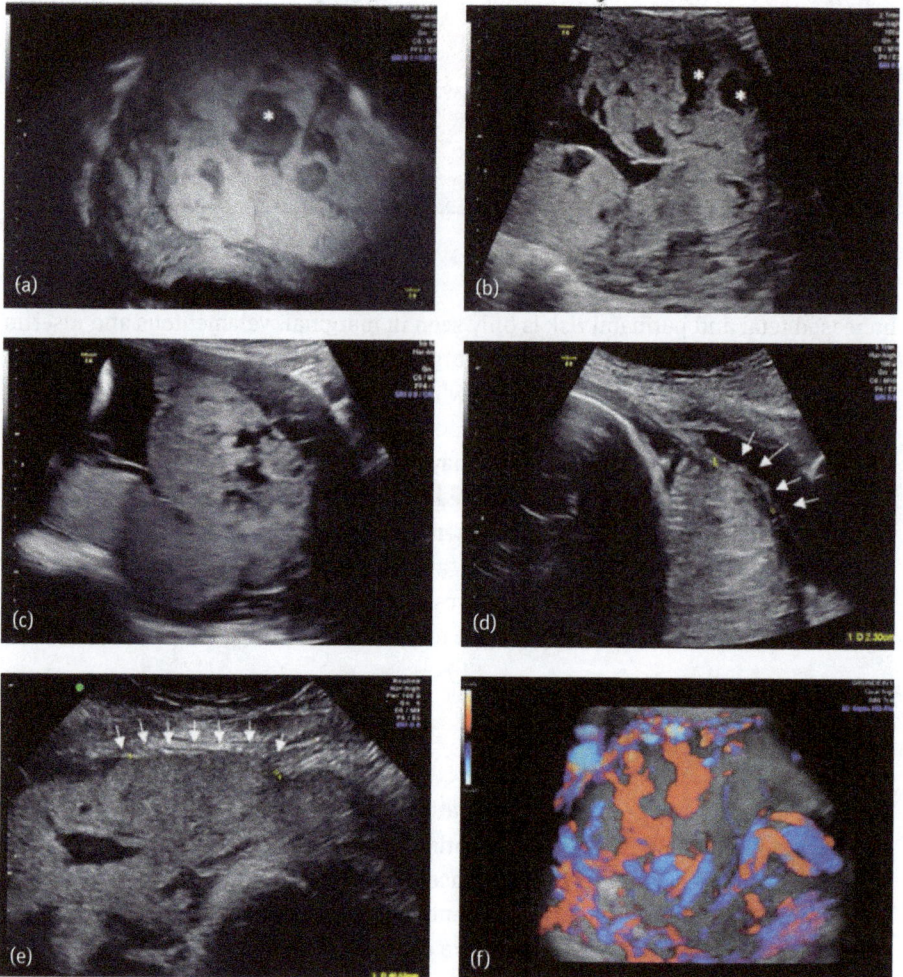

Fig. 5.15: (a, b, c) Ultrasound showing an abnormally invasive placenta (AIP). (d) Bladder wall interruption; (e) myometrial thinning; (f) uterovesical hypervascularity; (c) subplacental hypervascularity, loss of clearing zone, placental bulge and focal exophytic mass (by courtesy of Prof. Dr. Th. Braun, Department of Obstetrics, Charité Berlin, Germany).

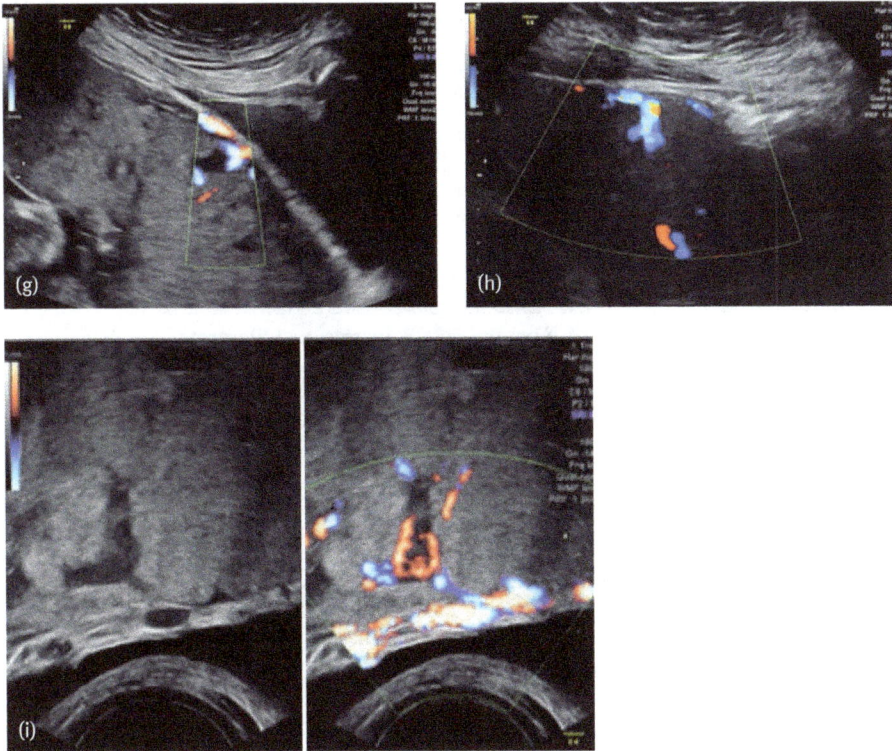

Fig. 5.15: (continued) (g, i) bridging vessels; (h) placental lacunae feeder vessels (by courtesy of Prof. Dr. Th. Braun, Department of Obstetrics, Charité Berlin, Germany).

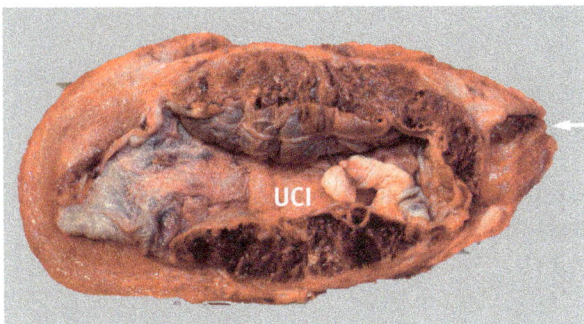

Fig. 5.16: Uterus with placenta previa, unfixated. Cervix (arrow marked); (UCI) umbilical cord insertion. Cesarean section in GW 34.

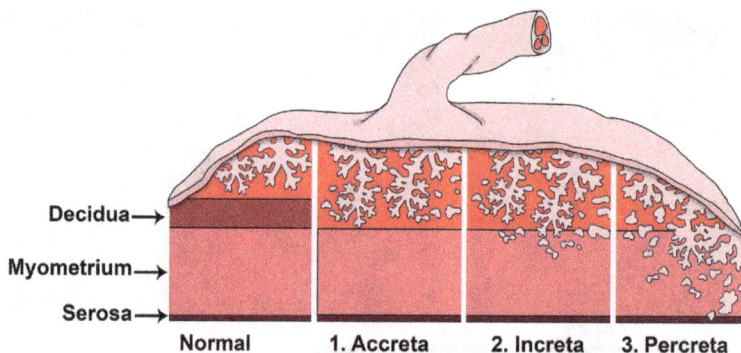

Fig. 5.17: Illustration. Normal and invasive placentas. Normally, placenta villi are separated from the myometrium by a thin decidual layer; (1) Accreta. Basal placental villi are lying close to the myometrium; (2) Increta. Placental villi and trophoblast islands are within the myometrium; (3) Percreta. Placental villi infiltrate the myometrium and extend through to the serosa (by courtesy of Kristin Berg-Eriksen, premed, University of Oslo).

For a definitive diagnosis, an adequate curettage specimen or uterine resection is required. The frequency of implantation disorders has increased up to 60-fold due to increased cesarean section rates in the last 40 years [21,22].

Pathogenesis

The most important factors in the development of implantation disorders are an insufficiently developed decidua and scar formations. Collagen may alter decidual development, and collagen types I and III are identified in higher proportions in the lower uterine segment, in the septum (not always anatomically present) and in the corneal region. These two areas, the septum and cornea, have the highest occurrence of abnormal placental adherence [23].

There are several risk factors for an increased implantation depth:
– previous cesarean sections, especially in anterior placenta,
– placenta previa,
– previous uterine curettage, especially after multiple procedures,
– endometrial infection with scar formation after abortion,
– age over 35 years (non-specific).

Typical complications are:
– total or partial placental retention,
– spontaneous uterine rupture, especially in placenta percreta.

Frequency

The incidence of placenta accreta has increased from ca. 0.8/1000 deliveries in 1980 to 3/1000 [24]; however, the incidence depends on the diagnostic criteria used and there is a discrepancy between the histological and clinical diagnosis of the condition [25]. In a 20 year study, which included additional clinical criteria, the incidence of placenta accreta increased to 1.87:1000 deliveries [26].

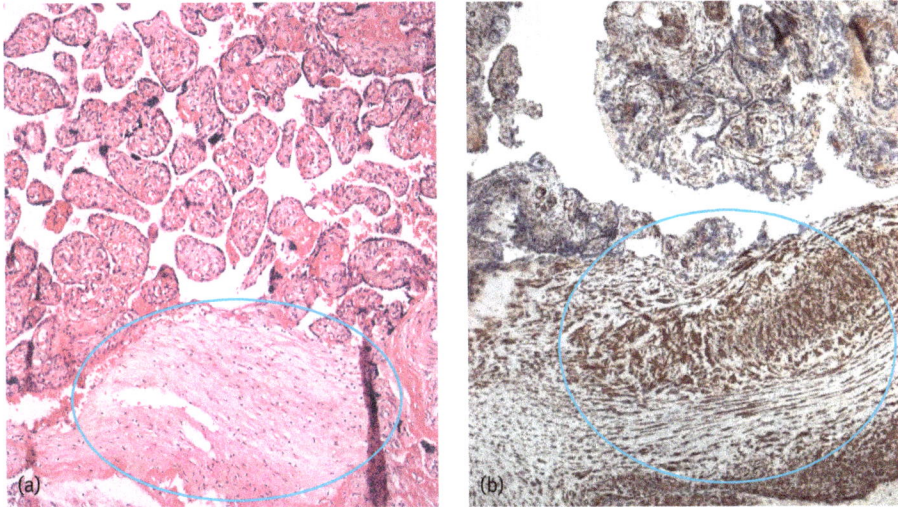

Fig. 5.18: (a) Placenta accreta. Placental villi lying close to the myometrium without a separating decidual layer (blue circle). (b) Actin immunostain. Placenta in Gestational Week 39 + 2, normal pregnancy. Attached villi to the myometrium (circled). The placenta was detached manually.

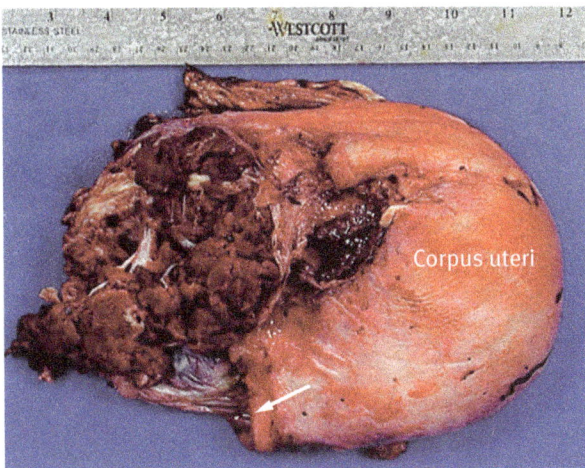

Fig. 5.19: Placenta percreta. Ruptured uterine wall (arrow) caused by placental villi infiltrating through the uterine serosa (by courtesy of Debra S. Heller, M.D., Department of Pathology and Laboratory Medicine, University Hospital (UH), Newark, NJ).

5.3 Pathological changes of the chorionic plate

Frequently encountered changes are:
– cystic lesions,
– varicosis,
– aneurysm,
– hematoma.

5.3.1 Cystic lesions

Cystic lesions on the surface of the chorionic plate consist of encapsulated fluid between the amnion and the connective chorionic tissue. They often develop nearby the umbilical cord insertion and can be up to the size of a chicken egg. They do not have an epithelial lining and hemorrhage into the cysts can sometimes be seen. The cysts are assumed to represent *rests* of the *amniotic-chorionic junctional layer* of the placenta or caused by tension between these layers. Cyst size is a result of fluid transudation into the cystic cavity.

Amniotic cysts may develop following withdrawal and constriction of the amnion; these cysts are lined by epithelium and increase if fluid is secreted into the cyst. Cysts of the chorionic plate are without pathological significance.

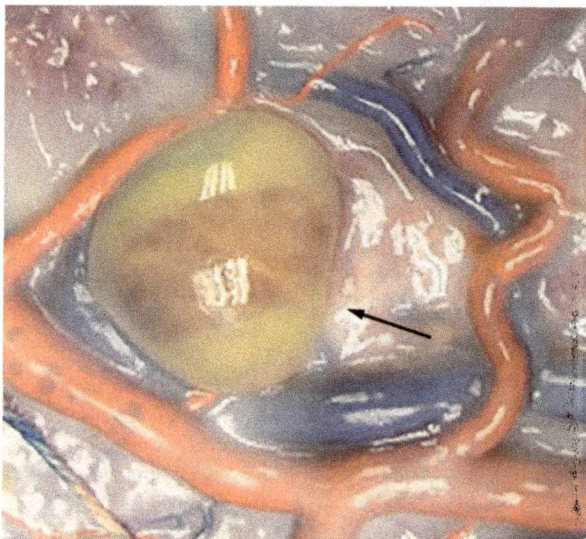

Fig. 5.20: Chorionic plate cyst (arrow). A 2 × 2 cm cystic lesion lies beneath the amniotic membrane. Incidental finding of an arterial varicosity in the arterio-venous anastomosis. Placenta in GW 36.

5.3.2 Varicosis

Varicoses are fusiform and serpentine dilatations of the venous fetal vessels. Varicoses in the chorionic plate are frequent and are without consequence for the fetus (varicoses of the umbilical cord, Ch. 4).

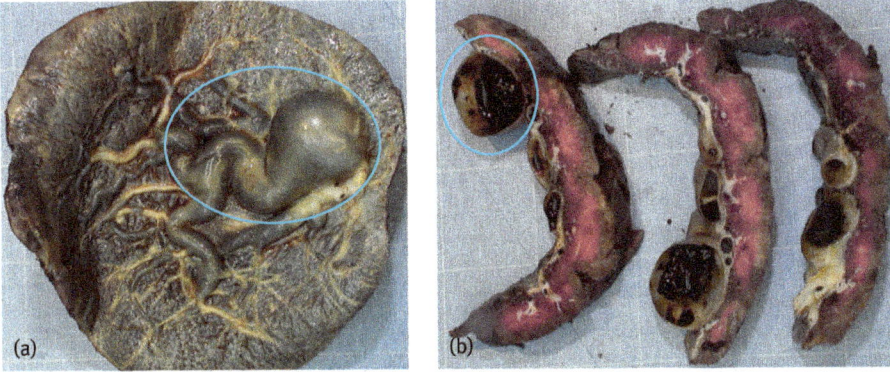

Fig. 5.21: (a) Formalin fixed placenta, chorionic/fetal surface. Sac-like and serpentine fetal vessel (circled). (b) Thrombosis (circle) on multiple cut sections, placenta in gestational week 39. Uncomplicated pregnancy with delivery of a healthy baby.

5.3.3 Aneurysm

Fetal aneurysms are a focal and circumscribed dilatation of the arterial branches of the central fetal vessels, and they can be found next to the chorionic plate and in the stem villi. They may be solitary or multiple and typically vary from a few millimeters to 2 cm in diameter. Larger aneurysms are more often found near the umbilical cord insertion while smaller aneurysms are found near the margo internus.

Histologically, hypoplasia of the tunica media is found in the dilated vessel [3,27,28].

Aneurysms in our archived material were found in 0.4 % of cases; however, a higher rate of 2.5 % is reported elsewhere [29]. Smaller aneurysms with collapsed vessel lumina are often difficult to see. Aneurysms do not usually confer an increased risk to the fetus, and an increased recurrence risk for developmental disorders of the allantois vessels has not been confirmed.

5.3.4 Hematomas

Hematomas typically lie on the superficial layer of the chorionic plate, below the amnion. Usually they are flat, often poorly demarcated and have sizes ranging from the tip of a finger to that of a hand.

They develop due to mechanical stress, such as tension on the chorionic plate, during delivery. They prevent fetal blood from reaching the end vessel branches of the chorionic tissue and, if of a sufficient size, may play a role in fetal anemia or fetal hemorrhagic shock [30].

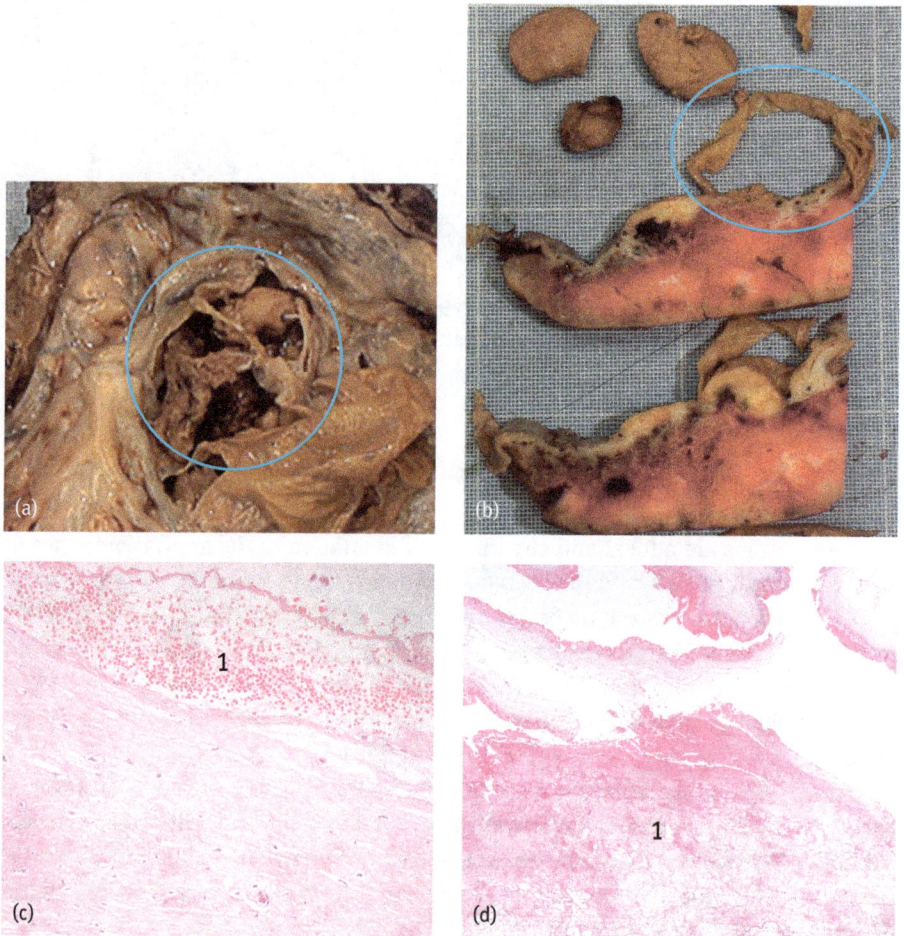

Fig. 5.22: (a) Formalin fixed placenta. Subamniotic cystic lesion (circle) 4 × 3 × 2.5 cm filled with necrotic material (fibrin and blood), representing episodic bleeding into an organized hematoma. Placenta in GW 38. (b) Cut sections through the cystic lesion (circled). (c) (1) Subamniotic erythrocytes, fresh blood. (d) (1) Subchorionic debris (old fibrin). Placenta in GW 38, child's weight 3280 g, APGAR 9-10-10. Normal pregnancy. Lesion was clinically suspected as a vanishing twin.

References

[1] Barker DJ, Osmond C, Thornburg KL, Kajantie E, Eriksson JG. The lifespan of men and the shape of their placental surface at birth. Placenta. 2011;32(10):783–787.

[2] Barker DJ, Osmond C, Thornburg KL, Kajantie E, Eriksson JG. The shape of the placental surface at birth and colorectal cancer in later life. Am J Hum Biol. 2013;25(4):566–568.

[3] Kloos K, Vogel. Pathologie der Perinatalperiode.: Thieme Stuttgart; 1974.

[4] Longtine MS, Nelson DM. Placental dysfunction and fetal programming: the importance of placental size, shape, histopathology, and molecular composition. Semin Reprod Med. 2011;29(3):187–196.

[5] Becker V, Schiebler TH, Kubli F. Allgemeine und spezielle Pathologie der Plazenta. Die Plazenta des Menschen. Stuttgart: Thieme; 1981. p. 251–393.

[6] Luque-Fernandez MA, Ananth CV, Jaddoe VW, et al. Is the fetoplacental ratio a differential marker of fetal growth restriction in small for gestational age infants? Eur J Epidemiol. 2015;30(4):331–341.

[7] Molteni RA, Stys SJ, Battaglia FC. Relationship of fetal and placental weight in human beings: fetal/placental weight ratios at various gestational ages and birth weight distributions. J Reprod Med. 1978;21(5):327–334.

[8] Roland MC, Friis CM, Voldner N, et al. Fetal growth versus birthweight: the role of placenta versus other determinants. PloS one. 2012;7(6):e39324.

[9] Eriksson JG, Kajantie E, Thornburg KL, Osmond C, Barker DJ. Mother's body size and placental size predict coronary heart disease in men. Eur Heart J. 2011;32(18):2297–2303.

[10] Misra DP, Salafia CM, Charles AK, Miller RK. Placental measurements associated with intelligence quotient at age 7 years. J Dev Orig Health Dis. 2012;3(3):190–197.

[11] Coletta JM, Lewin SN, D'Alton ME. Gestational trophoblastic disease. In: Copel JA DAM, Gratacos E, Platt LD, Tuschek B, Feltovich H., editor. Obstetric Imaging. 1. Philadelphia: Elsevier; 2012. p. 493–7.

[12] Torpin R, Mitchell JC. Placenta circumvallata associated with internal rupture of the membranes during pregnancy. J Med Assoc Ga. 1967;56(10):416–417.

[13] Lemtis H, Vogel M, Liedke K. Über die Ätiologie der Placenta circumvallata. In: Saling E DJ, editor. Perinatale Medizin. IV. Stuttgart: Thieme; 1973. p. 104–8.

[14] Benson RC, Fujikura T. Circumvallate and circummarginate placenta. Unimportant clinical entities. Obstetrics and gynecology. 1969;34(6):799–804.

[15] Fox H, Sen DK. Placenta extrachorialis. A clinico-pathological study. J Obstet Gynaecol Br Commonw. 1972;79(1):32–35.

[16] Lemtis H, Vogel M, Liedke K. Über die Ätiologie der Placenta circumvallata. In: Saling E DJ, editor. Perinatale Medizin. IV. Stuttgart: Thieme; 1973. p. 104–108.

[17] Krone HA. Die Bedutung der Eibettstörungen für die Enstehung menschlicher Missbildungen. Stuttgart: Fischer; 1961.

[18] Gavriil P, Jauniaux E, Leroy F. Pathologic examination of placentas from singleton and twin pregnancies obtained after in vitro fertilization and embryo transfer. Pediatr Pathol. 1993;13(4):453–462.

[19] Vogel M, Ahting U, , Hartung M, Saling E. CTG Befunde und ihre Beziehung zur Plazentamorphologie. Perinatale Medizin. 1974;V:144–146.

[20] Quek SP, Tan KL. Vasa Praevia. Aust N Z J Obstet Gynaecol. 1972;12(3):206–209.

[21] Khong Y, Brosens I. Defective deep placentation. Best practice & research Clinical obstetrics & gynaecology. 2011;25(3):301–311.

[22] Silver RM, Barbour KD. Placenta accreta spectrum: accreta, increta, and percreta. Obstetrics and gynecology clinics of North America. 2015;42(2):381–402.

[23] Chantraine F, Blacher S, Berndt S, et al. Abnormal vascular architecture at the placental-maternal interface in placenta increta. American journal of obstetrics and gynecology. 2012;207(3):188 e1-9.

[24] Flood KM, Said S, Geary M, et al. Changing trends in peripartum hysterectomy over the last 4 decades. Am J Obstet Gynecol. 2009;200(6).

[25] Palacios-Jaraquemada JM. Caesarean section in cases of placenta praevia and accreta. Best Pract Res Clin Obstet Gynaecol. 2013;Apr;27(2):221–232.

[26] Wu S, Kocherginsky M, Hibbard JU. Abnormal placentation: twenty-year analysis. Am J Obstet Gynecol. 2005;May;192(5):1458–461.

[27] Kloos K, Vogel M. [Placentation disorders]. Gynakol Rundsch. 1969;7(3):197–204.

[28] Wentworth P. Some Anomalies Of The Foetal Vessels Of The Human Placenta. J Anat. 1965;99:273–282.

[29] Lemtis H. On aneurysms of fetal vessels in the human placenta. Arch Gynakol. 1968;206(3):330–347.

[30] Friedmann W, Vogel M. Postpartale Beurteilung makroskopischer Plazentaveränderungen. In: G M, editor. Differentialdiagnose in Geburtshilfe und Gynäkologie. I. Stuttgart: Thieme; 1987.

6 Fetal circulatory disturbances

6.1 Fetal placental perfusion

The blood flow between the fetus and the placenta travels in the tunica media containing vessels of the umbilical cord, chorionic plate and stem villi. This circulatory system is regulated by the fetal vessels of the intermediate and terminal villi [1].

Feto-placental circulation is driven by the fetal heart, and the blood circulating between the umbilical cord arteries and the placenta is estimated to be between 40 % and 60 % of the total fetal heart volume. Umbilical cord circulation at term is ca. 110 ml/min/kg of fetal weight [2,3], and the blood is transported with a medium arterial blood pressure of ca. 53 mmHg; pressure in the intravillous capillaries and the umbilical vein is calculated to be ca. 35 and ca. 20 mmHg respectively.

There is some evidence of a peripheral regulation of the villous circulation, functioning like a villous pulse, which assists in venous return [4]. Desmin and actin positive muscle cells have been identified in the vessel walls of the stem villi and in the venules, precapillaries and capillaries of the intermediate villi. They are also seen in the stroma of both the stem and intermediate villi; however, actin positive cells have not been identified in the stroma of the terminal villi. Intravillous and intervillous blood flow fluctuates, with rapidly infused areas transitioning to areas with a relatively sluggish blood flow, and vice versa. These differences are regulated by muscle contractions occurring close to the arteries (reduced inflow) and veins (reduced venous outflow) and this results in relatively prolonged retention time for blood in the microcirculation.

Neural regulation of the feto-placental microcirculation does not occur; however, hormone regulation of the circulatory system by catecholamines, thromboxane, prostaglandin E2, angiotensin II, bradykinin and prostacyclin may occur, but this is, as of yet, unconfirmed [5,6].

6.2 Fetal circulatory disturbance

Fetal circulatory disturbances show morphology corresponding to acute or chronic disturbances of fetal arterial inflow or venous outflow. Vascular ectasia may indicate acute hypoxia.

Morphology
- villous stromal hemorrhage,
- villous stromal fibrosis,
- fetal thrombotic vasculopathy.

https://doi.org/10.1515/9783110452600-006

The 2015 Amsterdam workshop group consensus meeting statement recommends that fetal vascular malperfusion (FVM) is to be graded as high (global) or low (segmental) (Fig. 6.10, Table 6.1).

6.2.1 Villous stromal hemorrhage

Villous stromal hemorrhage may be seen at any gestational age. It is often seen in fetal abortion, especially if induced, and occurs close to villous groups with maturation arrest.

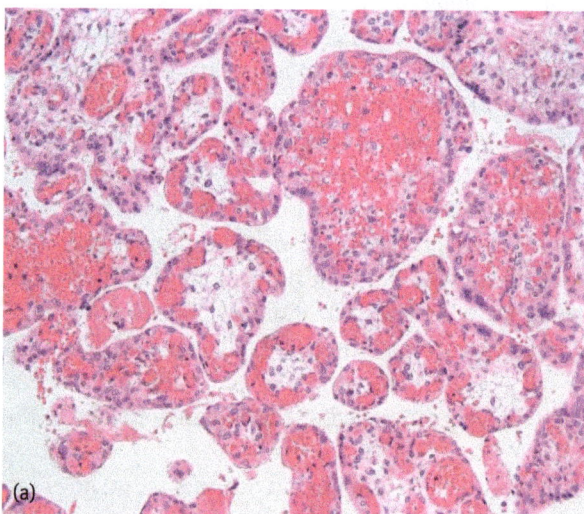

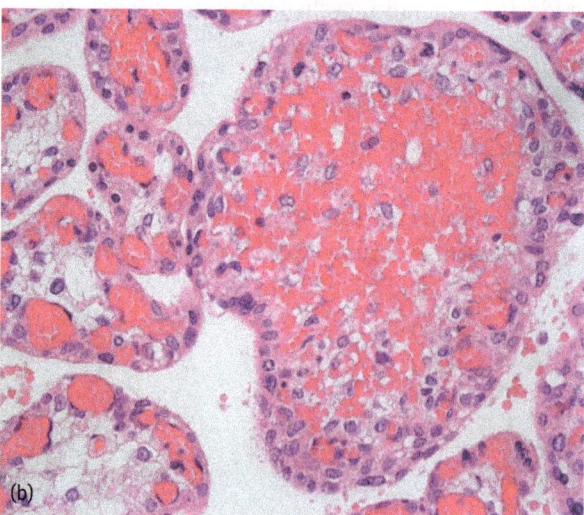

Fig. 6.1: Hyperemia in fetal vessels with focal stromal hemorrhage. Placenta in GW 29 + 0 with polyhydramnion, APGAR 3-4-6, child's weight 2000 g.

Hemorrhage is acute and can be seen, focally, in the surrounding parenchyma and in the periphery of infarcted areas. The superficial chorionic epithelium is normally preserved and is only rarely affected.

Pathogenesis
- hypoxia related diapedesis bleeding, thought to be influenced by prostaglandins,
- traumatic rhexis hemorrhage (vessel rupture) after diagnostic transplacental needle aspiration,
- trauma to the lower abdomen.

Consequences for the fetus
Stromal hemorrhage is believed to correlate with intrauterine hypoxia and anoxia. Sometimes siderophages, without any associated inflammatory response, can be seen in mid-pregnancy placentas, and they can be a residual indication of stromal hemorrhage.

Villous stromal hemorrhage, with a damaged chorionic epithelium, is found in feto-maternal transfusion (feto-maternal hemorrhage).

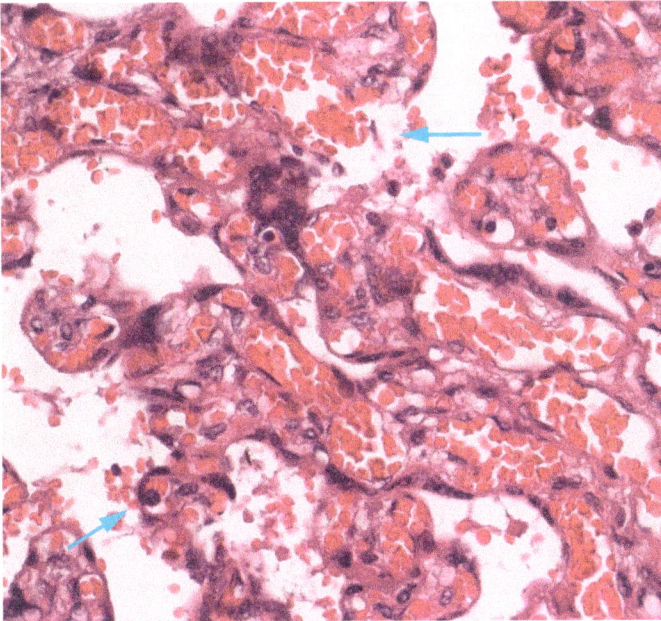

Fig. 6.2: Feto-maternal transfusion. Hemorrhage into the intervillous space due to a damaged chorionic epithelium (arrows). Placenta in GW 39 + 2, birth weight 4000 g. Child was limp and anemic following delivery.

6.2.2 Villous stromal fibrosis

Stromal fibrosis is an increase in the collagenous tissue content, and a reduction of the number of capillaries in the intermediate and terminal villi. It is seen in more than 20 % of risk pregnancies. Diffuse villous fibrosis, affecting up to 15 % of the total placental area, is seen in up to half of placentas from hypertensive pregnancies and arterio/arteriolopathy of other origins (diabetic angiopathy, nicotine abuse).

Morphology

The amount of collagenous tissue in the intermediate and terminal villi ranges from slightly increased to markedly increased with completely fibrotic villi. In the early stages, the collagenous stroma is cell rich (Fig. 6.3) but later becomes cell poor (Fig. 6.4). Capillaries are rare partly little lumen (Fig. 6.5). The endothelium of the vessels shows nuclear pyknosis and karyorrhexis. Endothelial markers may reveal, focally, negative immunohistochemistry for CD 31. Avascular villi are typically seen in the more advanced, fibrotic stages. The basement membrane of the capillaries and the trophoblasts is thickened [7] and the villous epithelium shows nuclear sprouts with well-preserved nuclei and regressive changes. A reduction, or total absence, of positive immunohistochemical staining for HCG and HPL may also be seen.

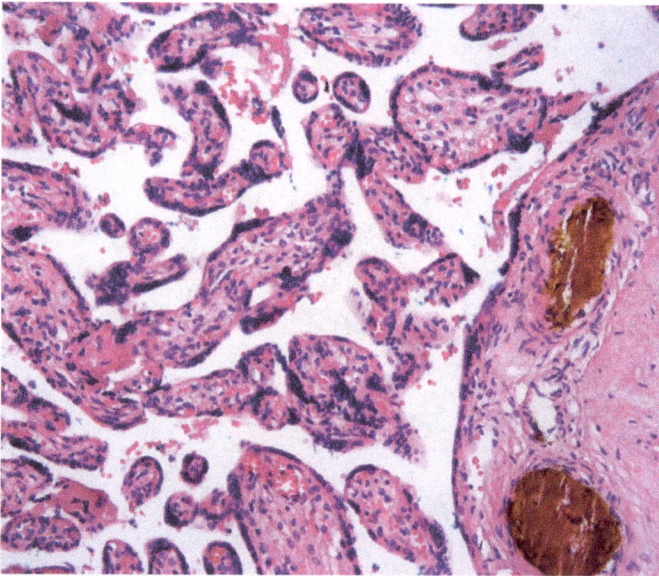

Fig. 6.3: Early stage of stromal fibrosis. Groups of intermediate and terminal villi with cell rich stroma, reduced number of fetal vessels and increased villous trophoblastic syncytial knots. Placenta in GW 38.

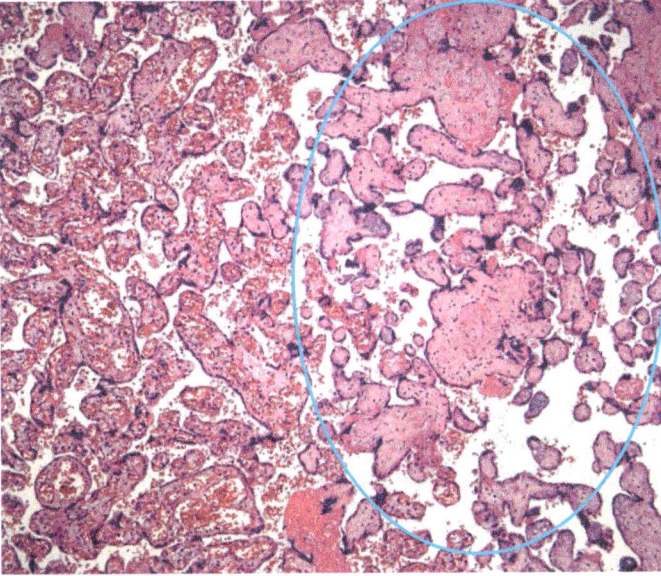

Fig. 6.4: Late stage of stromal fibrosis. Villous groups with stromal fibrosis and cell poor, homogenous and collagenous stroma with absent villous vessels. Collapse sclerosis of the stem villi vessels and hyperemia of the surrounding mature villi is apparent. Placenta in GW 41 + 3 with oligohydramnion and a pathological CTG, APGAR 2-5-7.

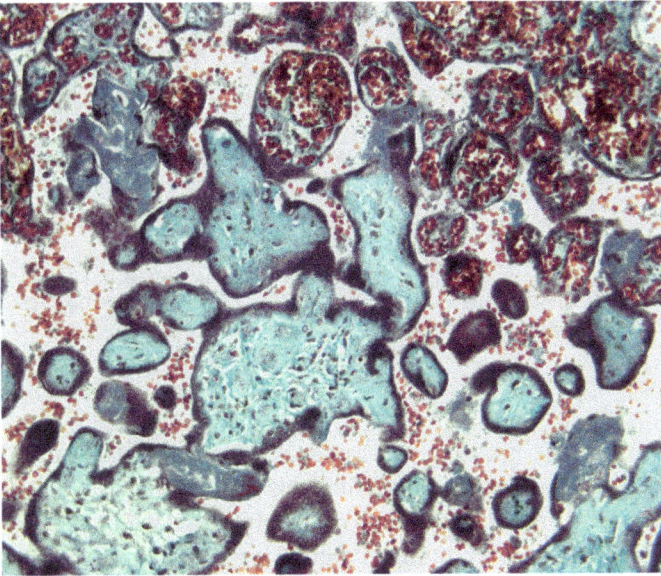

Fig. 6.5: Masson Trichrome stain (HPF) with regressive changes of the villous trophoblast. Placenta in GW 38 with fetal growth restriction, APGAR 5-8-8.

Avascular villi should be evaluated for their distribution in the parenchyma and subdivided into: small foci (3 or more foci of 2 to 4 terminal villi), intermediate foci (5 to 10 villi) and large foci (more than 10 villi) [8].

Pathogenesis

Villous stromal fibrosis affects immature and hypermature villi. Fibrosis is often closely related to increased intervillous and perivillous microfibrin depositions. It is caused by increased collagen synthesis, due to:

- *Chronic, relative ischemia* of the villi caused by stenosis, or occlusion, of the proximal artery in the stem villus. It is often associated with endangiopathia obliterans or organized thrombi.
- *Chronic hypoxic tissue damage;* secondary to decreased intervillous vascularization. Another theory suggests that inadequate oxygen uptake by fetal capillaries leads to increased oxygen in the villous stroma and that this stimulates collagen synthesis [9].

Consequences for the fetus

Fibrosis is a morphological change due to a disturbed villous vascular perfusion. It causes a disorder of capillary growth and sinusoidal dilatation of preexisting capillaries, with a subsequent decrease in the intravillous capillary blood volume.

Fetal risk depends on the grade and the extent of the fibrosis; small foci are clinically irrelevant.

6.2.3 Fetal thrombotic vasculopathy

Fibrin deposits may be luminal or mural, occlusive or non-occlusive and acute or chronic (8).

To be distinguished are:
- thrombosis of the stem villi vessels,
- microthrombosis of the terminal villi.

Thrombosis of stem villi vessels

Thrombosis of the stem villi vessels is characterized by stagnation of blood flow and a partial, occasionally occlusive, thrombosis. Quite often, this is associated with earlier endothelial cell damage and fibrinoid degeneration of the fetal vessel wall.

Thrombosis may show organization, if due to a prolonged duration of delivery [10]. Fetal thrombosis may cause acute or chronic circulatory disturbance in the downstream villi if there is complete occlusion of the functional end artery of the stem villus or the fetal arteries in the cotyledon.

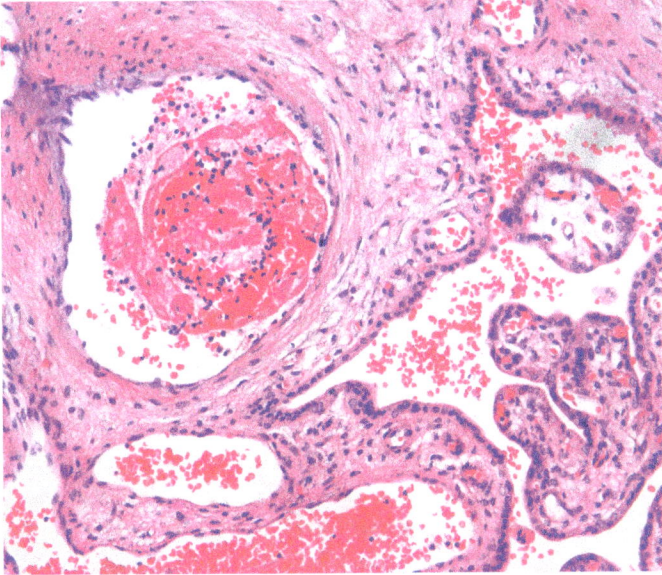

Fig. 6.6: Non occlusive thrombus in a stem villus vessel (very early stage) with stasis of the blood, erythrocyte cohesion, hemolysis and partial fibrin coagulation.

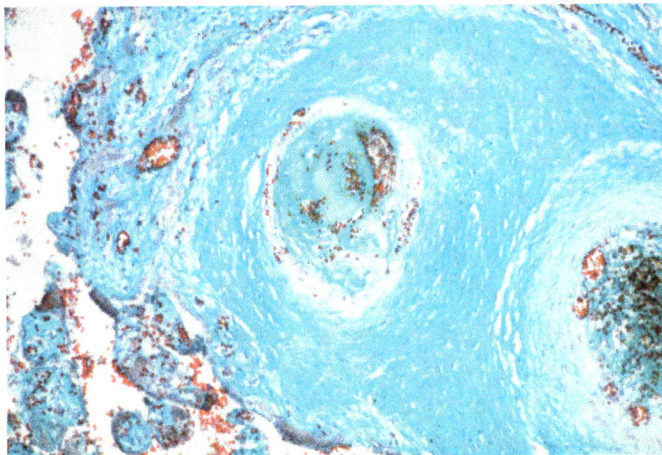

Fig. 6.7: Fetal thrombotic vasculopathy in a stem villus vessel (MG stained).

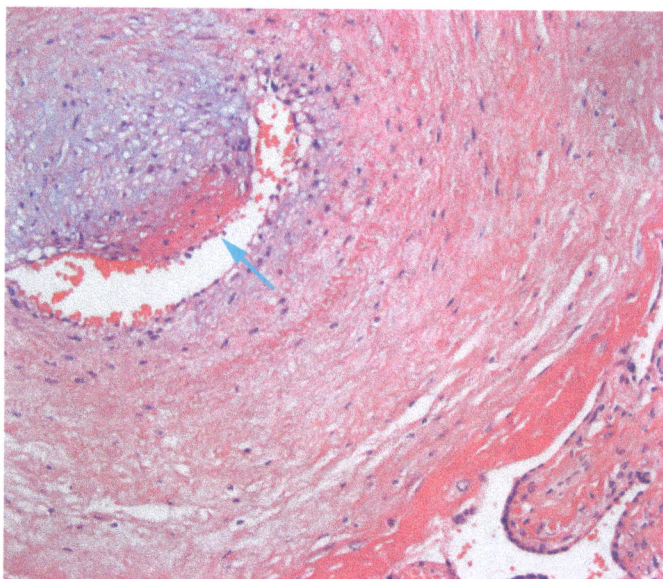

Fig. 6.8: Vessel in a stem villus with an acute and partially occlusive thrombus in a preexisting endothelial cushion, myxoid changes in the vessel wall and loss of endothelial cells (arrow). GW 37 + 1, APGAR 10-10-10, fetal weight 3280 g

Microthrombosis of the terminal villi

Fibrin rich thrombosis may be found in every vessel of the villous microvascular system. Fresh thrombosis may show luminal collapse, due to fetal circulatory disturbance, and is seen in: umbilical cord accidents (traction of the cord, strangulation and/or compression of the umbilical vessels), short umbilical cords, true knots, entanglement and umbilical prolapse with mechanical entrapment of the umbilical cord between the child and maternal pelvis. Disseminated intravasal coagulation (DIC) in intrauterine fetal distress (IUFD) and fetal abortion is considered to be an expression of a generalized circulatory disturbance in the microcirculatory system during shock [11]. Microthrombosis may also pinpoint a periplacental onset of respiratory distress syndrome [12,13].

6.3 Fetal vessel pathology

Pathology in the large vessels of the chorionic plate and stem villi is primarily caused by total/subtotal connective tissue occlusion and is classified as:
– endangiopathia obliterans,
– endangiitis obliterans,
– hemorrhagic endovasculopathy,
– collapse sclerosis.

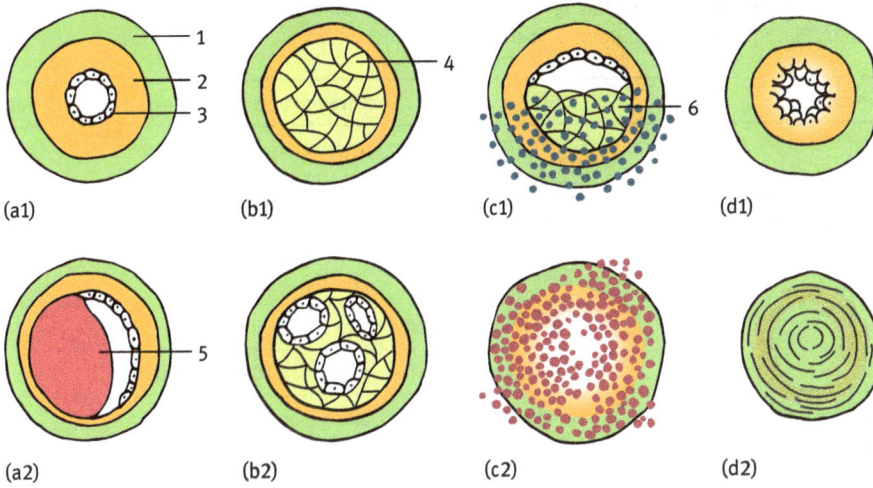

Fig. 6.9: Illustration of the classification of fetal vessel pathology. (a1) Normal structure of a fetal vessel with (3) endothelium, (2) thickened media and (1) collagen rich adventitia; (a2) (5) vessel thrombus; (b1) endangiopathia obliterans with (4) luminal obliteration by connective tissue; (b2) endangiopathia obliterans with luminal septation and revascularization; (c1) endangiitis obliterans with cellular exudate and (6) proliferation of connective tissue; (c2) hemorrhagic endovasculopathy; (d1) acute collapse of the vessel lumen with endothelial swelling and myocyte herniation; (d2) collapse sclerosis with a concentric connective tissue occlusion of the lumen.

Low Grade

segmental:
thrombotic occlusion
– of fetal vessels in the chorionic plate, or
– stem villous vessel obliteration downstream obstruction

global:
partially obstructed umbilical blood flow:
– venous ectasia, intramural fibrin deposition in large vessels, and/or
– small foci (5 villi per focus) of avascular or karyorrhectic villi

partial or intermittent obstruction

High Grade

more than one focus:
– ≥ 45 over 3 section avascular villi; or
– average of > 15 villi per section with or without thrombus, or
– 2 or more occlusive or non-occlusive thrombi

Fig. 6.10: Fetal vascular malperfusion classified as high and low grade changes; according to the Amsterdam Placental Workshop Group Consensus Statement. Table 6.1 recommended terminology [8].

Table 6.1: Recommended terminology and grading system for fetal vascular malperfusion; The Amsterdam Placental Workshop Group Consensus Statement.

Thrombosis	Grade	Thrombi location and extent of occlusion
		arterial
		venous
avascular villi	small foci	3 or more foci of 2 to 4 terminal villi with total capillary loss and hyaline stromal fibrosis
	intermediate foci	5 to 10 villi affected
	large foci	more than 10 villi affected
intramural fibrin deposition (intimal fibrin cushion)	isolated	one lesion per slide
	recent	large fetal vessels
	longstanding	calcification
	intramural	subendothelial, intramuscular occlusive, or non-occlusive
	calcification	with or without
villous stromal-vascular karyorrhexis (hemorrhagic endovasculitis)		3 or more foci of 2 to 4 terminal villi missing inflammatory component
stem vessel obliteration (stem vessel endovasculopathy)		stem vessel obliteration with marked thickening of the vessel wall
vascular ectasia		4x luminal diameter of the surrounding corresponding vessel

6.3.1 Endangiopathia obliterans

In endangiopathia obliterans the boundary between the tunica intima and media in the vessel wall disappears, and this loss of the elastic lamina favors a pannus-like, connective tissue proliferation in the vessel lumen. The original vessel circumference is demarcated by an outer adventitial collagen fiber ring which increases in size and is consistently larger when compared to the adventitial rings of unaffected vessels [11].

Completely occluded vessels, and vessels with septated erythrocyte filled spaces (indicating a continued, albeit reduced, blood flow due to re-endothelialization) may appear side by side.

Hypovascularity and/or avascularity *in* the downstream villi is caused by extreme vessel constriction or occlusion of the stem villi arteries. The consequences of this endangiopathy depend on the time of onset:

- If it occurs in the 1st half of pregnancy the villi appear focally immature with restricted branching and a reduced number of autochthon capillaries.
- If it occurs in the 2nd half of pregnancy the stroma of mature branched villi is fibrotic with an increase in cellularity and collagen fibers and occlusion of the fetal vessels.

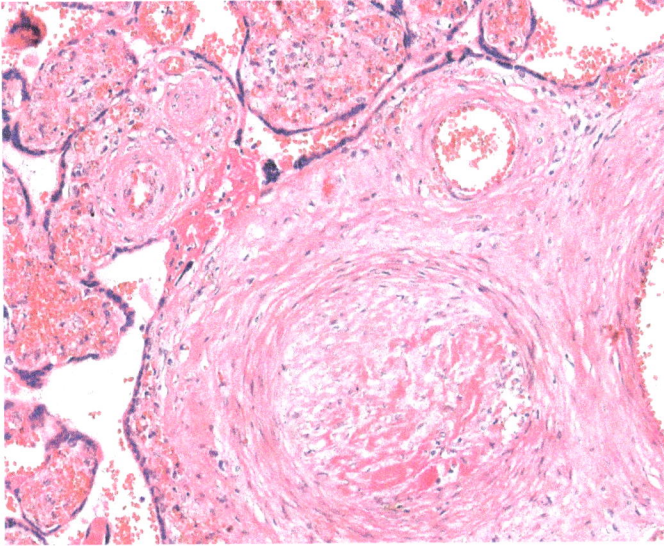

Fig. 6.11: Endangiopathia obliterans. Almost total occlusion of a stem villus vessel.

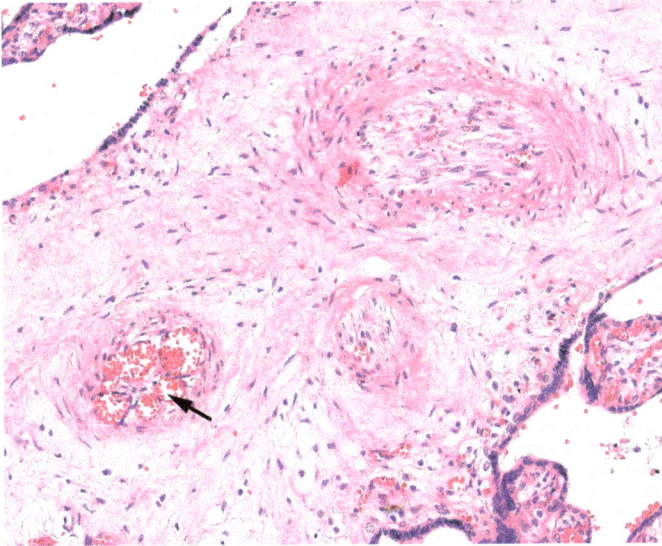

Fig. 6.12: Intraluminal septation and re-endothelialization (arrow) in a stem villus vessel with sub-total occlusive obliteration.

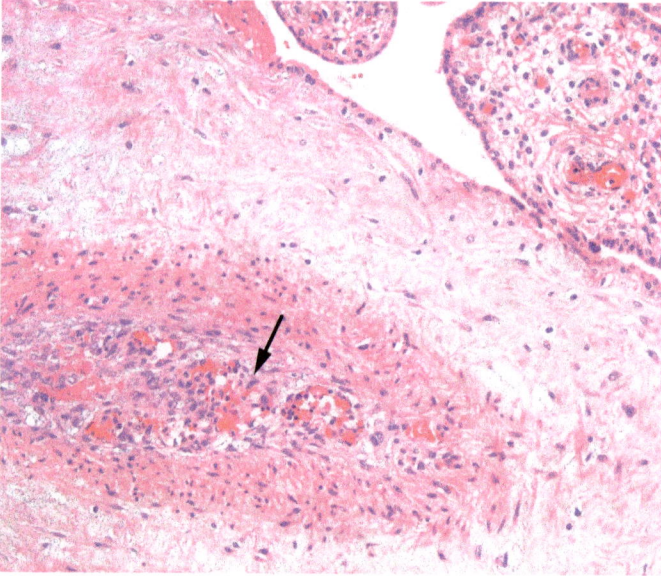

Fig. 6.13: Intraluminal septation and re-endothelialization (arrow) in an almost completely occluded stem villus vessel.

Endangiopathia obliterans frequency [14]:
- 4.5 % of placentas from at risk pregnancies and children,
- 30 % of placentas from IUFD (10 % show more than 50 % involvement of a MPF),
- 16 % of spontaneous abortions between gestational week 15 and 27 (multifocal involvement in ca. 8 %),
- 5 % of placental abruptions between gestational week 15 and 27.

Pathogenesis and causes

Endangiopathia obliterans is caused by a reactive connective tissue proliferation due to vessel wall damage. According to Becker, it is due to hypoxic endothelial cell damage, only sometimes seen as an inflammatory like process; however, an inflammatory cause can only be identified in a small number of cases.

Endangiopathia begins with endothelial cell damage and is followed by a reactive proliferation of the vessel wall cells, probably aided by loss of inhibiting growth factors. (Table 6.2)

Table 6.2: Differential diagnosis of endangiopathia obliterans and luminal collapse sclerosis.

endangiopathia obliterans	collapse sclerosis
focal	diffuse
large fetal vessels affected	concentric occluded lumen
live births	IUFD
short duration of retention	long duration of retention
villous maturation disorder/stromal fibrosis	villous branching occurs prior to death
vessel perfusion remains intact	loss of vessel perfusion

Endangiopathia obliterans is often seen in association with:
–   diabetes mellitus (possibly due to a metabolic mucopolysaccharide disorder of the vessel wall),
–   Rh-incompatibility (possibly due to antigen-antibody reaction),
–   preeclampsia, chronic hypertension (frequently with collapse sclerosis),
–   maternal collagenosis,
–   maternal nicotine use,
–   intrauterine infection,
–   retarded villous maturation,
–   villous stromal fibrosis,
–   fetal hypotrophy (FGR).

6.3.2 Endangiitis obliterans

Endangiitis obliterans is an obliterative inflammatory connective tissue proliferation with a cellular exudate and/or the presence of infectious agents.

Frequency
–   less than 1% of IUFD,
–   almost 2% of spontaneous abortions,
–   4% of placental abruptions (placental abruption caused by rubella infection).

Causes
–   in cases with proven rubella,
–   in congenital syphilis infection,
–   in maternal viral infection during middle pregnancy.
–   an early stage of this vessel change, described in placentas from HIV positive mothers [15], could not be confirmed.

6.3.3 Hemorrhagic endovasculopathy

Hemorrhagic endovasculopathy defines the vessel changes associated with endangiopathia obliterans. It is often described as hemorrhagic endovasculitis, and some recommend that it be referred to as villous stromal vascular karyorrhexis (Table 6.1) [16]. Acute endovasculopathy is characterized by intramural hemorrhage, necrosis of both endothelial cells and the tunica media and thrombosis. Older foci may show additional findings such as calcification. Hemorrhagic endovasculopathy is seen in less than 10 % of endangiopathy cases and has an estimated incidence of 0.67 %, from unselected material [17].

Pathogenesis and etiology of hemorrhagic endovasculopathy is not known, but in some cases it may be due to hypoxic vessel wall damage. An association with endangiopathia obliterans may indicate an infectious, toxic and/or immune mediated cause of damage to the vessel wall, whereas an association with non-immunological hydrops is frequently without a defined etiology [18,19].

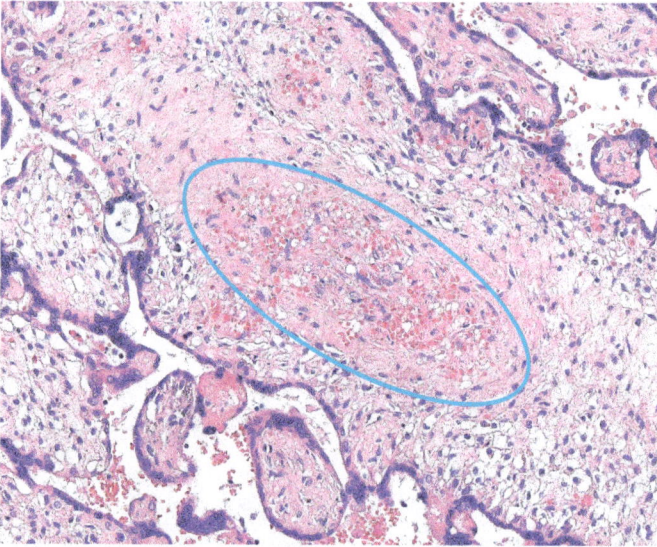

Fig. 6.14: Hemorrhagic endovasculopathy (circle). A loose inner vessel wall with endothelial cell necrosis and acute erythrocyte diapedesis into the outer vessel wall and surrounding tissue. Possibly due to hypoxic vessel wall damage.

6.3.4 Collapse sclerosis

Collapse sclerosis is seen in the vessels of the chorionic plate and stem villi. It is characterized by a concentric fibrous constriction with obliteration of the vessel lumen and loss of perfusion.

The preceding stage to the fibrous obliteration is assumed to be the concentric constriction of the vessel lumen by endothelial swelling and muscle herniation into the tunica intima. These changes cause a subacute loss of perfusion. Fixation artifacts can increase the impression of cellular vacuolization [20,21] (Figs. 6.15, 6.9 [d1]). At this stage the endothelial cells react positively for immunhistochemical markers, but this reactivity is lost during prolonged vessel underperfusion and concentric luminal constriction. In some cases the inner vessel wall is split and cell and fiber bridges, oriented towards the center of the lumen, are seen. This is in contrast to the septation seen in endangiopathia obliterans.

The final stage of this process is vessel occlusion by concentric collagen fibers; these fibers are negative for endothelial immunohistochemical markers. The original vessel diameter is no longer visible, and the boundary to the fibrous stroma outside the vessel is indistinct.

Collapse sclerosis is the result of an adaptive vessel wall change secondary to a chronic loss of perfusion. It is often diffuse but can occasionally be focal.

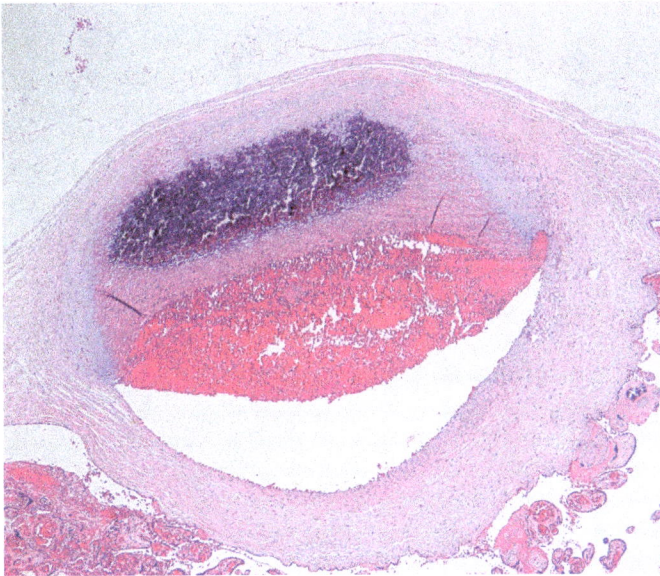

Fig. 6.15: Fibrotic vessel wall with secondary calcification and parietal thrombosis.

Diffuse collapse sclerosis is seen in:
- fetal loss,
- long term retention of products of conception,
- IUFD with advanced maceration.

Focal collapse sclerosis is seen:
- in both IUFD and live births:
  - above massive chronic infarcts,
  - close to villous fibrinoid necrosis.
- In occlusive thrombi of the distal umbilical cord, chorionic plate or stem villi vessels,

Distal to an aneurysm of the chorionic plate or large stem villus artery (rarely).

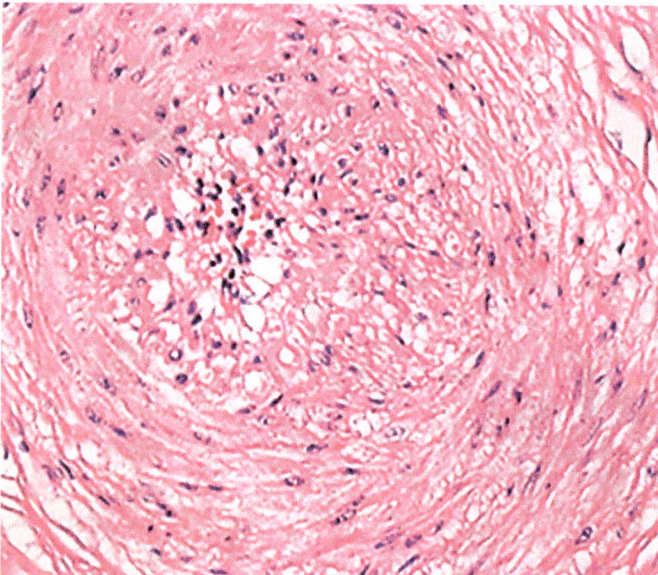

Fig. 6.16: Fetal vessel collapse with endothelial swelling (Fig. 6.9 [d1]).

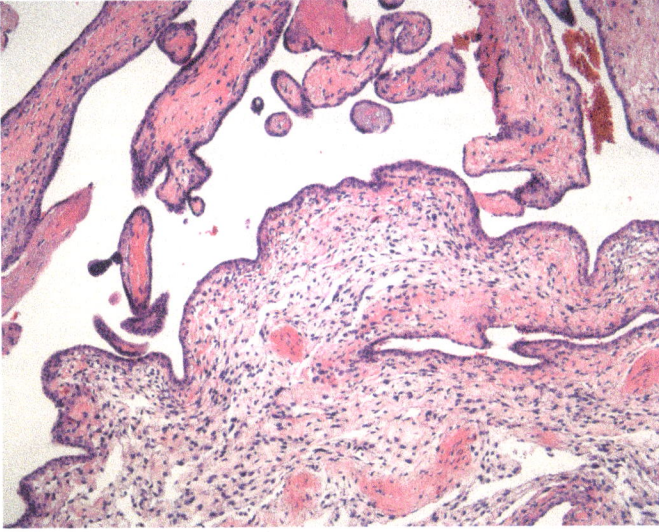

Fig. 6.17: Acute collapse sclerosis, end stage, in 2nd trimester placenta retention.

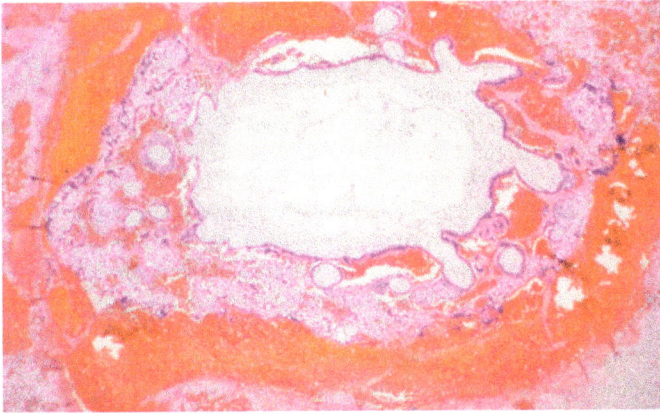

Fig. 6.18: An acute/chronic, massive and expansive hematoma of the chorionic plate with acute thrombosis, collapse of the chorionic plate vessels and anemia of the placental parenchyma. Late abortion in GW 17.

References

[1] Schiebler TH, Kaufmann P. Reife Plazenta. In: Becker V, Schiebler TH, Kubli F, editor. Die Plazenta des Menschen. Stuttgardt: Thieme; 1981. p. 51–100.

[2] Assali NS, Rauramo L, Peltonen T. Measurement of uterine blood flow and uterine metabolism. VIII. Uterine and fetal blood flow and oxygen consumption in early human pregnancy. American journal of obstetrics and gynecology. 1960;79:86–98.

[3] Stembera ZK, Hodr J, Ganz V, Fronek A. Measurement of umbilical cord blood flow by local thermodilution. American journal of obstetrics and gynecology. 1964;90:531–536.

[4] Ten Berge BS. [Blood flow in the placental villi]. Ned Tijdschr Geneeskd. 1955;99(32):2371–2377.

[5] Parisi VM, Walsh SW. Fetoplacental vascular responses to prostacyclin after thromboxane-induced vasoconstriction. American journal of obstetrics and gynecology. 1989;160(2):502–507.

[6] Wilkes BM, Mento PF. Bradykinin-induced vasoconstriction and thromboxane release in perfused human placenta. The American journal of physiology. 1988;254(6 Pt 1):E681-6.

[7] Emmrich P, Fuchs U, Heinke P, Jutzi E, Godel E. The epithelial and capillary basal laminae of the placenta in maternal diabetes mellitus. Lab Invest. 1976;35(1):87–92.

[8] Khong TY, Mooney EE, Ariel I, et al. Sampling and Definitions of Placental Lesions: Amsterdam Placental Workshop Group Consensus Statement. Arch Pathol Lab Med. 2016.

[9] Faye-Petersen OM, Heller D, Joshi VV. Placental Pathology. NY: Taylor & Francis; 2006.

[10] Fox H, Sebire NJ. Pathology of the placenta: Saunders Elsevier; 2007.

[11] Becker V, Schiebler TH, Kubli F. Allgemeine und spezielle Pathologie der Plazenta. Die Plazenta des Menschen. Stuttgart: Thieme; 1981. p. 251–393.

[12] Kloos K, Vogel M. Pathologie der Perinatalperiode. Stuttgart: Thieme; 1974.

[13] Bleyl U, Busing CM. [Disseminated intravascular coagulation and perinatal shock]. Verhandlungen der Deutschen Gesellschaft fur Pathologie. 1969;53:495–501.

[14] Vogel M. Atlas der morphologischen Plazentadiagnostik. 2 ed. Berlin: Springer; 1996.

[15] Jimenez E, Unger M, Vogel M, et al. [Morphologic studies of the placentas of HIV-positive mothers]. Pathologe. 1988;9(4):228–234.

[16] Sander CH. Hemorrhagic endovasculitis and hemorrhagic villitis of the placenta. Arch Pathol Lab Med. 1980;104(7):371–373.

[17] Shen-Schwarz S, Macpherson TA, Mueller-Heubach E. The clinical significance of hemorrhagic endovasculitis of the placenta. American journal of obstetrics and gynecology. 1988;159(1):48–51.

[18] Novak PM, Sander CM, Yang SS, von Oeyen PT. Report of fourteen cases of nonimmune hydrops fetalis in association with hemorrhagic endovasculitis of the placenta. American journal of obstetrics and gynecology. 1991;165(4 Pt 1):945–950.

[19] Sander CH, Stevens NG. Hemorrhagic endovasculitis of the placenta: an indepth morphologic appraisal with initial clinical and epidemiologic observations. Pathol Annu. 1984;19 Pt 1:37–79.

[20] Rockelein G, Hey A. [Ultrastructural studies of vacuole formation in arterial chorionic vessels of the mature human placenta]. Z Geburtshilfe Perinatol. 1985;189(2):65–68.

[21] van der Veen F, Fox H. The effects of cigarette smoking on the human placenta: a light and electron microscopic study. Placenta. 1982;3(3):243–256.

7 Maternal circulatory disturbances

The term maternal circulatory disturbance refers to the different mechanisms which may cause placental dysfunction in later pregnancy, such as high-velocity vascular disturbance due to placentation disorders in early pregnancy [1].

7.1 Maternal-placental perfusion

Maternal blood flows into the intervillous space via the wide spiral arteries in the decidua basalis and septa. It is assumed that each fetomaternal circulatory unit is supplied by one spiral artery (Fig. 7.1).

Maternal blood pressure in the basal arteries is measured in the endo-myometrial transition zone at 70–80 mmHg, in the spiral arteries close to the basal plate at 10–30 mmHg and in the intervillous space at 6–10 mmHg [2,3]. The pressure difference seems to be insufficient to create a blood supply from the spiral artery to the chorionic plate, indicating that the intervillous blood stream distribution and direction of flow in the fetomaternal unit is regulated by villous compactness instead [4]. For this to occur, loosely organised villi centrally in the fetomaternal unit are shaped like an umbrella, and this results in a decrease of blood flow velocity from the central region towards the periphery and subsequently from basal to chorionic plate by connecting zones arranged with densely organized villi.

The resulting balanced blood flow resistance achieves an equal perfusion of the intervillous space into the fetomaternal units.

Inflow into the units is inconstant and intermittent, with only some functionally active and opened spiral arteries. In keeping with this, intermittent blood flow vas-

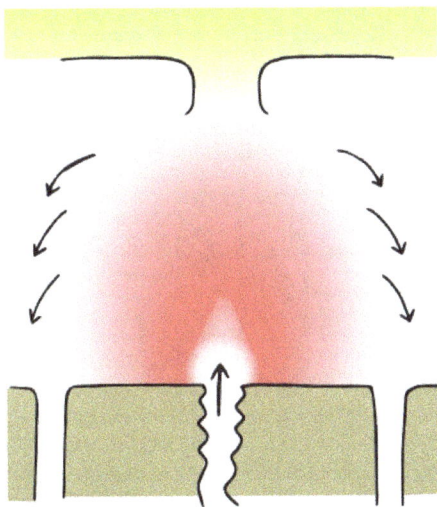

Fig. 7.1: Illustration. Feto-maternal circulatory unit: maternal blood inflow through spiral arteries; flow velocity is regulated by decreased villous density from basal to chorial and from central to the periphery; blood streams out at the marginal circulatory unit into maternal veins of the basal plate.

https://doi.org/10.1515/9783110452600-007

cularizes villous tufts [5]. Maternal blood downstream starts from the peripheral unit into decidual veins of the basal plate [3,6].

7.2 Maternal circulatory disturbance

The morphology of maternal circulatory disturbance may correlate with clinically diagnosed, acute or chronic, disturbances of the arterial inflow and venous outflow in maternal placental circulation.

The *morphological diagnosis* of a maternal vascular disturbance may be given, in the presence of:

–   placental infarct (massive and cotyledon infarct),
–   microfibrin deposition,
–   Gitterinfarct,
–   maternal floor infarct,
–   subchorionic pseudoinfarct,
–   intervillous thrombus,
–   placental hematoma.

7.2.1 Infarct

An infarct is a circumscribed area of parenchymal necrosis, caused by interrupted, maternal, arterial blood inflow.

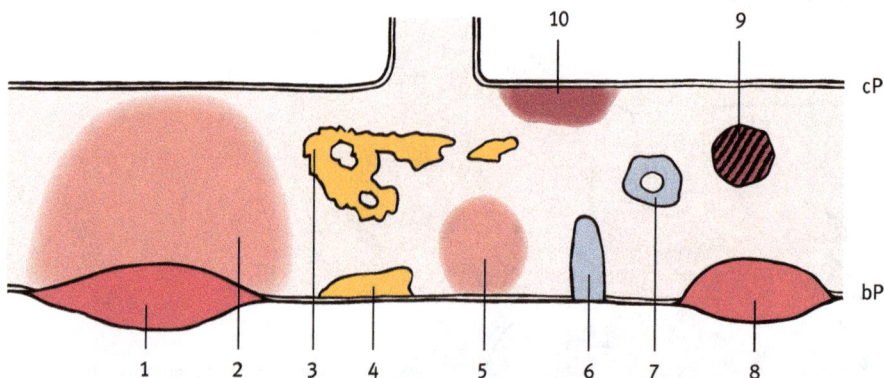

Fig. 7.2: Illustration of pathology due to maternal circulatory disturbances: (Cp) Chorionic plate; (Bp) Basal plate. (1) Retroplacental hematoma with basal plate hollow; (2) acute hemorrhagic infarct with basal hematoma; (3) Gitterinfarct; (4) maternal floor infarct with basal pseudoinfarct; (5) cotyledoninfarct; (6) septum; (7) decidual island; (8) basal hematoma; (9) intervillous thrombus; (10) subchorionic thrombus.

It may be classified due to:
– depending on the extent:
  – massive infarct,
  – votyledon infarct,
– depending on the age:
  – acute-red infarct,
  – subacute-brown infarct,
  – chronic-white infarct.

Massive infarct

Compact necrosis of several adjacent feto-maternal units. Massive placental infarcts were seen in less than 10 % of placentas from eutrophic newborns and in nine of ten cases of chronic type.

These infarcts are twice as likely to be seen in placentas from risk pregnancies, especially in hypertension and utero placental vessels diseases.

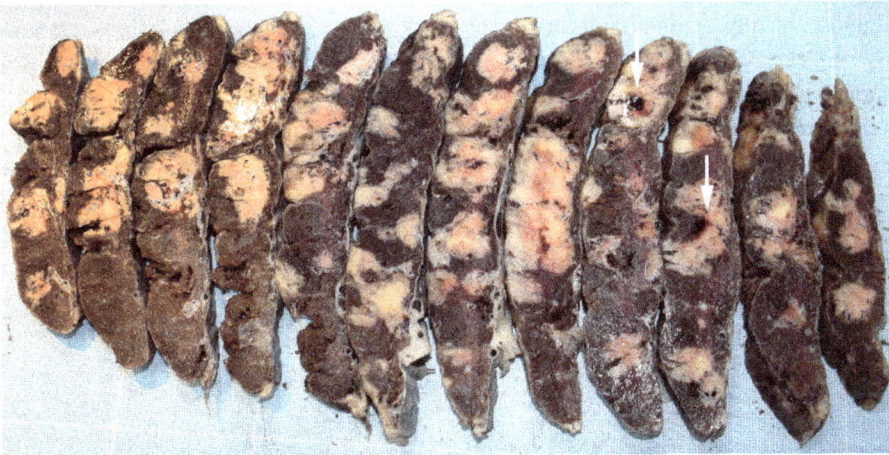

Fig. 7.3: Massive chronic infarct: macroscopic slices showing infarcted, adjacent grey-whitish feto-maternal units. There is also some fresh, acute thrombus (arrow). Placenta in Gestational Week 35 + 6, 391 g net weight, clinical bleeding.

Cotyledon infarct

Parenchymal necrosis limited to one cotyledon [7]. Cotyledon infarcts were seen in ca. 10 % of placentas from eutrophic newborns. In risk pregnancies cotyledon infarcts were seen in ca. 20 % and in 75 % of these cases, one to three cotyledons were affected [8].

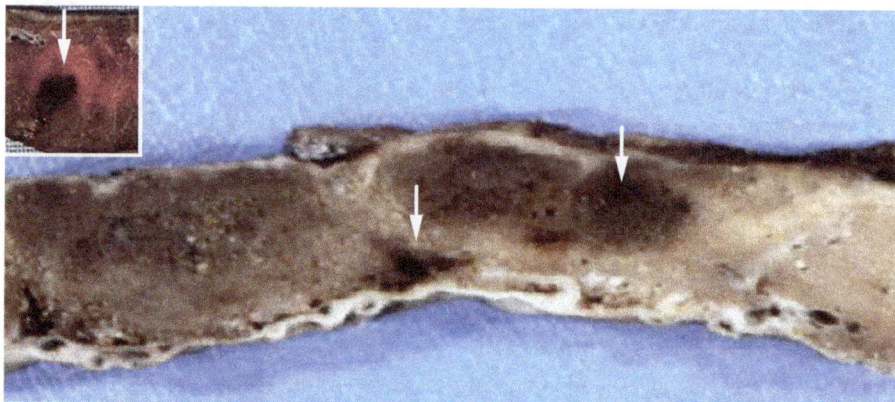

Fig. 7.4: Acute cotyledon infarcts: Several brownish lesions, broadly circumscribed and well defined in relation to non-infarcted areas. Inlay: acute cotyledon infarct; inadequately fixed placenta

Acute infarct

Macroscopically, acute infarcts are of any size and appear as dark red lesions, circumscribed and demarcated from neighbouring areas. While poorly defined in unfixed mature placentas, they are easy visible after formalin fixation.

Microscopically the area of infarction is demarcated by:

– Increased villous diameter with irregular constriction of the intervillous space and villous agglutination.

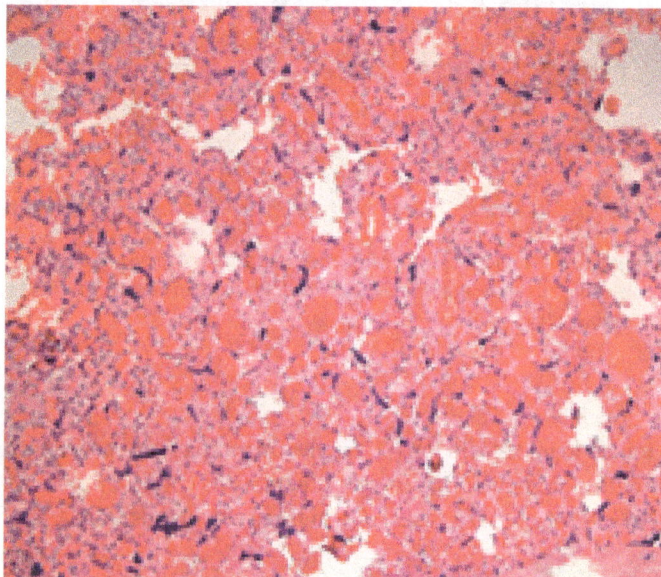

Fig. 7.5: Early acute infarct with villous capillary congestion in the villous stroma.

- Dilated villous vessels and capillary congestion.
- Flattened chorionic epithelium, nuclear pyknosis and karyorrhexis.
- Hemorrhage in the villous stroma and intervillous space.

Subacute infarct

Macroscopically, a brown-reddish cut surface is seen with corresponding chorionic epithelial necrosis, villous stromal necrosis and intra and intervillous fibrin depositions microscopically. In addition, chorionic epithelial knots (nuclear pyknosis) in the periphery of infarcts and from cellular to chronic organized necrosis in the transition zone are also seen. Occasionally maternal neutrophilic granulocytes demarcate the infarct edge to the intervillous space. Rarely, complete leucocytic demarcation of the necrosis is seen.

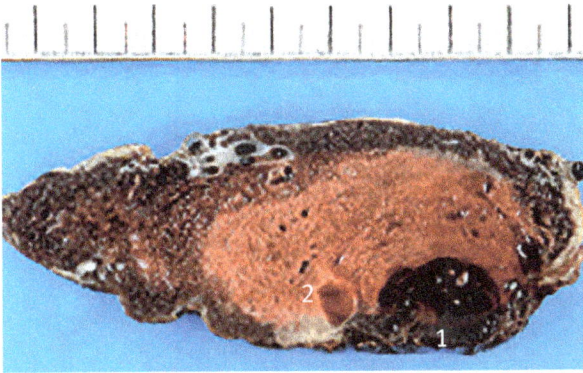

Fig. 7.6: Massive subacute infarct: (1) basal hematoma with extention into the basal plate (premature placental abruption); (2) basal pseudocyst with bleached hemolytic content.

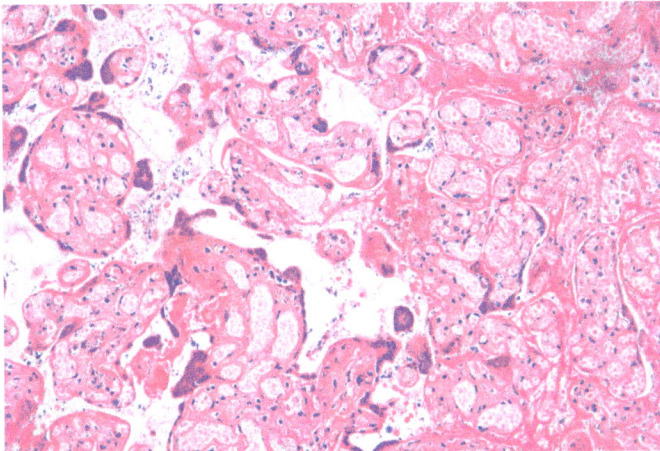

Fig. 7.7: Subacute infarct: Agglutinated villi by microfibrin with necrotic epithelial cells, pale tissue and fetal vessels with hemolytic erythrocytes. Chorionic epithelium partly condensed. Growth restricted placenta in gestational week 38, live birth.

Centrally, subacute infarct areas are characterized by loss of dehydrogenase activity, as well as endocrine chorionic epithelial activity (HCG, HPL). In peripheral zones and adjacent necrosis, ferment and hormones are decreased, while they are increased in areas of developing nuclear sprouts.

Chronic infarct

Chronic infarct is the final stage of an acute infarct. Macroscopically, it is a well circumscribed grey-whitish firm lesion. Histologically, total villous necrosis with formation of ghost villi is seen. Peripheral stem, intermediate and terminal villi, including fetal vessels, are necrotic. In contrast, the muscle containing stem villous vessels may be less affected and retain blood.

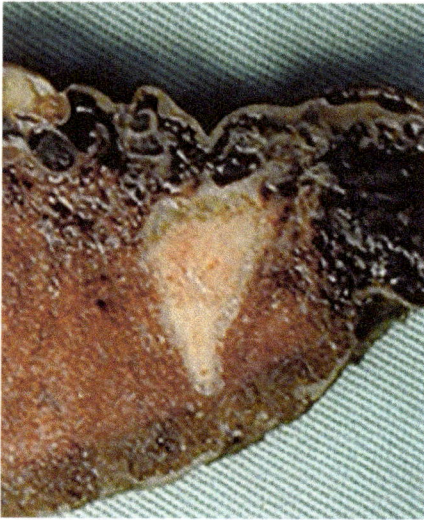

Fig. 7.8: Chronic cotyledon infarct. Circumscribed grey-white and firm lesion.

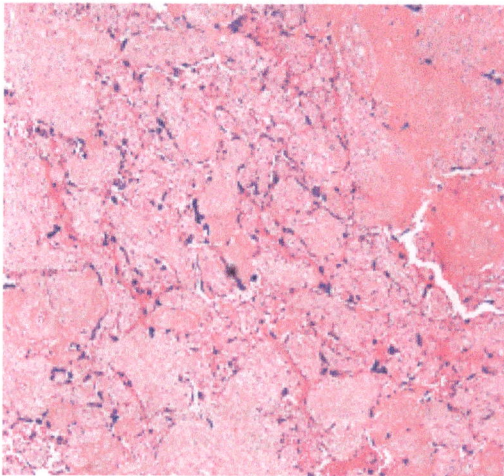

Fig. 7.9: Chronic infarct. Villous necrosis and formation of ghost villi in a placenta in Gestational Week 38, live birth, 3280 g weight, Apgar 9-10-10.

The timeline of infarct development

The chronological sequence of a placental infarct is not fully known in detail. Simian placentas, 24 h after ischemic collapse of the intervillous spaces, show nuclear pyknosis and necrosis of the chorionic epithelium and leucostasis in necrotic adjacent villi. After 48 h all macroscopic and microscopic criteria of a hemorrhagic placental infarct were seen, ghost villi were seen after 7 days [9].

Guinea pig placentas demonstrate focal hemorrhagic necrosis after 4–5 h and macroscopically fulfills all the criteria for a hemorrhagic infarct after 12 h [10]. After 2–5 days the necrosis is infiltrated by fibrin depositions and resorptive trophoblast activity in infarct edges could be seen from day 6. In contrast to hemorrhagic placentas, necrosis in labyrinth placentas is partly resorbed and demarcated by connective tissue.

Close monitoring of pregnancy suggests, that ca. 5–6 hours are lying between clinical infarct onset and macroscopic and morphological visible infarct in human placentas [11].

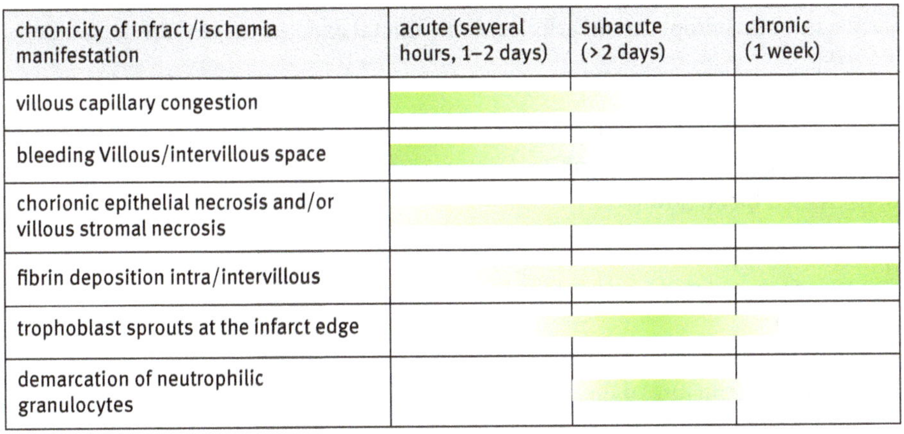

chronicity of infract/ischemia manifestation	acute (several hours, 1–2 days)	subacute (>2 days)	chronic (1 week)
villous capillary congestion			
bleeding Villous/intervillous space			
chorionic epithelial necrosis and/or villous stromal necrosis			
fibrin deposition intra/intervillous			
trophoblast sprouts at the infarct edge			
demarcation of neutrophilic granulocytes			

Fig. 7.10: Manifestation of ischemic changes correlated with chronicity [11].

Causes and pathogenesis of infarction

In the placenta, the maternal and fetal circulation are anatomically distinct from one another. Functionally they are tightly connected and both provide feto-maternal exchange of nutrition and waste products. However, nutrition of the villous tissue depends on the maternal circulation, and this is supported by the following findings:
- the chorionic epithelial proliferates without embryonic implantation, after embryonic abortion, and without functional embryonic-placental circulation,
- placenta fetalis persists after fetal death in middle and late pregnancy,

- the endocrine activity of the chorionic epithelium persists several days after fetal death,
- villous chorionic epithelium is active, though the supplying stem villous vessels are occluded,
- animal experiments of the simian placenta show no villous tissue necrosis after 50 days of continuous fetal vessel ligature [12].

Infarction is caused by interrupted maternal blood supply, seen as morphological stenosis or obliteration of the pre-placental vessels and may be due to:
- atherosclerosis, parietal thrombosis or aneurysm of the spiral arteries, predominantly myo-endometrial vessel transition [13,14],
- arterio/arteriolopathy and thrombosis in diabetes mellitus with vascular involvement, Lupus erythematodes and other immunological disorders, vessel wall diseases due to exogenous damage,
- increased, intrinsic arterial resistance due to functional constriction of the uteroplacental vessels [15],
- preterm placental abruption,
- ligature of uteroplacental arteries, from animal experiments in Rhesus monkeys [16].

Only a slight correlation between decreased uteroplacental blood flow and placental infarcts have been noted in studies. Infarcts manifested after several days and weeks of decreased blood flow [17].

Consequences of the infarcts for the fetus
Depends on:
- extent and age of the infarct,
- preceding structural damage of the placenta.

7.2.2 Micro fibrin deposition

Difference between fibrin and fibrinoid
Depositions in the human placenta from gestational week 8 may be differentiated into fibrin and fibrinoid. Fibrin refers to coagulation products, whereas fibrinoid refers to products of another origin [18]. Immunohistochemical studies demonstrate fibrin reactivity with fibrin antibodies and fibrinoid, matrix type, reacting with oncofetal fibronectin (antibody BC-1) [19].
    Zones of normal fibrin and fibrinoid depositions:
- Langhans fibrinoid: subchorionic,
- Rohr fibrinoid: basal plate in the transition zone to the intervillous space,

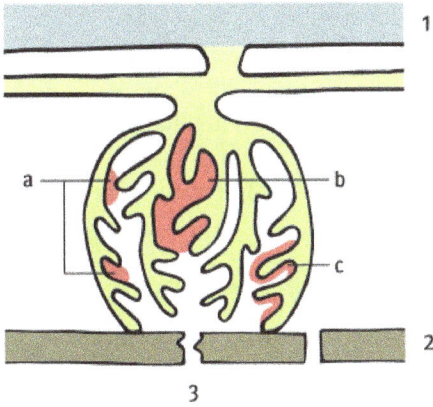

Fig. 7.11: Most frequent localization of fibrin depositions: (a) intervillous and perivillous between neighbouring villi; (b) fibrinous obturation of the intervillous space with villous inclusion; (c) perivillous areal: on the villous surface. Lesions are fibrinolytic treatable. (1) Chorionic plate; (2) basal plate; (3) spiral artery inflow.

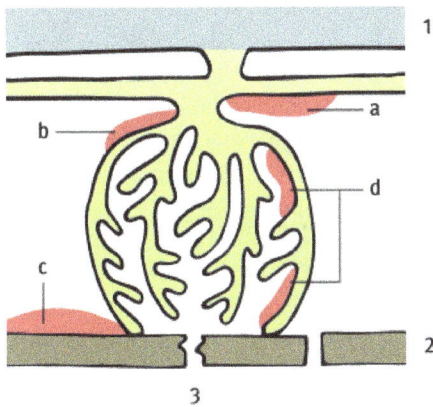

Fig. 7.12: Most frequent localization of fibrin and fibrinoid depositions: (a) subchorionic space; (b) along stem villi; (c) basal, close to islands and septs; (d) periphery of feto-maternal units. Lesions are fibrinolytic treatable. (1) Chorionic plate; (2) basal plate; (3) spiral artery inflow.

- Nitabuch fibrinoid: deep basal plate,
- placental septa and islands.
  Intra and intervillous fibrin depositions:
- fibrin depositions sometimes leading to fibrinoid villous necrosis,
- inter and perivillous fibrin depositions between the villi or on the villous surface.

Controversial aspects of the origin and significance of normal fibrin/fibrinoid depositions:
- degeneration of the placental tissue [20],
- belonging to placental structure with stream giving function in the intervillous space [21],
- facilitating placental stability [22],
- immunological protection for fetus and mother.

Consequences of pathological microfibrin deposition

Depending on quantity of fibrin depositions, gradual displacement of the intervillous flow can occur and compensatory processes, such as accelerated villous maturation, increased sinusoidal dilatation of villous capillaries and differentiation into vasculo-syncytial membranes are seen (chorangiosis type II)

Increased microfibrin depositions with more than 50 % MPF cause:
- decreased intervillous volume,
- secondary reduction in intravillous flow,
- villous fibrosis occurring within several weeks [23].

Pathologically increased fibrin depositions are the histological precursor of macro-scopic gitterinfarcts. Fibrin depositions are primarily mesh and bandlike diffuse depositions on the villous surface or between adjacent villi which impede villous transport, mainly of maternal origin [24,25]. Several types of deposition could be identified [26]:
- *Intervillous fibrin:* ball and cone like fibrin deposition between the villi.
- *Perivillous fibrin:* fibrin covering the villous surface and displacing small villi.
- *Fibrinous obstruction of the intervillous space and* merging of inter and perivillous fibrin with encasement of villous groups leading to a micro infarct.
- *Intravillous fibrin(-oid)* with fibrinoid villous degeneration.

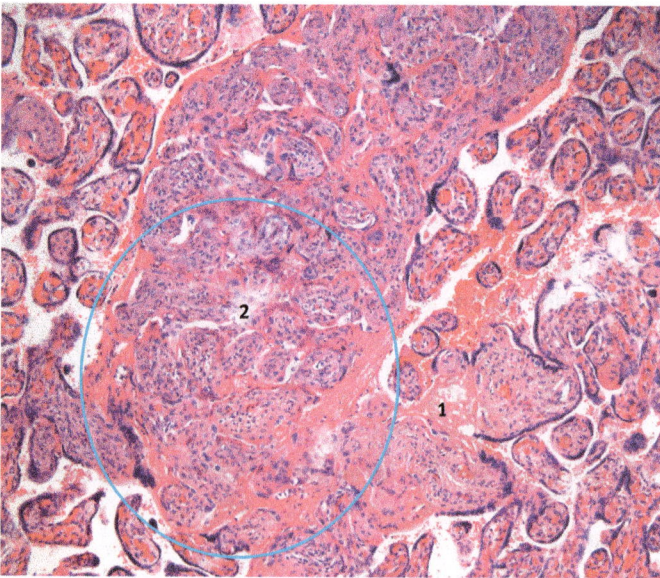

Fig. 7.13: Fibrinous obturation of the intervillous space (so called microinfarct): (1) inter and (2) perivillous microfibrin deposition. Increased villous capillarization in the periphery.

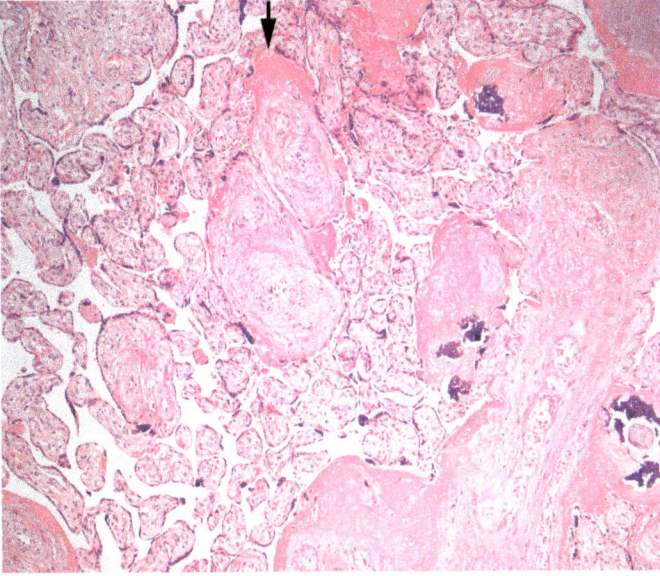

Fig. 7.14: Intervillous fibrin depositions cone like (arrow) on the stem villous surface: Placenta in Gestational Week 38, clinically manual detachment from implantation bed.

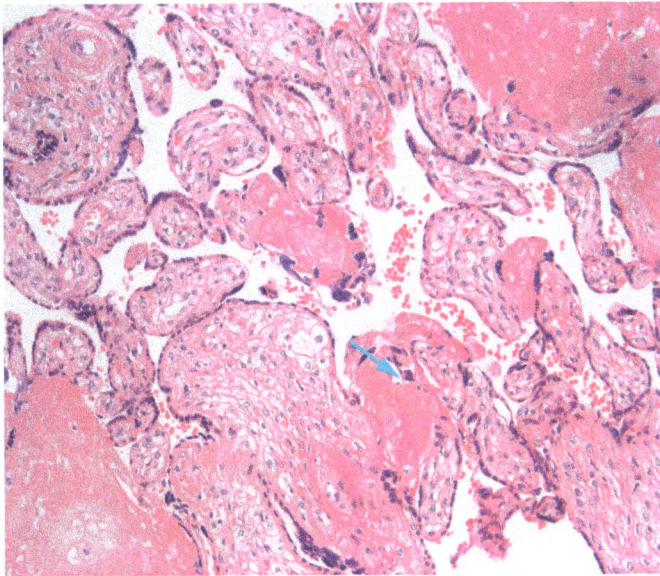

Fig. 7.15: Intervillous fibrin depositions. Obstruction of the intervillous space with villi entrapped within fibrin.

Pathogenesis

Inter and perivillous microfibrin deposition with villous encasement is a consequence of reduced intervillous circulation. This is caused by stenotic preplacental vessels which results in hypoxic cell damage of the chorionic epithelium and localized hyper-coagulability [27]. Following this, intervillous flow leads to microfibrin depositions in the periphery of the feto-maternal unit [28].

Massive fibrin depositions may impress macroscopically, appearing as irregularly demarcated grey-white and firm lesions, covering the central parts of the circulatory unit.

Apart from hyopoxic chorionic epithelium cell damage, other toxic or infectious damage to the epithelium may cause increased fibrin deposition of the same type on the villous surface.

Heparin therapy over several weeks may prevent pathological deposition of inter-villous microfibrin. This was shown by a histometric placental study which measured

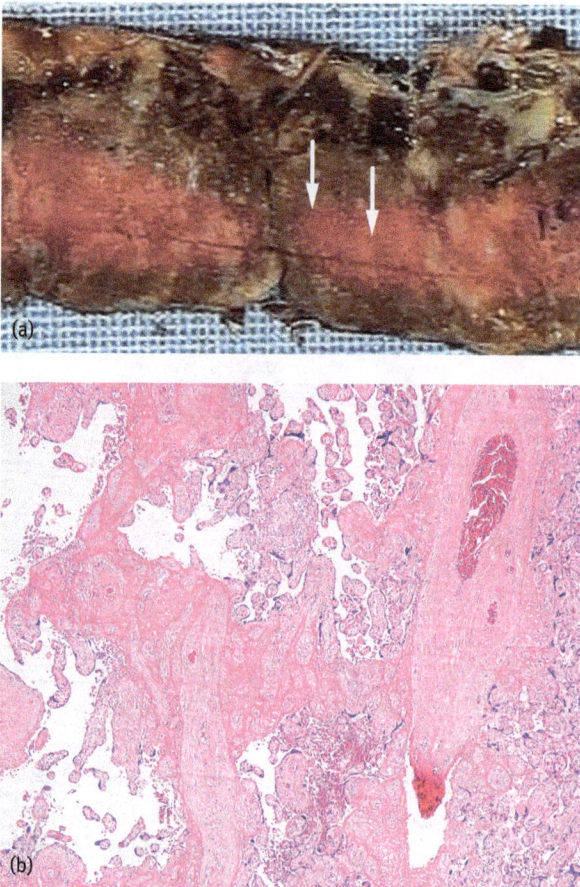

Fig. 7.16: (a) Fibrin deposi-tions. Firm and irregular grey-white cut surface. (b) Confluent perivillous fibrin depositions. Gestational Week 42 + 1, fetal weight 5535 g.

less fibrin in heparin treated pregnancies, duration of treatment > 6 weeks, when compared to untreated patients [18].

Recurrence risk
Microfibrin deposition and Gitterinfarct in 1rst pregnancy recur in 36.5 % of subsequent pregnancies. If fibrin was inconspicuous in the 1st pregnancy, it will be inconspicuous in ca. 85 % of following pregnancies.

7.2.3 Gitterinfarct

Gitterinfarcts are described as sclerotic areas of varying size without a direct relation to, or demarcation from, fetomaternal units. Macroscopically they are white-grey, firm and irregularly circumscribed lesions which measure from a few millimeters up to a near total distribution throughout the whole placenta. If more than 20 % of the total area are affected, the placenta is defined as infarct placenta.

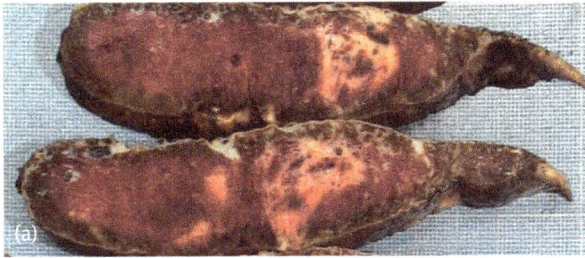

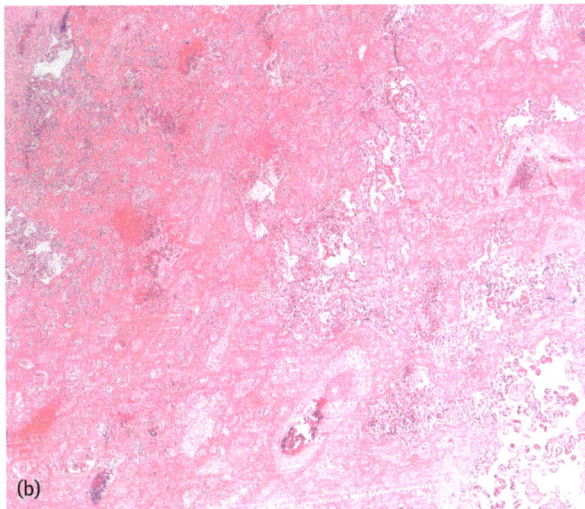

Fig. 7.17: (a) Gitterinfarct. Grey-colored, firm, and irregularly circumscribed lesions. Placenta in Gestational Week 32 + 6, child's weight 1595 g, Apgar 9-10-10; pathological Doppler Flow examination on ultrasound. (b) Gitterinfarct. Eosinophilic necrotic villi, trapped within fibrin masses, minimal irregular intervillous space.

Microscopically, the villi are embedded in fibrin masses and they show every stage of infarction, from regressive changes of the epithelium, vessels and stroma to complete necrosis with ghost villi.

Gitterinfarcts are clinically related to materno-placental circulatory disturbance and maternal thrombophilia and are seen, in small foci, in ca.20 % of the placentas in newborns without risk factors. In placentas with associated fetal growth restriction (FGR) an increased amount of scattered gitterinfarcts can be seen in 33 % to 50 % of placentas.

7.2.4 Maternal floor infarct

Maternal floor infarcts are 3 mm or more areas with an irregularly demarcated thickening of the basal plate [29]. Due to this, the intervillous space is almost completely obliterated along the basal plate, in keeping with the earlier used term "basal pseudoinfarct". Macroscopically the placental base is firm, yellow-white and thickened. Histology shows obliteration of the intervillous space between the connecting villi and septa along the basal plate. Additionally amorphic eosinophilic fibrinoid, matrix type, depositions are seen along the placental bed and septa and inflammatory cells can be found nearby [30].

Consequences for the fetus
Fibrin depositions, grade 3, are associated with expanded gitterinfarcts and may lead to FGR, fetal hypoxia and intrauterine fetal death (IUFD).

Isolated maternal floor infarcts are usually of no pathological significance.

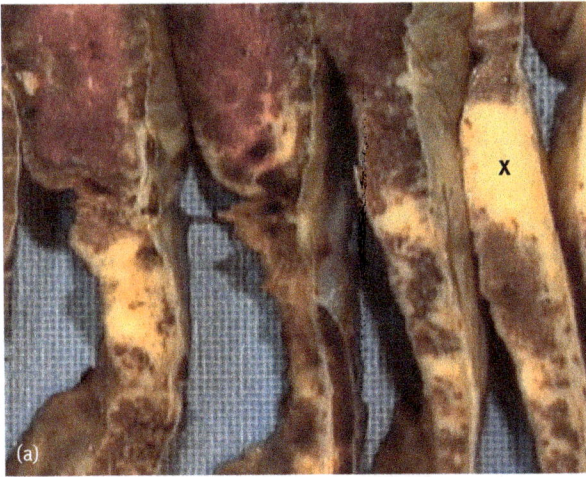

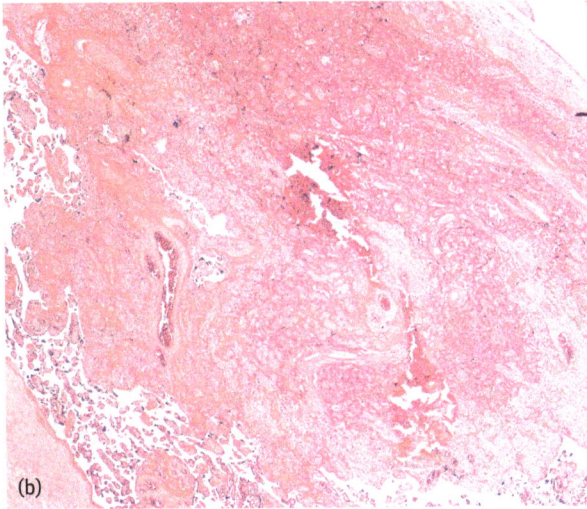

Fig. 7.18: (a) "Gitterinfarcts". Thick, firm and white lesions **X** confluence to chronic massive infarct in Gestational Week 40 + 6, child's birthweight 3077 g, Apgar 2-4-5; acute caesarian section because of fetal asphyxia. (b) Maternal floor infarct. Amorphous eosinophilic fibrin located in the decidua and adjacent villi.

7.2.5 Subchorionic pseudoinfarction

Subchorionic pseudoinfarction is characterized by increased fibrin deposition in the subchorionic space [31]. Stem villi, as well as decidual and trophoblast islands, are trapped in fibrin masses.

Irregular, thick and firm deposits directly under the chorionic plate are seen macroscopically which cause constriction of the physiological placental "dead zone" which leads to a decreased intervillous blood flow [7]. This is supposed to act as a physiological regulatory mechanism to improve blood circulation through constriction of the intermediate zone.

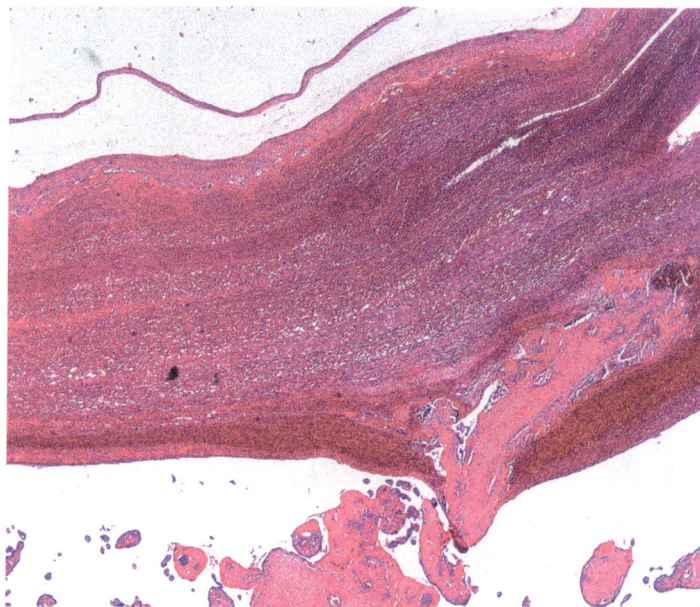

Fig. 7.19: Gestational week 36 + 4. Subchorionic subacute thrombosis. An eosinophilic and multi layered lesion expanding into the intervillous space.

7.2.6 Intervillous thrombus

An intervillous thrombus shows coagulation and aggregation in the intervillous space and are found in 25 % of all placentas.

Macroscopically, thrombus is well defined/circumscribed and usually 5 to 10 mm in size, in rare cases they can reach up to 5 to 10 cm. The color changes on the cut surface corresponds to the age and to the amount of organization in the thrombus.

Coagulation related thrombosis shows a typical structure microscopically with extension into the intervillous space and villous displacement. Acute intervillous hemorrhage in a villous free zone is considered to be the precursor. Chronic with old dense fibrin (aged) fibrin slats.

Pathogenesis
- penetration of a retroplacental hematoma through the basal plate into the inter-villous space with subsequent coagulation,
- venous flow turbulence and stasis of the maternal blood in the feto-maternal unit at the placental base with massive intervillous blood clots centrally in the feto-maternal unit and adjacent placentons,
- irregular architecture of the intervillous space, related to villous maturation dis-orders with enlarged intervillous space and circulatory stasis,

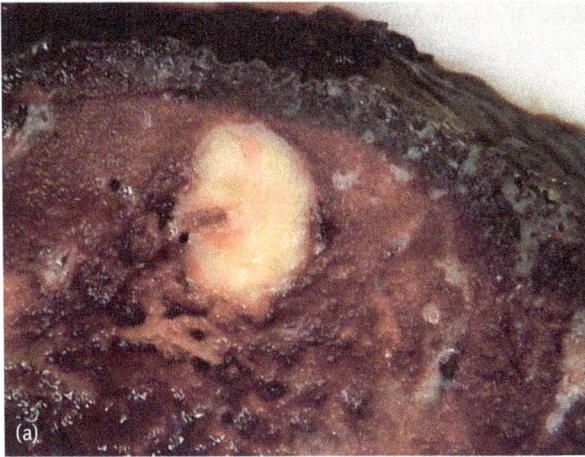

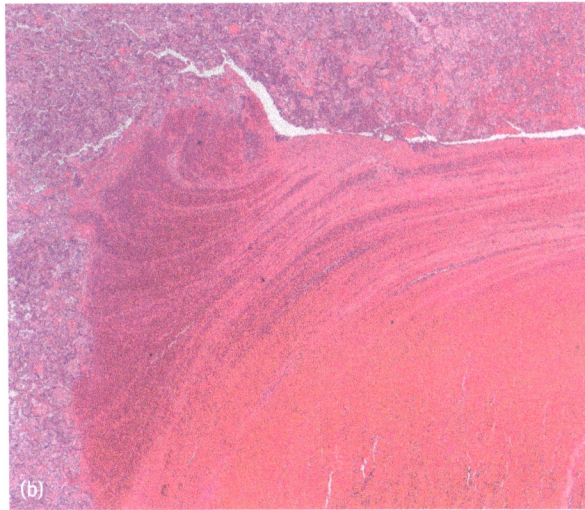

Fig. 7.20: (a) Chronic intervillous thrombus. Demarcated, firm and yellow-whitish lesion. (b) Intervillous subacute thrombosis, acute in the center part. Lesion with a laminar structure, partly acute and partly organized.

– rupture of intravillous vessels and villous surface due to villous necrosis or trauma and premature placental abruption.

Intervillous thrombosis may be differentiated from *subchorionic thrombosis* by location, last one with typical laminated architecture in the subchorionic space. Slender and small depositions are common, large thrombosis is rare.

Consequences of thrombosis for the fetus

In the majority of cases, thrombosis is of no clinical relevance. However, massive thrombosis may be related to premature placental abruption with rupture of the basal plate, and may represent a threat to the fetus. In exceptional cases, a longstanding subchorionic thrombosis, of several weeks duration, with compression of the surrounded villi may cause fetal growth restriction. Such thrombosis is visible on ultrasound.

7.2.7 Placental hematoma

Hematomas in the placenta are defined as hemorrhage outside the intervillous space and include hemorrhage adjacent to the chorionic plate, basal plate and placental margins; referred to as chorionic plate hematoma, marginal hematoma and retroplacental hematoma respectively. Marginal and retroplacental hematomas may cause premature placental abruption.

Retroplacental hematoma
Retroplacental hematomas are localized between the basal plate and the uterine wall and are adherent to the basal plate, these are to be differentiated from basal plate clots which can detach during delivery and easy to brush away without residual traces remaining on the decidua.

The size of the hematoma ranges from 1–2 cm in diameter to hematomas covering nearly the whole of the basal plate.

Acute hematomas are soft and dark red, whereas old hematomas are red-brown or dirty yellow and consist of brown-red to yellow-brown compact laminations. The basal plate may become hollowed out due to the hematoma. Retroplacental hematomas with corresponding changes in the basal plate are a morphological clue to premature placental abruption.

Marginal hematoma
Hematomas located towards the edge of margo internus and externus. Macroscopically they show a triangular symmetry.

Marginal placental hemorrhages are caused by bleeding from thin-walled, maternal veins [32]. Hematomas are often seen in placenta extrachorialis circumvallata, low implanted placentas or premature placental abruptions of normally implanted placentas.

Small marginal hematomas do not have any risk for the mother or the fetus [33] but larger hematomas, as part of a premature placental abruption or incorrectly implanted placentas, may have risk of adverse outcome.

Premature placental abruption
Abruption is defined as a partial or total detachment of the normal implanted placenta before and during delivery.

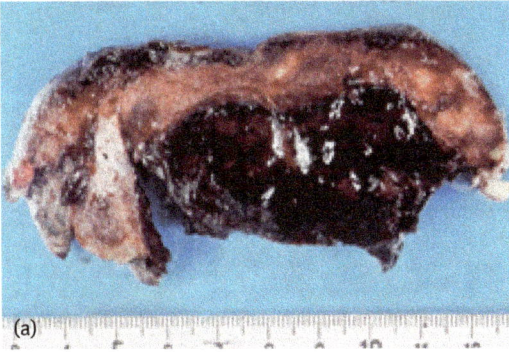

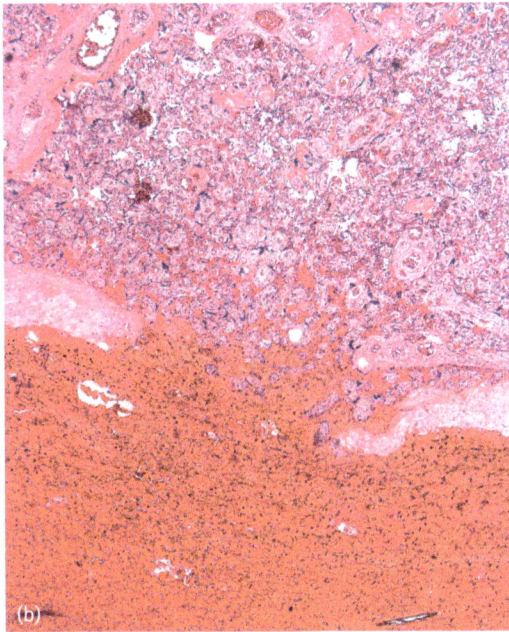

Fig. 7.21: (a) Retroplacental hematoma. Dark red blood clot close to the marginal zone of the placenta. (b) Intervillous hemorrhage with bleeding into the intervillous space supplying it from the basal plate. Gestational Week 36, IUFD due to massive acute retroplacental hematoma.

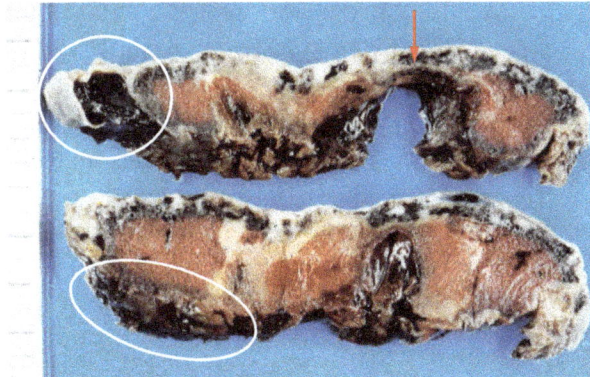

Fig. 7.22: Marginal and retroplacental hematoma (rings) combined with intervillous defect due to multiple hemorrhage along the basal plate. IUFD in Gestational Week 36, due to multiple premature placental abruption.

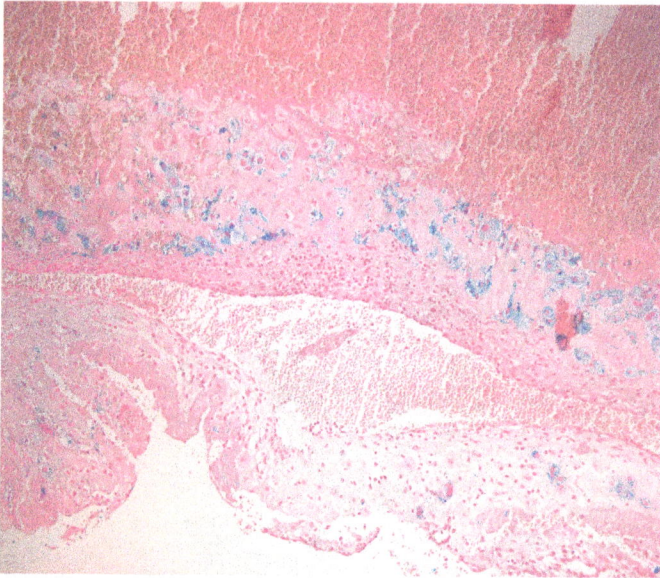

Fig. 7.23: Retroplacental hematoma. Perl stained sidero macrophages, consistent with organization in hematomas. IUFD in Gestational Week 30 + 2 due to old premature placental abruption.

Morphological signs of premature placental abruption are seen as:
- retroplacental hematoma (RH) with a well circumscribed impression on the basal plate,
- RH with basal plate abruption, with hemorrhage from and into adjacent placental parenchyma, also observed in cases of prostaglandin induced abortion,
- RH with corresponding circulatory disorders of same duration as infarct and/or intervillous thrombosis.

Early premature placental abruption may be organized into retroplacental hematomas with infarcts and circumscribed hollow with compression of neighbouring villi close to the basal plate with parenchymal necrosis.

Fresh hematomas show, microscopically, blood and fibrin. The basal plate may be affected or even destroyed so that the bleeding involves the intervillous space.

In chronic hematomas erythrocytes, fibrin, neutrophilic granulocytes, macrophages, and sidero macrophages may be seen microscopically in the adjacent basal plate.

The morphological features that correspond to a premature placental abruption are missing in cases with:
- short intervals between abruption and delivery,
- partial abruption and marginal bleeding, without involvement of the basal plate.

Clinically, a placental abruption with classical symptoms are only seen in 2–5 % of cases. Mild to asymptomatic abruptions are seen in 0.5–1 % of cases. Morphological evidence following premature placental abruption in livebirths can be seen in 1.1 %, without any risk factors, and in 4–26 % placentas of risk babies. Prematurely born children with premature abruption have a 20-fold higher risk than mature live births without risk factors. Premature placental abruption is seen as cause of fetal death after gestational week 35.

Pathogenesis and cause
- etiology is unknown in more than 50 %,
- vasculopathy of the pre-placental vessels, associated with hypertension,
- sudden decrease of uterine volume:
  - caused by decreased amniotic fluid in polyhydramnion
  - after delivery of the 1st twin in multiple pregnancy
- reduced venous downstream pressure and intervillous increased pressure in vena cava compression syndrome,
- shortened umbilical cord,
- trauma to the lower body. Premature placental abruption due to traumatic events, such as a fall or impact, car accidents in the 2nd trimester have been reported however, a direct correlation between trauma and abruption has not been established. Furthermore, intraplacental hematomas can be seen after accidents without premature abruption. Villous and fetal vessel rupture subsequent feto-maternal

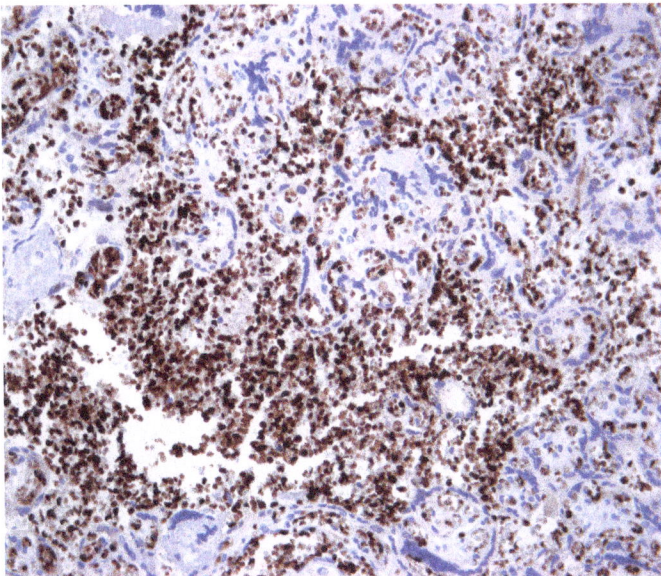

Fig. 7.24: Feto-maternal transfusion. HbF stained fetal erythrocytes in the intervillous space in Gestational Week 40, associated with placental abruption.

transfusion is the most serious fetal threat due to premature placental abruption and seen in less than 10 % of cases following trauma in late pregnancy [34].

Clinical meaning: Clinically, three grades of placental abruption can be distinguished, due to:
- quantity of the bleeding,
- fetal impairment,
- maternal shock.

Fetal risk is due to:
- Intrauterine hypoxia and anoxia dependent on time interval between abruption and fetal development, size of the abruption and structural placental damage. Premature abruption affecting 20 % or more of placental tissue will causes intrauterine hypoxia. An abruption affecting more than 40 % of the total placental area is associated with IUFD.
- Anemia – Fetal hemorrhage due to feto-maternal micro- and macrotransfusion into the intervillous space following villous abruption is independent from size of the ruptured tissue. Morphological evidence is given by HbF immunostained fetal erythrocytes in the intervillous space. Clinically, a feto-maternal blood transfusion can be identified by the presence of maternal and fetal blood cells in the hematoma and maternal serum. The risk to the fetus risk can only assessed though clinical correlation of the histological findings.

References

[1] Khong TY, De Wolf F, Robertson WB, Brosens I. Inadequate maternal vascular response to placentation in pregnancies complicated by pre-eclampsia and by small-for-gestational age infants. British journal of obstetrics and gynaecology. 1986;93(10):1049–1059.
[2] Boyd JD. Hamilton WJ. The Human Placenta. Cambridge: Heffer; 1970. 365 p.
[3] Ramsey EM, Donner MW. Placental vasculature and circulation. Stuttgart: Thieme; 1980.
[4] Moll W. Physiologie der Plazenta. In: Becker V, Schiebler TH, Kubli F, editor. Die Plazenta des Menschen. Stuttgart: Thieme; 1981. p. 120–206.
[5] Lemtis H. [Physiology of the placenta]. Fortschr Geburtshilfe Gynakol. 1970;54:1–52.
[6] Freese UE. The uteroplacental vascular relationship in the human. American journal of obstetrics and gynecology. 1968;101(1):8–16.
[7] Kloos K, Vogel M. Pathologie der Perinatalperiode. Stuttgart: Thieme; 1974.
[8] Vogel M. Pathologie der Plazenta der mittleren und der späten Schwangerschaft. In: Vogel M, editor. Atlas der morphologischen Plazentadiagnostik. 2nd ed. Berlin: Springer; 1996. p. 50–68.
[9] Wallenburg HCS. On the morphology and pathogenesis of placental infarcts. Groningen: Van Denderen; 1971b.
[10] Jimenez E, Vogel M, Hohle R, Ferszt R, Hahn H. Age determination of infarcts in the guinea pig-placenta. Advances in pathology. 2. Oxford: Pergamon; 1982. p. 397–400.
[11] Vogel M. Klinische Pathologie der Embryonal- Fetal und Perinatalpathologie. In: Dudenhausen JW, editor. Praxis der Perinatalmedizin. Stuttgart: Thieme; 1984. p. 413–454.

[12] Myers RE, Fujikura T. Placental changes after experimental abruptio placentae and fetal vessel ligation of rhesus monkey placenta. American journal of obstetrics and gynecology. 1968;100(6):946–951.

[13] Brosens I, Renaer M. On the pathogenesis of placental infarcts in pre-eclampsia. J Obstet Gynaecol Br Commonw. 1972;79(9):794–799.

[14] Robertson WB, Brosens I, Dixon HG. The pathological response of the vessels of the placental bed to hypertensive pregnancy. J Pathol Bacteriol. 1967;93(2):581–592.

[15] Kubli F, Wernicke K. Plazentainsuffizienz. In: Becker V, Schiebler TH, Kubli F, editor. Die Plazenta des Menschen. Stuttgart: Thieme; 1981. p. 395–470.

[16] Wallenburg HC. On the morphology and pathogenesis of placental infarcts. Groningen: Van Dederen; 1971b.

[17] Jimenez E, Vogel M, Arabin B, Wagner G, Mirsalim P. Correlation of Ultrasonographic Measurement of the Utero-Placental and Fetal Blood Flow with the Morphological Diagnosis of Placental Function. In: Kaufmann P, Miller RK, editors. Placental Vascularization and Blood Flow: Basic Research and Clinical Applications. Boston, MA: Springer US; 1988. p. 325–334.

[18] Hoffbauer H, Vogel M: Pathologische Fibrinierung der Plazenta und ihre Bedeutung für den feto-maternen Stoffaustausch. In: Dudenhausen JW, Schmidt E, editor. Perinatale Medizin, Stuttgart: Thieme; 1975. p. 155–156.

[19] Frank HG, Malekzadeh F, Kertschanska S, et al. Immunohistochemistry of two different types of placental fibrinoid. Acta Anat (Basel). 1994;150(1):55–68.

[20] Horn V, Horalek F. [On so-called fibrinoid substance in the placenta]. Zentralbl Allg Pathol. 1961;102:514–521.

[21] Hormann G. [An attempt to systematize disorders of placental development]. Geburtshilfe Frauenheilkd. 1958;18(4):345–349.

[22] Becker V, Schiebler TH, Kubli F. Allgemeine und spezielle Pathologie der Plazenta. Die Plazenta des Menschen. Stuttgart: Thieme; 1981. p. 251–393.

[23] Schuhmann R, Geier G. [Histomorphologic placenta findings in pregnancy toxemias. Contribution to the morphology of placenta insufficiency]. Arch Gynakol. 1972;213(1):31–47.

[24] Baergen RN. Placental Malperfusion. Manual of Benirschke and Kaufmann's Pathology of the human placenta. 1 ed. New York: Springer; 2005. p. 232–350.

[25] Ludwig KS. [The role of fibrin in formation of human placenta]. Acta Anat (Basel). 1959;38:323–331.

[26] Gerl D, Ehrhardt G. [Quantitative determinations of fibrinoid in the human placenta]. Zentralbl Gynakol. 1970;92(20):617–624.

[27] Ludwig KS. Pathologische Fibrinierung bei der Spätgestose. In: Ripmann ET, editor. Die Spätgestose. Basel: Organisat Gestosis Press; 1969. p. 69–94.

[28] Wigglesworth JS. Vascular anatomy of the human placenta and its significance for placental pathology. J Obstet Gynaecol Br Commonw. 1969;76(11):979–989.

[29] Katzman PJ, Genest DR. Maternal floor infarction and massive perivillous fibrin deposition: histological definitions, association with intrauterine fetal growth restriction, and risk of recurrence. Pediatric and developmental pathology : the official journal of the Society for Pediatric Pathology and the Paediatric Pathology Society. 2002;5(2):159–164.

[30] Benirschke K., Burton G, Baergen RN. Pathology of the Human Placenta. 6 ed. Heidelberg, NY, London: Springer; 2012 2012.

[31] Thomsen K. [Morphology and genesis of so-called placental infarct]. Arch Gynakol. 1954;185(2):221–247.

[32] Schiebler TH, Kaufmann P. Reife Plazenta. In: Becker V, Schiebler TH, Kubli F, editor. Die Plazenta des Menschen. Stuttgart: Thieme; 1981. p. 51–100.

[33] Martius J. Fieber sub partu (Amnioninfekstionssyndrom). Extragenitales Fieber. In: Martius G, editor. Differentialdiagnose in Geburtshilfe und Gynäkologie. I. Stuttgart: Thieme; 1987. p. 94–7.

[34] Hof K, Wobbe HD. Intrauterine Schädigung durch Verkehrsunfall. Gynäkol Prax 7. 1983:197–200.

8 Villous maturation disorders

Definition

Maturation disorders are characterized as disorders of villous branching (ramification) and villous stromal development. These disorders may be focal or diffuse and may display qualitative and quantitative deviations from the normal villous development at a given gestational age

Villous maturation disorders may occur at every stage of pregnancy after development of the placenta (Ch. 1). Changes in the villous structure are more significant if they occur in early pregnancy. Maturation disorders in the 2nd half of the pregnancy only affect the timing of normal maturation and present as retarded or accelerated maturation disorders.

A histological diagnosis should document the type and the extent of the disorder; subtyping may be of clinical relevance and should also be included in the histology report. Additionally, semi-quantitative grading may aid in the estimation of placental function (Ch. 15)

Classification

A common classification system for villous maturation disorders does not currently exist. Our proposed classification system is based on the following histological findings [2]:

- arrest of villous maturation
- retardation of villous maturation
- chorangiosis type I
- chorangiosis type II
- deficiency of the intermediate villi (Distal Villous Hypoplasia)
- peripheral villous immaturity
- preterm (accelerated) villous maturation

Subtyping may be of diagnostic value for:
- the child's wellbeing,
- maternal disease,
- pregnancy follow up.

The *grading of villous maturation disorders* and microfibrin deposition is based on the percentage of tissue involved at a medium power field (MPF) magnification:
- grade I: up to 10 %
- grade II: > 10 % to < 50 %
- grade III: > 50 %

https://doi.org/10.1515/9783110452600-008

Grade 1 maturation disorders are assumed to be without functional significance, whereas diffuse changes affecting more than 50 % of a MPF, grade 3, are considered to be pathophysiologically relevant [1].

Morphology

Manifestation of maturation disorders are predominantly seen in two areas of the villous tree:

1. the transition zone between stem villi and central intermediate villi (immature type)
2. the transition zone between peripheral intermediate villi (mature type) and terminal villi.

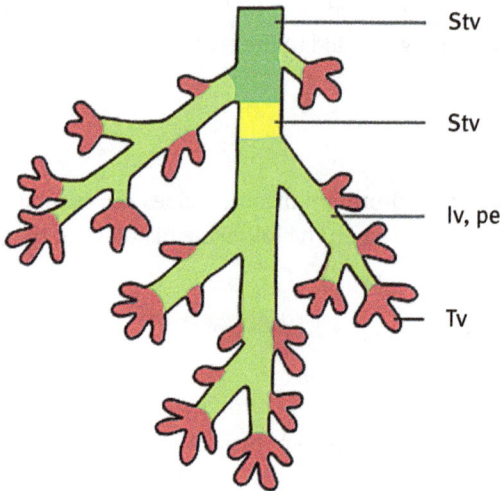

Stv

Stv

Iv, pe

Tv

Fig. 8.1: Illustration of the villous tree. (Stv) Stem villi, (Iv, ce) central intermediate villi (immature type), (Iv, pe) peripheral intermediate villi (mature type), (Tv) Terminal villi.

Table 8.1: Histometric data of the different villous maturation disorders (%) and their relationship to the values of mature villous structures.

0		mature	A–C	100 %
Nr		maturation disorder	measurement	%
1	AVM	arrest of villous maturation	A	52
			B	23
			C	29
2	RVM	retardation of villous maturation	A	65
			B	45
			C	41
3	CH I	chorangiosis type I	A	62
			B	187
			C	37
4	CH II	chorangiosis type II	A	70
			B	173
			C	56
5	DIV	deficiency of the intermediate villi (distal villous hypoplasia)	A	71
			B	67
			C	35
6	PVI	peripheral villous immaturity	A	85
			B	49
			C	46
7	PrVM	preterm (accelerated) villous maturation	A	87
			B	91
			C	89

A: villous surface density = value of ramification; B: surface density of the intravillous vessels = value of vascularization; C: proportion of vasculosyncytial membranes on the villous surface = value of epithelial differentiation. Measurements of villous maturation and maturation disorders performed in standardized, well selected MPFs, with qualitative histological diagnosis [3,4].

Villous maturation disorders
- categories 1–5 are characterized by deficient or defective villous branching
- categories 6 and 7 show normal villous branching for gestational age
  - in category 6 the villous subtypes show immaturity in the periphery
  - in category 7 preterm accelerated villous maturation is seen

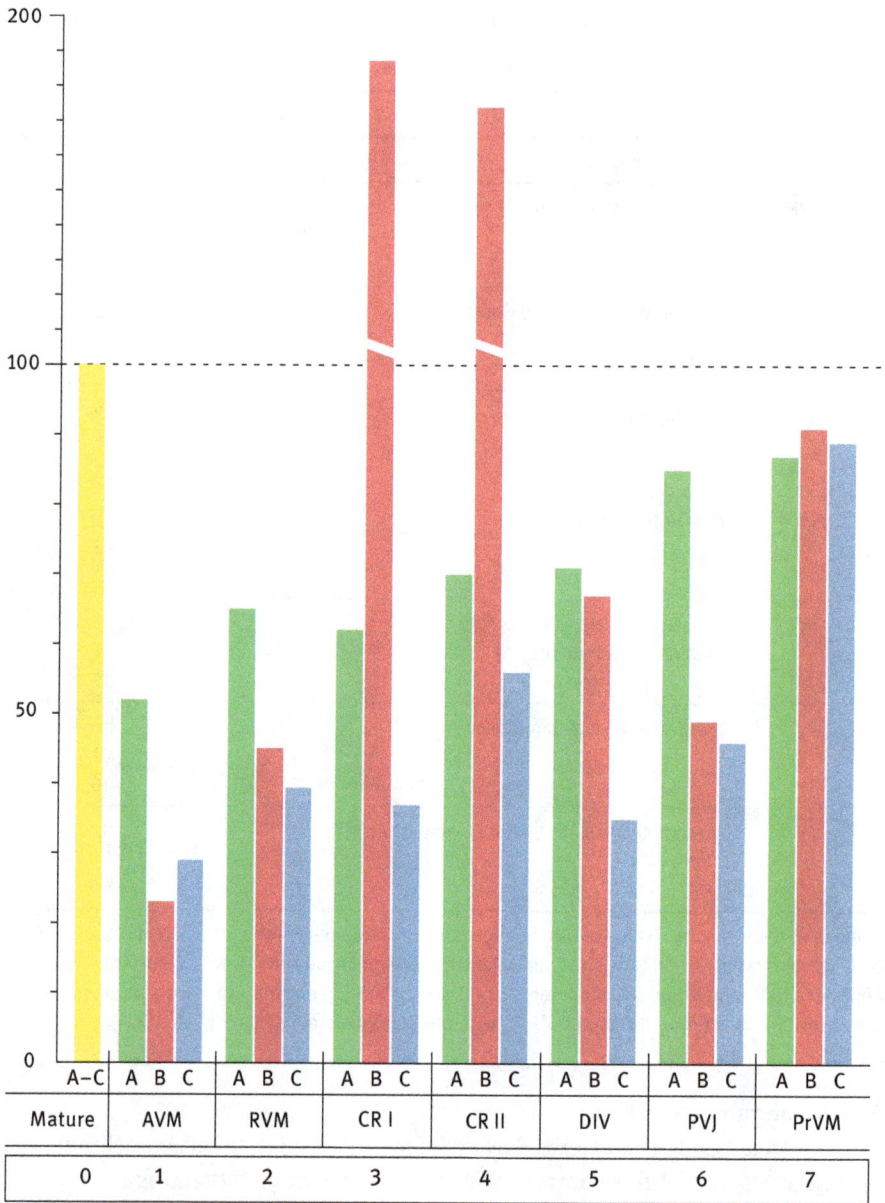

Fig. 8.2: Diagram of histometric values (Table 8.1). A–C (yellow) = 100 %; normal villous maturation according gestational age 0 = mature. Villous maturation subtypes 1–7: A (green): villous surface density = value of ramification; B (red): surface density of the intravillous vessels = value of vascularization; C (blue): proportion of vasculosyncytial membranes on the villous surface = value of villous trophoblast differentiation.

Table 8.2: Villous maturation disorders of the placenta in eutrophic term pregnancies without any known risk factors. N = 1022. Frequency in % [3,4].

maturation disorder	%
arrest of villous maturation	2.1
retardation of villous maturation	6.2
chorangiosis type I	1.3
chorangiosis type II	2.9
deficiency of intermediate villi (distal villous hypoplasia)	4.3
peripheral villous immaturity	8.1
preterm (accelerated) villous maturation	32.4

8.1 Arrest of villous maturation

Definition
Arrest of villous maturation is characterized by a combination of reduced branching of intermediate villi of the central immature type and incomplete transformation into stem villi. Stem villi are enlarged with immature embryonic stroma and with an irregularly developed villous trophoblast.

Diagnostic characteristics (Figs. 8.3–8.5)
– villous groups with increased diameters
– embryonic and mesenchymal stroma or a loose reticular stroma
– vessels of stem villi have a slender tunica media (hypoplastic)
– paravascular fiber rings inconspicuous, with a decreased number of α smooth actin positive cells
– few capillaries with rare connections to the villous surface
– flat single-layered villous trophoblast, lacking nuclei in the epithelium and with few vasculosyncytial membranes

Pathogenesis
Arrest of villous maturation may begin in the 1rst trimester and is caused by maternal and fetal diseases. The ability of the placenta to adapt to noxious stimuli results in a pattern of villous maturation that is relatively monomorphic. Growth of immature villi and cellular regeneration is limited by the villous trophoblast; this occurs at the expense of villous diameter, stromal maturation, vascular proliferation and epithelial differentiation.

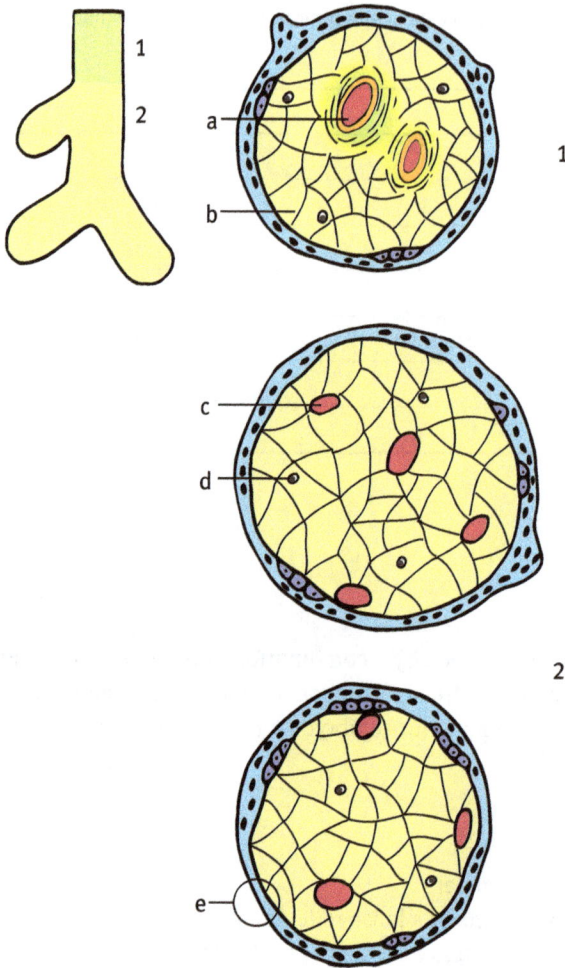

Fig. 8.3: Illustration. Histological characteristics of villous maturation arrest. The villous tree, on the left, illustrates reduced villous branching. (1) Stem villus, (2) intermediate villi of the central immature type. Cross sections: (a) inconspicuous paravascular fibrous rings; (b) loose, embryonic stroma; (c) few capillaries; (d) Hofbauer cells; (e) flattened, partly single-layered and nuclear free epithelium.

Occurrence

Arrest of villous maturation is seen in both early and late pregnancy and is associated with:

- chronic diabetes or insulin dependent maternal diabetes mellitus with a limited metabolic regulation (Ch. 14)
- severe Rh-incompatibility
- alpha thalassemia
- non hemolytic hydrops fetalis
- congenital nephrotic syndrome (Finnish subtype)
- syndromic diseases; chromosome aberrations, skeletal dysplasia
- anencephaly, craniorachischisis
- intrauterine infection; rubella, cytomegalovirus, toxoplasma, syphilis
- implantation disorders (local, hormonal)

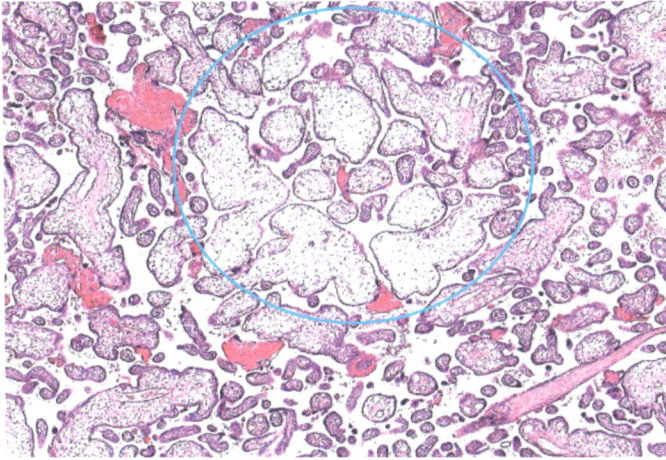

Fig. 8.4: Arrest of villous maturation. Groups of immature intermediate villi with embryonic stroma containing few capillaries and an irregular single- and double-layered villous epithelium (circle).

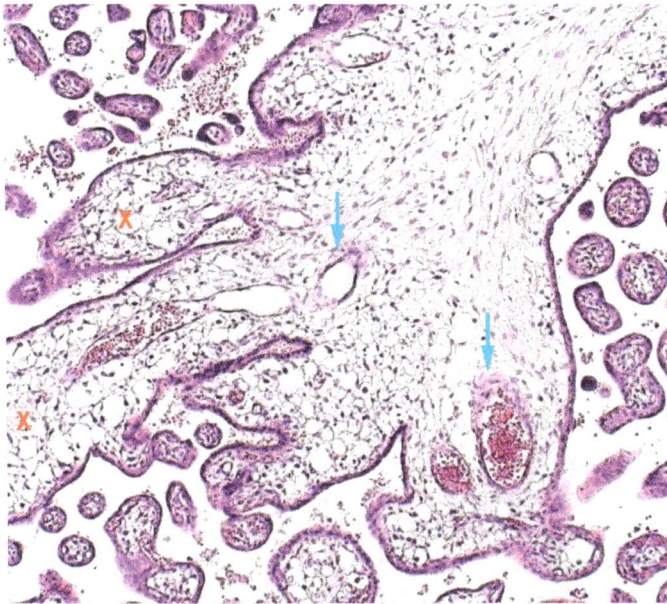

Fig. 8.5: Arrest of villous maturation. Stem villi with tunica media hypoplasia (arrows) and the transition into immature intermediate villi with an embryonic stroma (X).

Risk and consequences for placental function

– increased risk of recurrence in subsequent pregnancies is more often seen when there is a clinical manifestation of disease (cases such as chronic diabetes and in metabolic syndrome with maternal adiposity) (Ch. 14)

- limited diffusion capacity is seen in medium and high grade maturation arrest (grade 2 and 3)
- seldom: associated placental growth restriction with reduction in the absolute villous surface area and an increased risk of chronic placental insufficiency (Ch. 15).

8.2 Retardation of villous maturation

Retardation of villous maturation is characterized by a villous branching disorder of the intermediate villi and a focal, or diffuse, stromal and epithelial immaturity.

Diagnostic criteria (Figs. 8.6–8.8)
- predominantly groups of villi of medium sized diameter (5 villi/MPF)
- deficient villous branching into intermediate subtypes
- reticular stromal variation with increased collagenous tissue and small to medium sized cells
- few capillaries
- single layered, nuclear rich villous trophoblast with decreased number of vasculosyncytial membrane.
- reduced number of nuclear sprouts on the villous surface

Pathogenesis
While the etiology is of retarded villous maturation is unknown, the onset is believed to occur in the beginning of the 2nd half of pregnancy.

Occurrence
Retarded villous maturation may be seen in:
- term or late deliveries (frequent)
- following intrauterine infections, most frequently virus infection in late early pregnancy (rubella, EBV, Coxsackie B).
- frequently associated with endangiopathia obliterans (Ch. 5)
- intrauterine hypoxia in mature newborns and IUFD without identifiable cause
- post term pregnancy (> 10 days), accompanied chorangiosis type II
- chronic diabetes mellitus
- unknown causes

Consequences for placental function
1. maturation disorders (grades 2 and 3) with normal placental size may cause a limitation of placental diffusion capacity (Ch. 15)
2. associated with placental growth restriction: chronic placental insufficiency

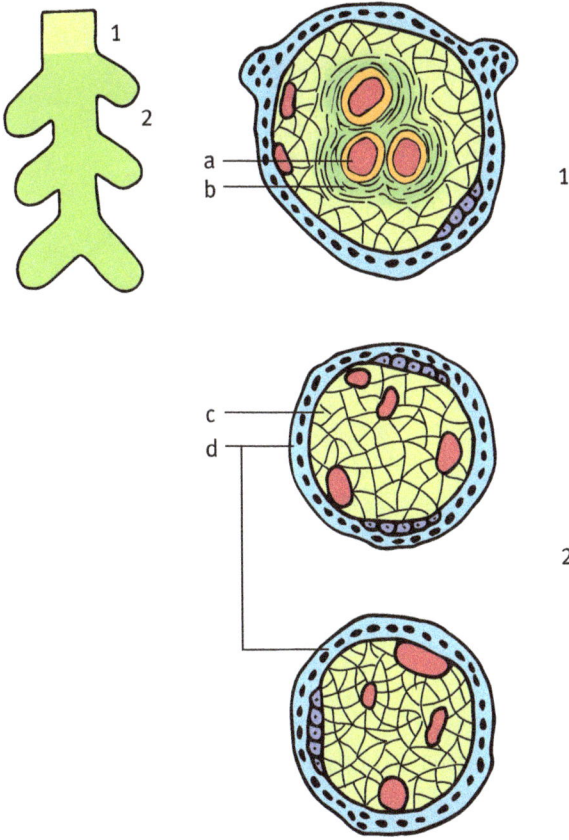

Fig. 8.6: Illustration. Histological characteristics of retarded villous maturation with the villous tree, on the left, illustrating a deficiency of branching into the intermediate subtypes. (1) Stem villus, (2) intermediate villi of the peripheral mature type. Cross sections: (a) central fetal vessels and a subepithelial reticular stromal hem between the peripherally lying vessels; (b) paravascular fibrous rings; (c) reticular stroma, characterized by a variable cellular and fibrous content and few capillaries; (d) nuclear rich villous epithelium.

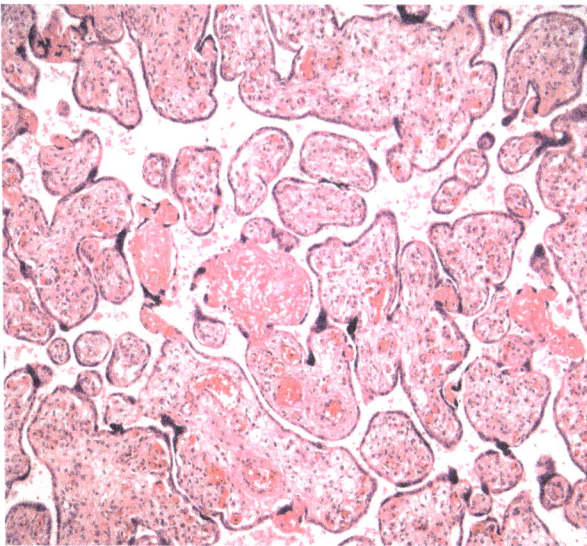

Fig. 8.7: Retarded villous maturation. Villi with irregular and medium sized diameters containing a reticular and capillary poor stroma. The nuclear rich villous epithelium only shows rare vasculosyncytial membranes.

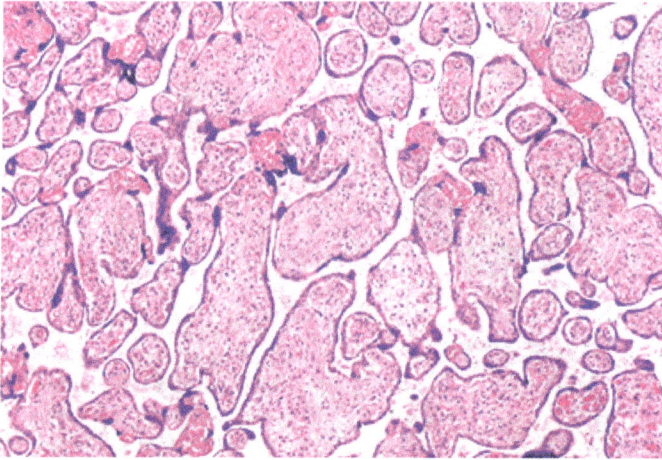

Fig. 8.8: Retarded villous maturation. Villi with irregular and medium sized diameters containing a reticular and capillary poor stroma. The nuclear rich villous epithelium only shows rare vasculosyncytial membranes.

8.3 Chorangiosis type I

Definition
A focal villous maturation disorder characterized by reduced villous branching, increased capillary proliferation, more than 10/villus [5] and lack of vasculosyncytial membranes.

Diagnostic criteria (Figs. 8.9–8.11)
– groups of large and medium sized villi (5 villi per MPF),
– many irregular adjacent capillaries of variable size and maturity
– more than 10 capillaries per villus, partially immature.

Pathogenesis
This category of maturation disorder can be diagnosed at any gestational age, 1st trimester included. It is considered to be a primary angiogenic response to hypoxia; however, a genetic cause cannot be excluded. Histologically, increased capillary growth with an associated decrease in stromal maturation and deficient differentiation of the villous trophoblast are seen. VEGF and cytokine expression by the trophoblast results in an increase in capillary proliferation and is believed to stimulate this process [6].

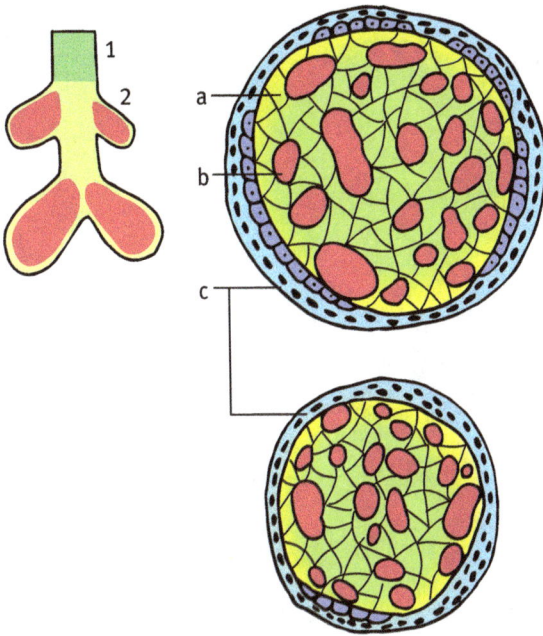

Fig. 8.9: Illustration. Histological characteristics of type I Chorangiosis with the villous tree on the left illustrating deficient branching. (1) Stem villus; (2) intermediate villus. Cross sections of Intermediate villi: (a) reticular, partly embryonic stroma; (b) hypervascularization with more than 10 capillaries per villus; (c) a nuclear rich villous epithelium.

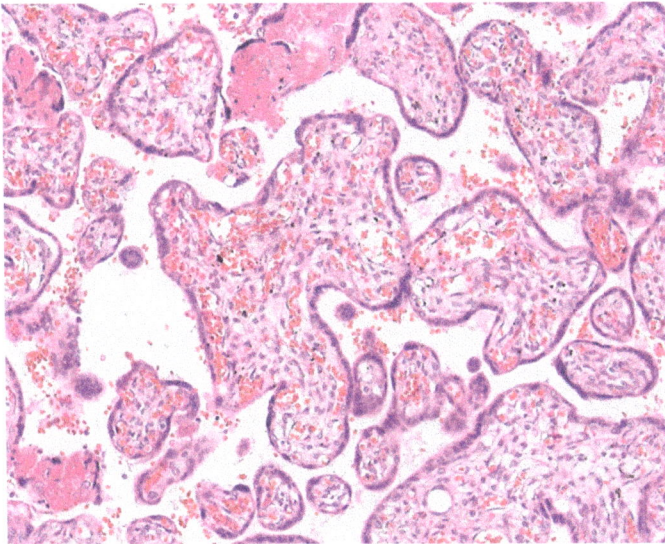

Fig. 8.10: Chorangiosis type I. Group of villi with enlarged diameters, reticular stroma, hypervascularization and a nuclear rich epithelium which is deficient in vasculosyncytial membranes.

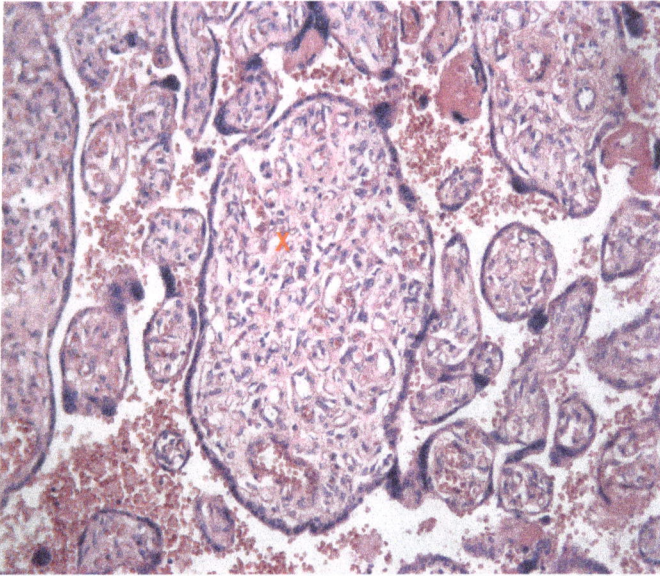

Fig. 8.11: Chorangiosis type I. Villus (X marked) with a cellular, capillary rich stroma and a nuclear rich chorionic epithelium.

Occurrence

– rh-incompatibility, associated with retarded villous maturation
– non-immunological hemolytic anemia and fetal hydrops occurring in combination with arrested villous maturation
– alpha thalassemia
– insulin dependent diabetes mellitus with vasculopathy
– maternal cardiac disease
– placental mesenchymal dysplasia
– unknown causes.

Consequences for placental function

1. placental growth restriction is associated with grade 2 disorders
2. decreased placental diffusion capacity is associated with grade 3 disorders

8.4 Chorangiosis type II

Definition
Type II chorangiosis is characterized by slender to medium sized villi, usually focally, with numerous mature capillaries and numerous vasculosyncytial membranes in close proximity to each other.

Diagnostic criteria (Figs. 8.12, 8.13):
– villi (5 villi per MPF) with medium sized diameters
– > 10 capillaries in each villus cross section
– numerous vasculosyncytial membranes.

Pathogenesis
The increased angiogenesis and branching seen in type II chorangiosis is interpreted as a compensatory response to uteroplacental hypoxemia and intervillous circulatory deficiency in the late fetal period [7]. The capillary diameter in each villus and the proportion of vasculosyncytial membranes is increased; these adaptations increase feto-maternal gas and nutrition transfer.

Type II chorangiosis is associated with:
– foci of chronic maternal vascular disturbance
– foci of villous fibrosis and chronic proliferative villitis

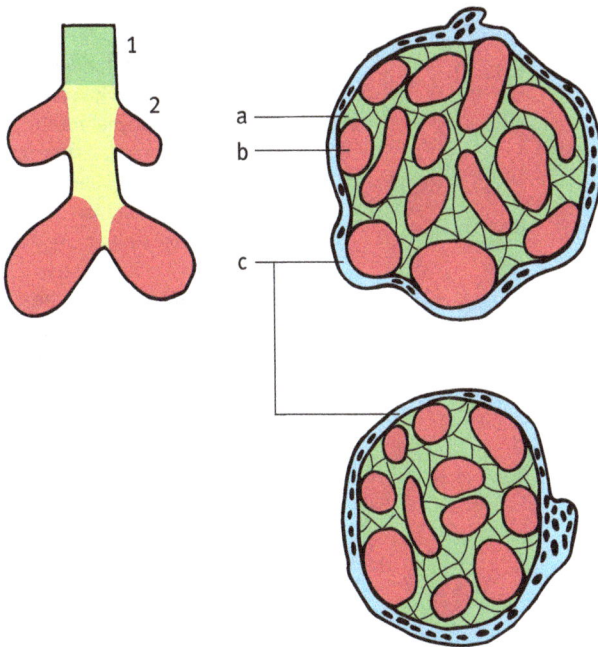

Fig. 8.12: Illustration. Histological characteristics of type II chorangiosis. (1) Stem villus, (2) intermediate peripheral and terminal villi. Cross sections of intermediate and terminal villi: (a) stroma with more than 10 capillaries; (b) fetal capillaries close under the chorionic epithelium; (c) nuclear poor chorionic epithelium with numerous vasculosyncytial membranes.

– retarded villous maturation in post-term placentas
– maternal vitium cordis

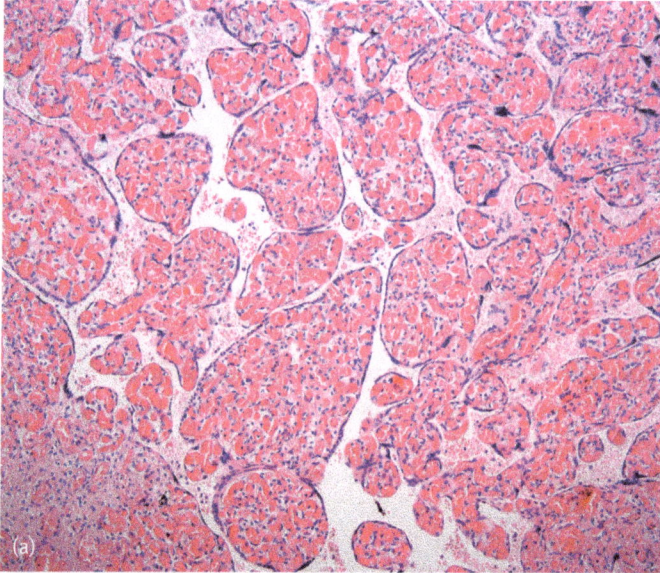

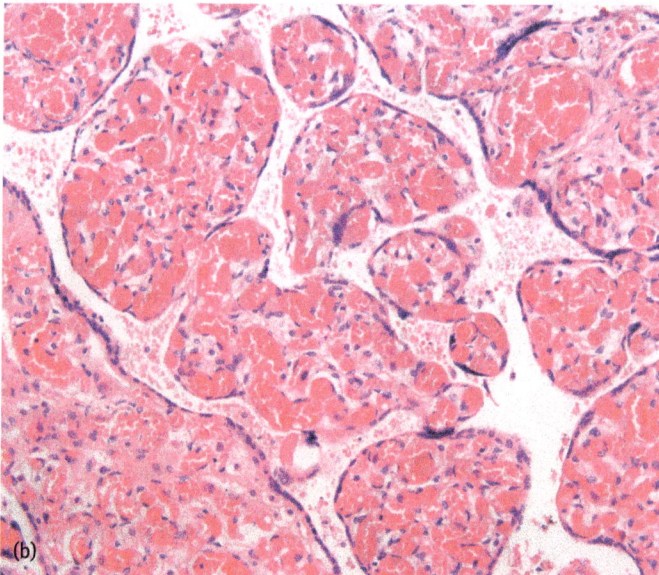

Fig. 8.13: (a) Chorangiosis type II LPF. Groups of intermediate villi of the peripheral type with medium sized diameters and a capillary rich stroma. (b) chorangiosis type II HPF. Capillary rich stroma with more than 10 capillaries, centrally located in the stroma of each villus, and vasculosyncytial membrane formation. Macrosomic placenta in gestational week 38, known maternal GDM.

8.5 Deficiency of intermediate villi (distal villous hypoplasia

Definition
A villous maturation disorder characterized by deficient branching and a decreased number of intermediate villi.

Diagnostic criteria (Figs. 8.14–8.15)
- diffuse developmental deficiency of the intermediate villi
- stem villi and slender terminal villi are adjacent to one another
- terminal villi have sometimes reduced vasculosyncytial membranes and a partially fibrous stroma
- sinusoidal capillaries in terminal villi
- increased syncytial sprouts and knots with regressive nuclear changes.

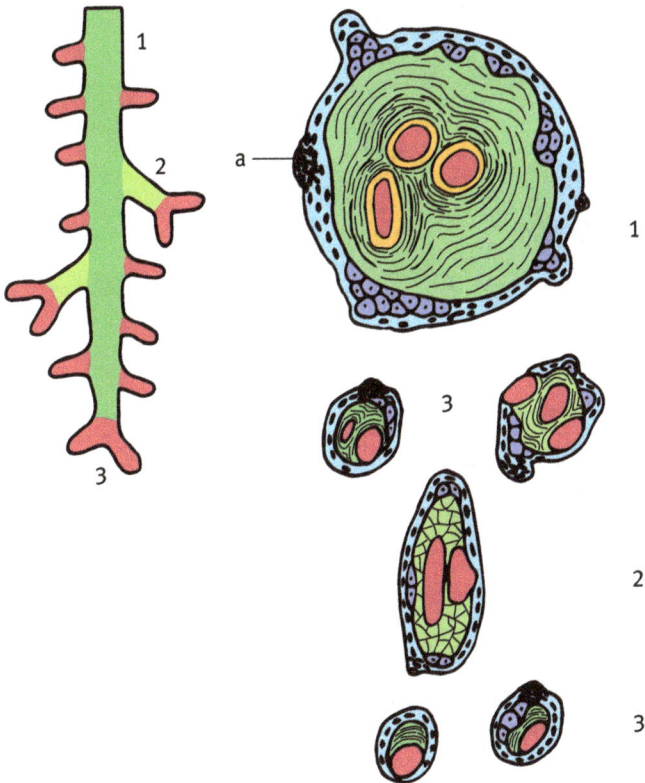

Fig. 8.14: Illustration. Histological characteristics of a deficiency of the intermediate villi. (1) Stem villus; (2) intermediate villi of the peripheral mature type; (3) terminal villi. Cross sections: (a) stem villus with nuclear sprouts and regressive knots; (2, 3) slender terminal villi admixed with intermediate villi.

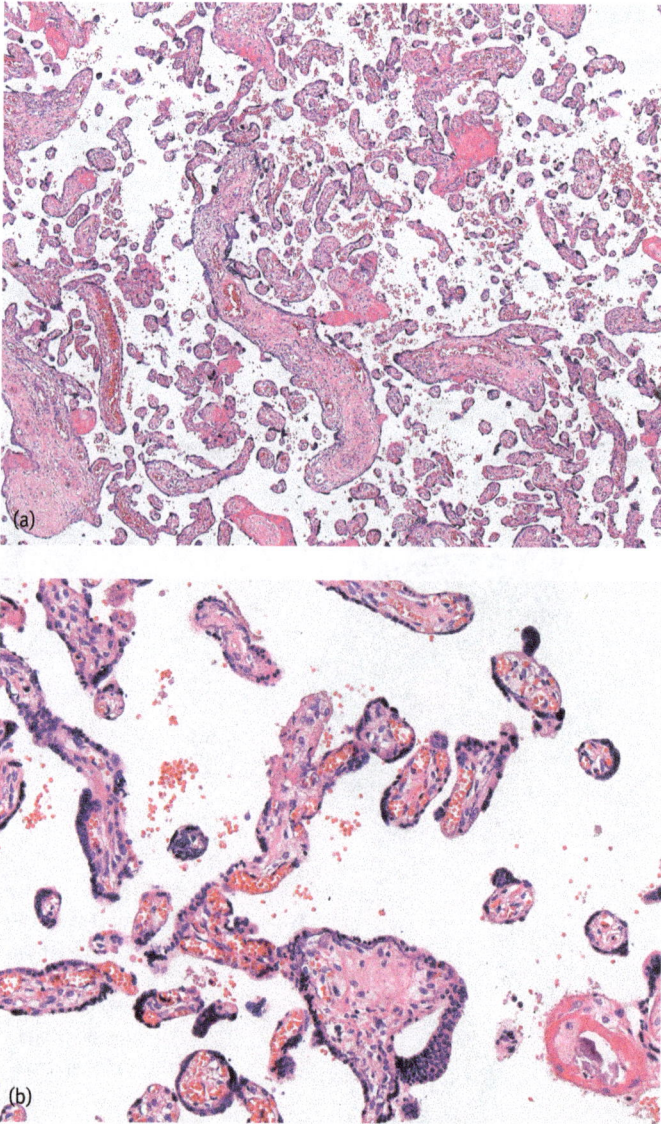

Fig. 8.15: (a) Deficiency of the intermediate villi (LPF). Stem and terminal villi with a large, open intervillous space. Elongated and slender terminal villi, non-branching vasculogenesis and stromal fibrosis. (b) Deficiency of the intermediate villi. Regressive cellular and epithelial knots in stem and terminal villi. Placenta in GW 35 + 5 with normal growth and area. Maternal preeclampsia (hypertensive 183/104 mmHg), proteinuria. Acute cesarean section, APGAR 6-4-8.

Pathogenesis

It is hypothesized that stenosis in the uteroplacental vessels develops in early pregnancy (decidual stenosed vasculopathy) and causes decreased intervillous circulation. Placental growth restriction, due to a reduced number of spiral arteries in the basal plate, cannot be excluded as cause; however, the maternal and fetal blood circulations are intimately intertwined in the feto-maternal unit and so any disturbance in the intervillous circulation affects both. The extent to which this stimulates terminal villi development, directly from stem villi, by elongated, non-branching angiogenesis remains unclear. This villous growth response favors terminal villi formation at the expense of intermediate villous development; this may represent an extreme variant of accelerated villous maturation.

An analogous physiological model of this maturation disorder may be illustrated in villous ramification in the subchorionic space (dead fluid zone) of the placenta [8].

Consequences of intermediate villi deficiency
- reduced placental weight with growth restriction of the basal plate (placental hypoplasia)
- pre-term and term births with FGR
- pregnancy related hypertension
- chronic maternal hypertension
- HELLP syndrome
- SLE in fetal abortion
- unknown cause.

Consequences for placental function
Inadequate development of the intermediate villi causes a reduced fetal vessel volume and a disturbed microcirculatory environment, leading to decreased perfusion capacity. This is associated with pre-term delivery, fetal hypoxia and fetal death. Doppler ultrasound shows a reduced diastolic flow close to umbilical cord arteries in growth restricted newborns.

8.6 Peripheral villous immaturity

Definition
A villous maturation disorder characterized by a regular villous branching into the villous subtypes but with reticular stroma and only few capillaries and syncytiovascular membranes.

Diagnostic criteria (Figs. 8.16–8.18)
- peripheral villi with reticular stroma
- villi with reduced capillaries
- decreased number of vasculosyncytial membranes

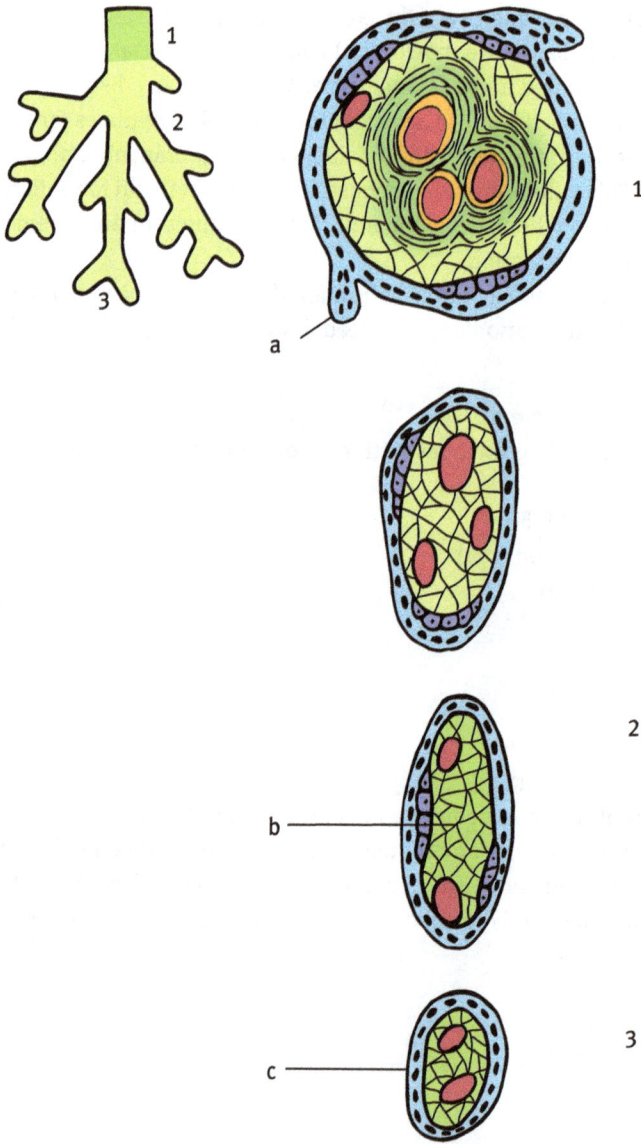

Fig. 8.16: Illustration. Histological characteristics of peripheral villous immaturity. The villous tree shows regular branching of the villous tree with small peripheral villi but with reticular stroma and few capillaries. Cross sections: (1) *stem villi* with reticular stroma and (a) epithelial sprouts; (2) *intermediate villi* with (b) with a reticular stroma of variable cellularity, few capillaries and (3) *terminal villi* with condensed nuclear epithelium, missing vasculo-syncytial membrans.

Combinations and transitions between disorders of retarded villous maturation are common. The diagnosis of peripheral immaturity is limited to the last trimester.

Occurrence

Similar to that of "retarded villous maturation", but without a defined prevalence. Frequently without an identifiable cause.

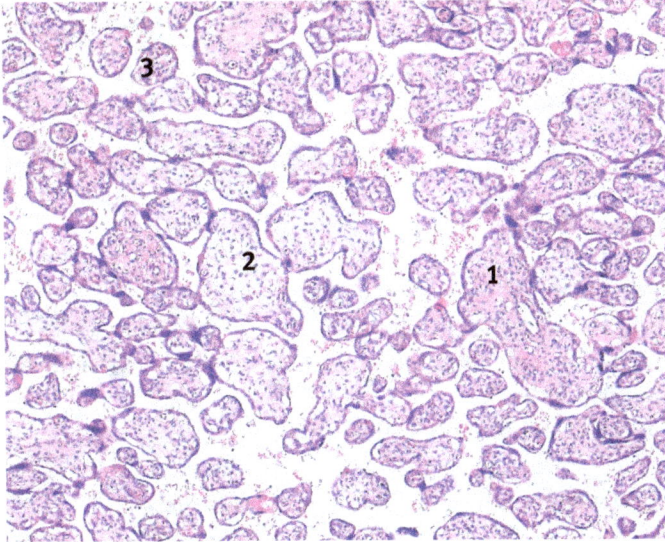

Fig. 8.17: Peripheral villous immaturity (MPF). (1) Stem villi with reticular stroma; (2) intermediate villi with reticular stroma, varying cellularity and fibrous content; (3) terminal villi with few capillaries and missing vasculosyncytial membranes.

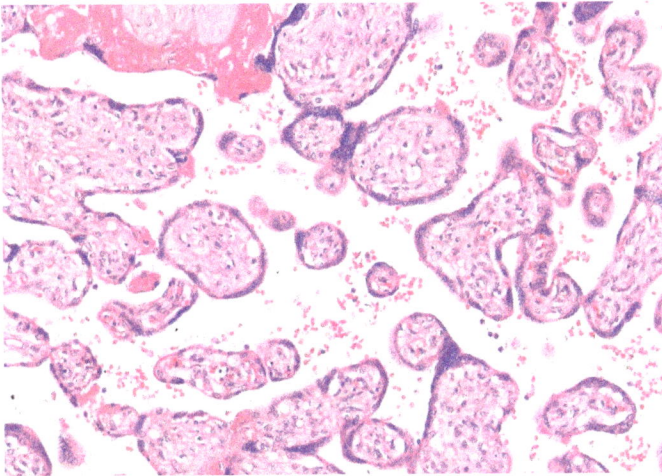

Fig. 8.18: Peripheral villous immaturity (HPF). Peripheral (distal) villous immaturity with regularly branched villi in the periphery, loose reticular stroma; Terminal villi with few capillaries, a nuclear rich villous epithelium and rare vasculosyncytial membranes.

Consequences for placental function
In small placentas, the placental diffusion capacity is limited (Ch. 15).

8.7 Preterm (accelerated) villous maturation

Definition
An accelerated villous maturation when compared to gestational age and fetal maturation.

Diagnostic criteria (Figs. 8.19, 8.20)
- gestational age is essential
- regular villous branching into the four villous subtypes
- premature terminal villi with capillaries and vasculosyncytial membranes
- stem villi with collagenous stroma surrounding the fetal vessels, but subepithelial often hem of loose reticular stroma
- central intermediate villi may show embryonic stroma.

The diagnosis is made in premature deliveries, up to gestational week 32.

Pathogenesis
A compensatory process in small for gestational age placentas, such as those due to an early onset of chronic maternal vascular disturbance [9].
    Preterm (accelerated) villous maturation is associated with:
- young primagravida
- hypoplasia uteri
- athletic constitution and low body weight [10]
- working women [11]
- pregnancy induced hypertension
- multiple pregnancies.

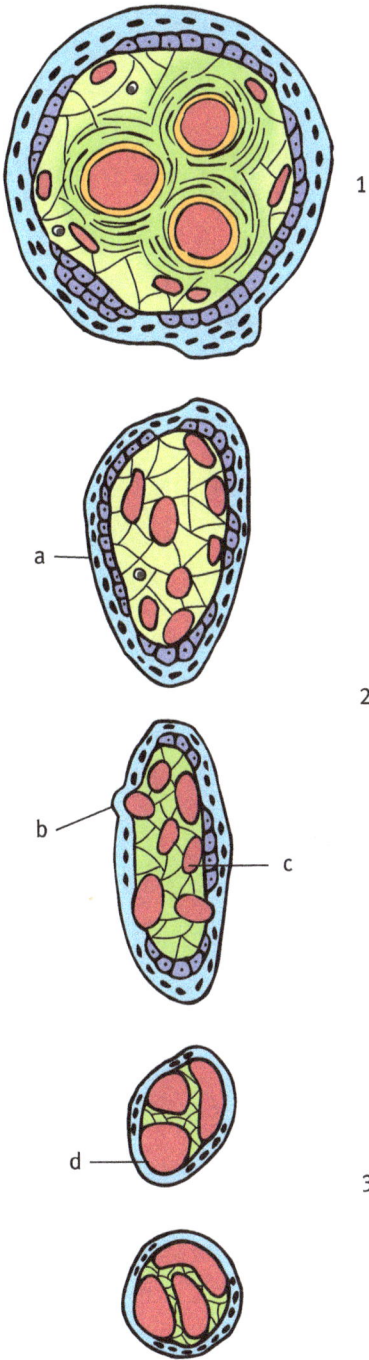

Fig. 8.19: Illustration. Histological characteristics of preterm villous maturation on cross sections: (1) *Stem villi* with dense collagenous stroma surrounding capillaries, close to the chorionic epithelium; (2) *intermediate villi* with loose stroma, numerous capillaries and few vasculosyncytial membranes; (3) *terminal villi* with sinusoidal capillaries;
(a) nuclear rich epithelium; (b) vasculosyncytial membrane; (c) capillary; (d) numerous vasculosyncytial membranes.

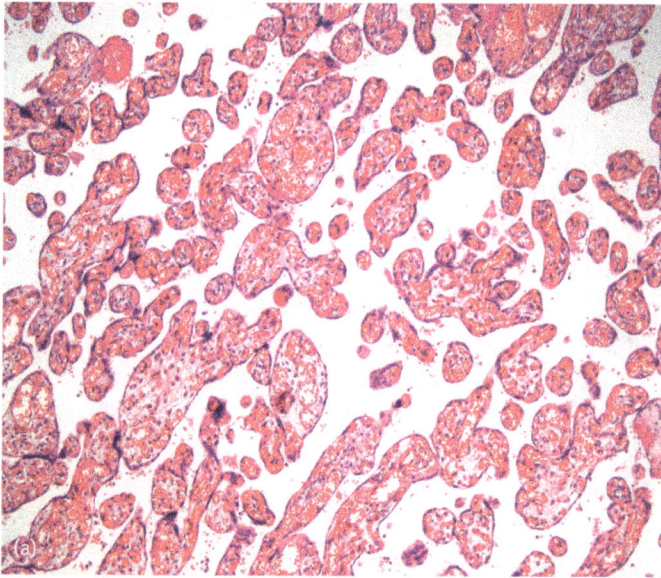

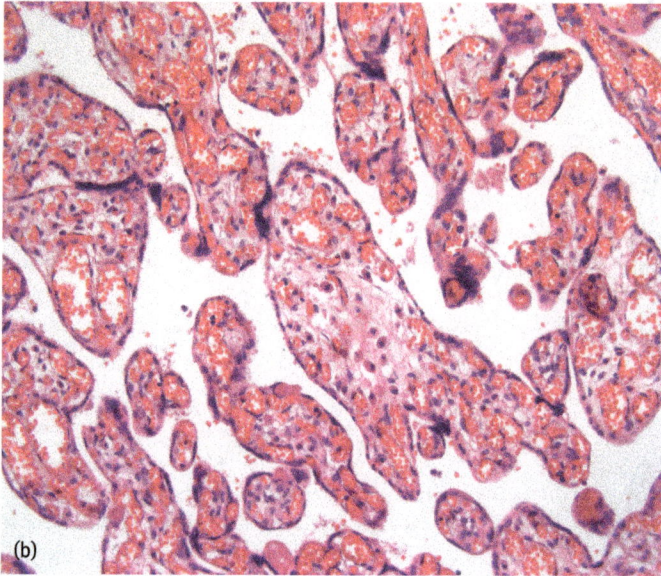

Fig. 8.20: (a) Preterm (accelerated) villous maturation (LPF). Increased villous branching, increased diameter of the villi, numerous sinusoidal capillaries and vasculosyncytial membranes. Hyperemic capillaries. (b) Preterm (accelerated) villous maturation (HPF). Residual, loose connective tissue in the peripheral intermediate villi. Placenta in GW 30.

8.8 Recurrence risk of villous maturation disorders

A normal and mature, when compared to gestational age, placenta in a 1^{rst} pregnancy recurs in the 2nd and 3rd pregnancies in 60 % of cases; however, retarded villous maturation in the 1st pregnancy recurs twice as often as expected in the next pregnancy. The recurrence of arrested villous maturation depends on the severity of maternal and fetal disease (metabolic disorder, syndromes, incompatibility disease).

References

[1] Vogel M. Morphological placental findings and fetal outcome. In: Merten UP LJ, editor. Pathology, a medical speciality. Cologne: News Bull World Assoc Soc Pathol; 1979. p. 72–75.
[2] Vogel M. Pathologie der Schwangerschaft, der Plazenta und des Neugeborenen. In: Remmele W, editor. Pathologie. 3. Berlin: Springer; 1984. p. 510ff.
[3] Vogel M. Plazentagrösse und -struktur als Voraussetzung für den Wachstumsstand des reifgeborenen Kindes bei der Geburt, mit besonderer Berücksichtigung der Plazentationsstörungen. Berlin: Freie Universität (FU); 1975.
[4] Vogel M. Zur Biometrie der Plazenta eutropher Reifgeborener aus risikofreier Schwangerschaft und Geburt. VerhDtschPath. 1974;58.
[5] Altshuler G. Chorangiosis. An important placental sign of neonatal morbidity and mortality. Arch Pathol Lab Med. 1984;108(1):71–74.
[6] Kraus FT, Redline RW, Gersell DJ, Nelson DM, Dicke JM. Placental Pathology: American Registry of Pathology Washington, DC; 2004.
[7] Benirschke K, Burton G, Baergen RN. Pathology of the Human Placenta. 6 ed. Heidelberg, NY, London: Springer; 2012.
[8] Kloos K, Vogel M. Pathologie der Perinatalperiode. Stuttgart: Thieme; 1974.
[9] Arabin B, Jimenez E, Vogel M, Weitzel HK. Relationship of utero- and fetoplacental blood flow velocity wave forms with pathomorphological placental findings. Fetal Diagn Ther. 1992;7(3–4):173–179.
[10] Raiha CE, Kauppinen M. An attempt to decrease perinatal mortality and the rate of premature births. Dev Med Child Neurol. 1963;5:225–232.
[11] McNicol GP, Douglas AS. Treatment of Peripheral Vascular Occlusion by Streptokinase perfusion. Scand J Clin Lab Invest. 1964;16:Suppl 78:23–29.

9 Inflammatory disorders

Inflammation in the placenta may be seen during every stage of pregnancy; however, the type of response depends on gestational age [1]:
- cell/tissue necrosis,
- exudation,
- fibrin deposition,
- connective tissue proliferation.

Necrosis and proliferation are reactive inflammatory processes of equal importance in the embryonic and fetal period. Exudation, at its earliest, is seen at 15 days of gestational age with a cellular exudate in the umbilical cord [2,3].

Pathological findings following inflammation are variable and are dependent on the causative inflammatory pathway. Inflammation of the amniotic type (amnion, chorionic plate and umbilical cord) is different from that of the parenchymatous type (villi and intervillous space). Involvement of the basal plate may be seen in both types.

Amniotic placental inflammation is characterized by distinct maternal and fetal reaction patterns as a result of the maternal infection. The maternal response is seen as inflammation in the chorioamniotic membranes, while the fetal response manifests as inflammation in the fetal vessels of the umbilical cord, chorionic plate and placental villi [4,5].

9.1 Inflammation of amniotic type

Chorioamnionitis (amniotic infection syndrome) [3,6] is inflammation of the amnion, chorionic plate and/or umbilical cord with an infiltrate of, predominantly, neutrophil granulocytes. Rarely, this may be seen in combination with tissue necrosis [7].

Classification
Chorioamnionitis may be subclassified on the basis of the localization and extent of the inflammatory infiltrate and on the density of the cellular infiltrate (Table 9.1):
- amnionitis,
- chorial placentitis, with/without fetal vascular inflammation,
- omphalovasculitis,
- funiculitis.

https://doi.org/10.1515/9783110452600-009

Table 9.1: Histological staging and grading of acute chorioamnionitis [6,7].

stage of expansion		grading of infiltrate density	
minimal infil- tration	cellular infiltration of the am- nion without chorionic plate affection (basal)	minimal grade	few granulocytes (< 5) in a single HPF
partial infiltration	cellular infiltration in 2 regions: 1. membrane and/or chorionic plate (subamniotic) 2. and/or umbilical cord	moderate grade	several granulocytes in several adjacent HPFs
full infiltration	cellular infiltration in 3 regions: 1. amniotic membrane 2. chorionic plate 3. umbilical cord	high grade	many granulocytes in several HPF

Incidence

From the literature, the incidence of amniotic inflammation/chorioamnionitis is variable and ranges from 4 to 30 %, in unselected material [8,9] and can reach up to 50 % in selected preterm placentas [10]. In a study of 7,000 singleton placentas, the incidence of acute diffuse chorioamnionitis decreased from 94 %, between gestational weeks 20 and 24, to 3.8 % between gestational weeks 27 and 40 [11]. Other studies reported an incidence of 10 % in gestational week 40 [12] and in term placentas, from uncomplicated pregnancies, amnionitis was seen in 1.2 % and inflammation of the chorionic plate in 4 % [13]. In prospective studies of unselected singleton placentas, from gestational week 28 to 42, amnionitis was seen in 11 [14] to 25 % [15] and histologically graded into:
– minimal grade: 25 %,
– moderate grade: 44 %,
– high grade: 31 %.

Amniotic inflammation is frequently seen in defined risk groups. In 1,834 singleton placentas: acute chorioamnionitis was seen in 66 % between gestational week 20 and 26, in 22.5 % of pre-terms between gestational week 33 and 36 and in 19 % of term placentas [16]. Others have found amnionitis in preterm placentas twice as often as term placentas [17].

Amnionitis increases the risk of pre-term birth and mortality and morbidity in early pre-term deliveries. It was diagnosed in 48.6 % of hospitalized pre-term deliveries with a birth weight less than 1,500 g (n = 463) and in 29.3 % of those over 1,500 g (n = 208). Even in placentas from preterm IUFD, before gestational week 28, amniotic infection was seen twice as often as in older preterm IUFDs [18].

In 2nd trimester miscarriages (gestational week 13–27) amnionitis was seen in 58.2%, in IUFD (gestational weeks 28–42) in 12.9% and in perinatal deaths (GW 26–41) in 27.8% [19].

The variation in reported frequency is due to the differing definitions of amniotic infection. Some, for example, include isolated deciduitis in the definition [12,20]; however, according to Fox, this 'acute deciduitis' is of no pathological significance [21].

Additionally, the subclassification of amniotic infection varies with some studies defining inflammatory cells in the amniotic stroma as minimal, if 4 polymorph nuclear leucocytes are seen in two or more HPFs [17], whereas other authors define it as a minimum of 10 granulocytes in at least 10 adjacent HPFs, or a focal aggregation of 5 granulocytes in several HPFs in one area [13]. Others suggest defining grade 1 (mild–moderate) as single cells, or small clusters, of neutrophil granulocytes in the amnion, chorionic plate, chorion leve and/or subchorionic fibrin. Grade 2 (severe) is defined as 3 or more chorionic microabscesses (10–20 cells) lying between the chorion and decidua in the membranes and/or under the chorionic plate, or continuous bands (> 10 cells) of confluent chorionic polymorphonuclear leukocytes (PMN) affecting more than half of the subchorionic fibrin or the membrane. Chronic or subacute chorioamnionitis is characterized by mononuclear cells in the chorionic plate and is often seen with coexisting acute chorioamnionitis [22].

Macroscopy and histomorphology

Macroscopically, a characteristic granulocyte rich exudate and a grey to yellow color of the chorionic plate and amnion are seen. Additionally miliary pathogenic foci can be seen on the umbilical cord or the amniotic membrane (seen in fungal, listeria and Staphylococcus infections).

Placentas in mid to late pregnancy, and in immature preterm deliveries, may additionally show amniotic and marginal hematomas due to deciduitis parietalis or basal placentitis with vessel rupture. Marginal and retroplacental hematomas may merge and can be associated with a distinct pathogenesis of placental abruption due to chorioamnionitis [23].

The microscopic characteristics of amniotic inflammation due to infection are mainly determined by granulocyte amniotropism in the different phases [6] (Fig. 9.1).

Pathogens pathways of inflammation

Pathogens reach the amniotic surface either directly from the amniotic sac, if there is rupture, or by intra/transmembranous infiltration from the inner cervix, if the amniotic membranes are preserved. The amniotic epithelium is altered in the early stages of infection and changes such as: cytoplasmic condensation, nuclear pyknosis, epithelial desquamation and amniotic epithelial erosion may be seen.

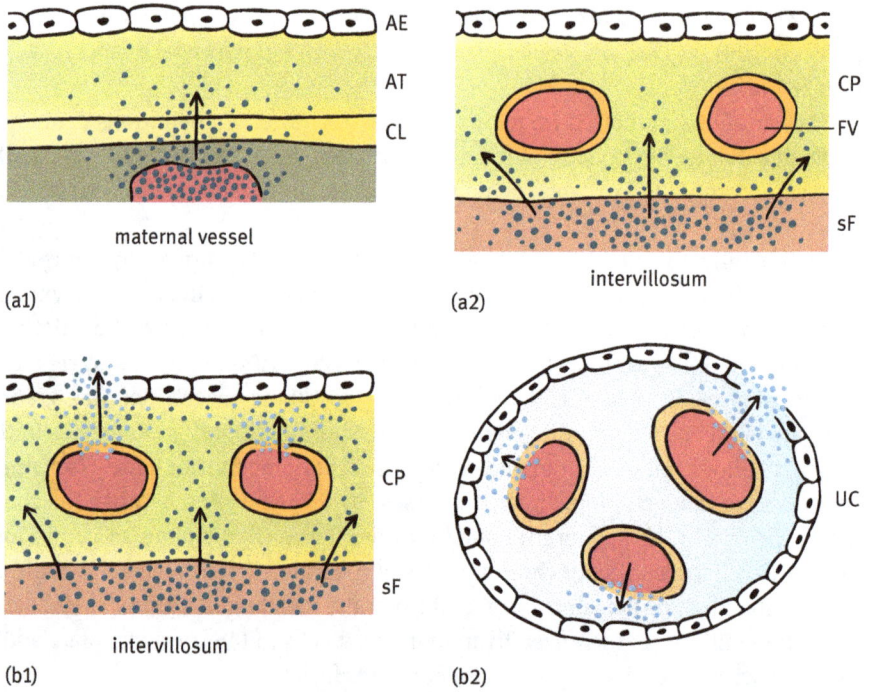

Fig. 9.1: Illustration of inflammation of the amniotic type. (a): Maternal cellular reaction. (a1) Amnionitis: inflammatory cells from decidua parietalis (Dp) extend into the chorion leve (CL) and the amniotic connective tissue (AT). (a2) Chorionic placentitis: inflammatory cells from the intervillous space extend into subchorionic fibrin (sF) and the chorionic plate (CP). (b): Fetal cellular reaction. (b1) Chorionic placentitis and vasculitis: maternal and fetal cellular reaction with inflammatory cells from the intervillous space extending into subchorionic fibrin (sF) and the chorionic plate (CP); fetal granulocytes infiltrate into fetal vessel wall, into the chorionic plate (CP) and through the amniotic epithelium (AE). (b2) Omphalovasculitis/funiculitis: fetal granulocytes pass from the fetal vessels (FV) into Wharton's Jelly, and sometimes through the amniotic epithelium.

Maternal granulocytes are the first cells to react to infection, via leucotactic stimulation, and migrate from the decidual vessels (parietalis sive capsularis) towards the amniotic surface and into the decidua, chorion leve and amniotic connective tissue.

The maternal inflammatory response is characterized by intraplacental granulocytes in the subchorionic space and subchorionic fibrin, also often seen in fetal deaths as part of a localized and well circumscribed inflammation.

The fetal inflammatory response is characterized by fetal granulocytes infiltrating from the fetal vessels into the chorionic plate. This begins focally, subsequently expands and becomes more diffuse, depending on the amount of pathogens and their pathogenicity. Maternal and fetal granulocytes collectively infiltrate into the chorionic plate and into the amniotic sac causing damage to the amniotic epithelium.

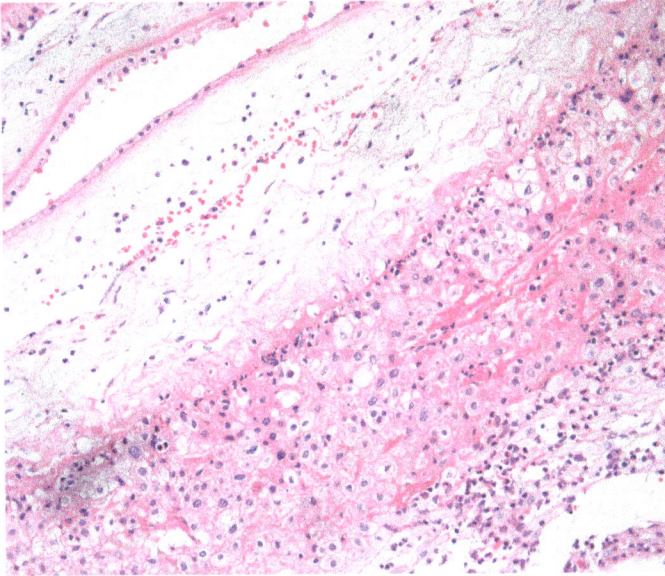

Fig. 9.2: Amnionitis, minimal grade. Maternal granulocyte infiltration in the decidua (deciduitis), chorion leve and amniotic connective tissue. Emergency cesarean section in GW 38 + 5, APGAR 7-8-10.

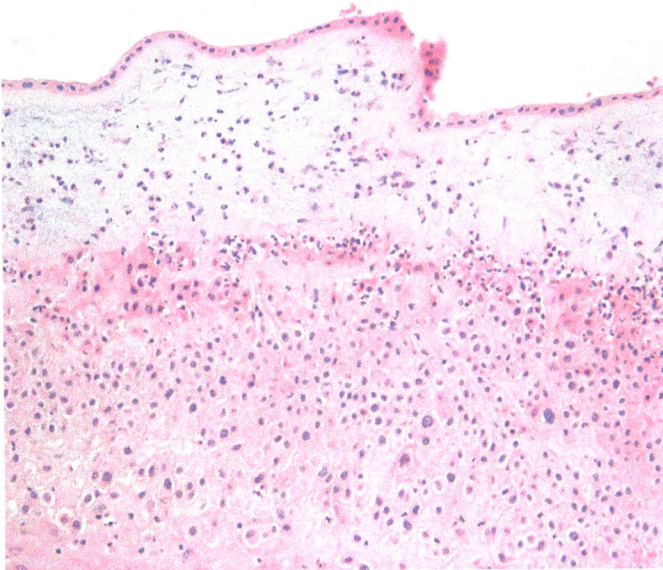

Fig. 9.3: Amnionitis. Maternal granulocyte infiltration in the decidua, chorion leve and amniotic connective tissue.

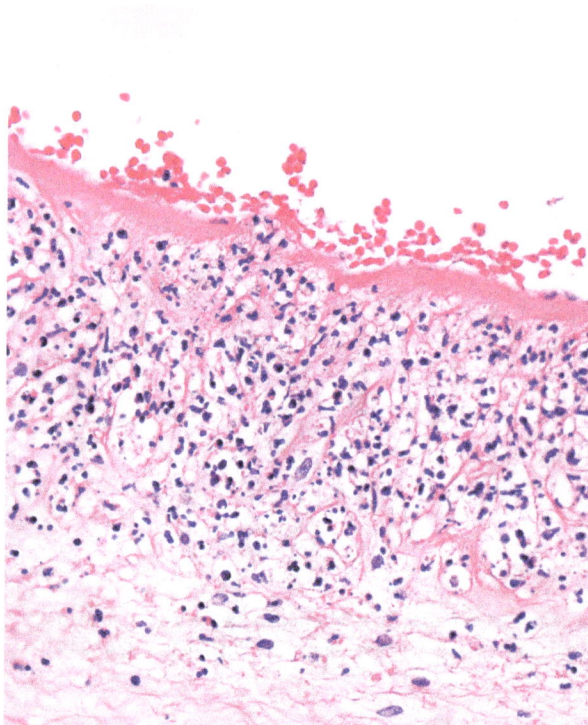

Fig. 9.4: Amnionitis, high grade. A dense maternal granulocyte infiltration in the amniotic stroma with disseminated epithelial erosion. Maternal infection in GW 23 + 0 with delivery in GW 23 + 6 and fetid amniotic fluid.

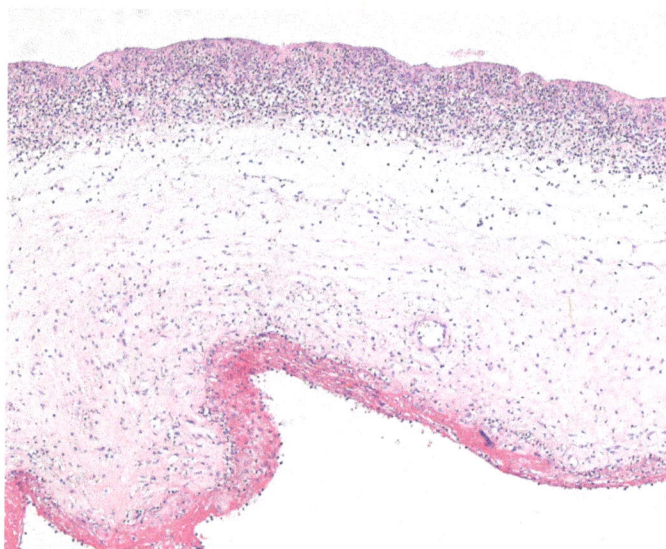

Fig. 9.5: Chorionic placentitis with only a maternal cellular reaction. Granulocyte invasion of the subchorionic fibrin and the basal part of the chorionic plate (high grade) with phlegmonous cellular invasion of the subepithelial stroma and widespread necrosis of the amniotic epithelium with nuclear loss.

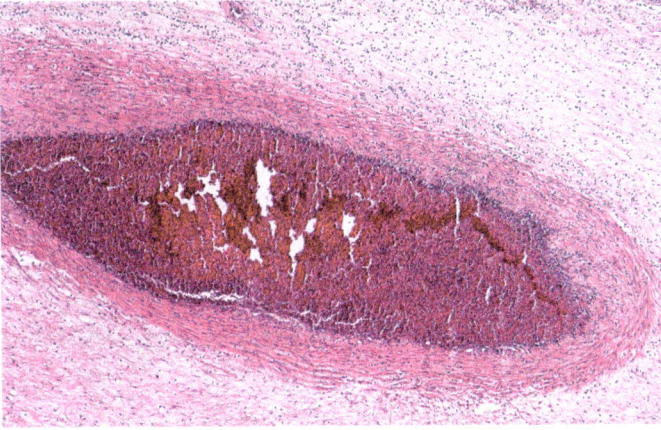

Fig. 9.6: Vasculitis and chorionic placentitis. Disseminated fetal granulocytic exudate extending through the fetal wall and into the surrounding chorionic stroma. PROM in GW 23 + 3.

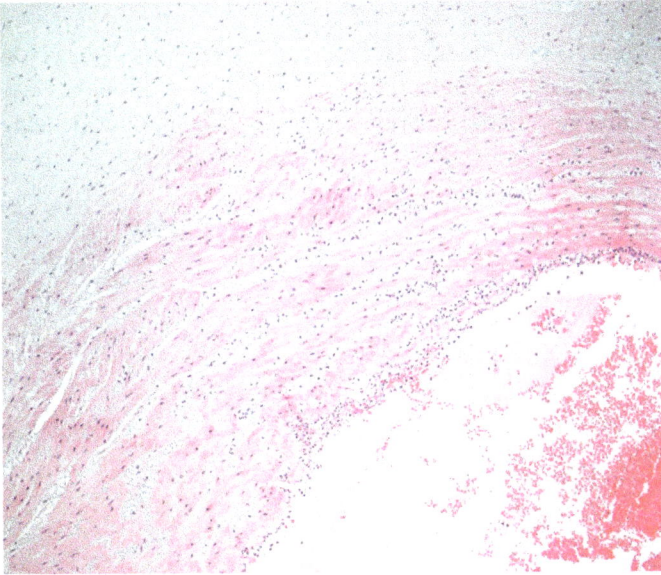

Fig. 9.7: Acute omphalovasculitis with granulocytic infiltration through the vessel wall and into the Wharton's Jelly.

The inflammatory reaction is unmistakable when an infiltrate of fetal granulo-cytes is seen in the umbilical cord vessel wall and in Wharton's Jelly. Initially the cells are seen in the vein and then in the arteries.

Independent of gestational age, the maternal inflammatory reaction is seen ear-lier and at a greater intensity than the fetal inflammatory reaction. An intense fetal reaction was exclusively seen in combination with high grade maternal inflammation [7,24,25].

Special processes in amnionitis

Massive inflammation, such as in abscesses with focally dense aggregates of neutrophilic granulocytes and necrotic exudates in the chorionic plate, subchorionic space and adjacent stem villi, is seen in ascending inflammation with listeriosis and campylobacter infections, as well as maternal staphylococcal and Escherichia coli sepsis [26].

Herpes infection typically shows necrosis in the amniotic membrane [27], whereas chlamydia and mycoplasma infections cause necrosis in the amniotic stroma and amniotic cells [28].

In perinatal mycoplasma infections, an ascending inflammation with acute granulocytic deciduitis, chorioamnionitis and funiculitis was seen (Ureaplasma urealyticum, Mycoplasma hominis et genitalium) [29].

On the other hand, a different intensity of inflammatory reaction in the amniotic sac is seen in candida infection.

Funiculitis is characterized by a circular necrosis and granulocytic aggregation around the umbilical cord vessels, especially the vein. Residually, these may be apparent as concentric calcifications in the Wharton's Jelly. The etiology of necrotizing

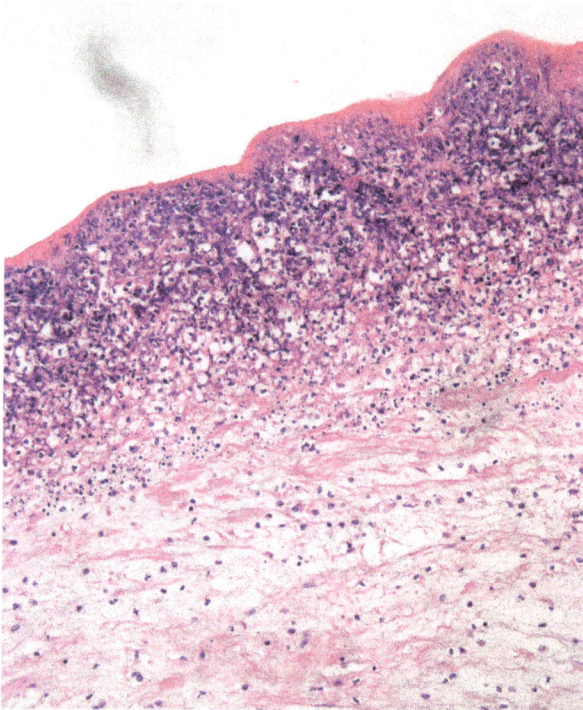

Fig. 9.8: Necrotizing amnionitis. Widespread loss of amniotic epithelial cells with massive neutrophilic infiltration. Placenta in GW 23 + 3, APGAR 1-5-6. No pathogens identified.

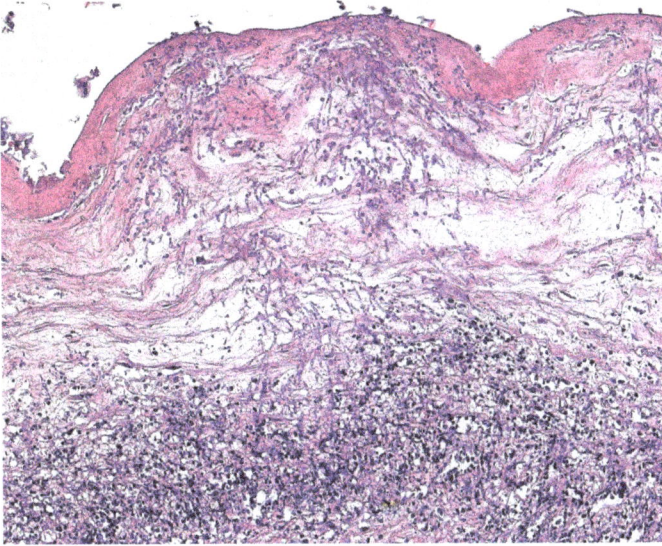

Fig. 9.9: Candida Chorioamnionitis with superficial and extensive epithelial necrosis and deep invasion by active candida mycelia with bot spores. Basal high grade necrotic inflammation. GW 19, intrauterine device (IUD), ascending infection, spontaneous abortion.

funiculitis is frequently unknown. In more than 90 % it is seen in conjunction with chorioamnionitis and assumed to represent an immunoreaction, triggered by different bacterial and viral antigens, such as those described in congenital syphilis infections [30,31].

Thrombi in the umbilical cord and larger vessels of the chorionic plate may be rarely seen in very immature pre-term deliveries after several days of membrane rupture and high grade amniotic inflammation. The thrombi may cause peripheral fetal thromboembolism.

Chronic amniotic inflammation
Chronic amniotic inflammation is very rare and the detailed pathogenesis of it remains unknown. On histology, a moderate lymphocyte-rich infiltrate may be seen in the amniotic membrane, and rarely in the chorionic plate tissue. Plasma cells and macrophages may also be found. Amniotic epithelial necrosis is absent, but if present the chronic process is associated with an acute granulocytic infiltration. In PROM, of more than one week duration, amniotic inflammation is not present but instead dense collagen deposition may be seen by the fibrotic connective tissue of the amnion. Chronic villitis may be associated with chronic amnionitis and is considered to be of viral origin. Single cases have been reported associated with toxoplasma, rubella and herpes simplex infections in the literature [32].

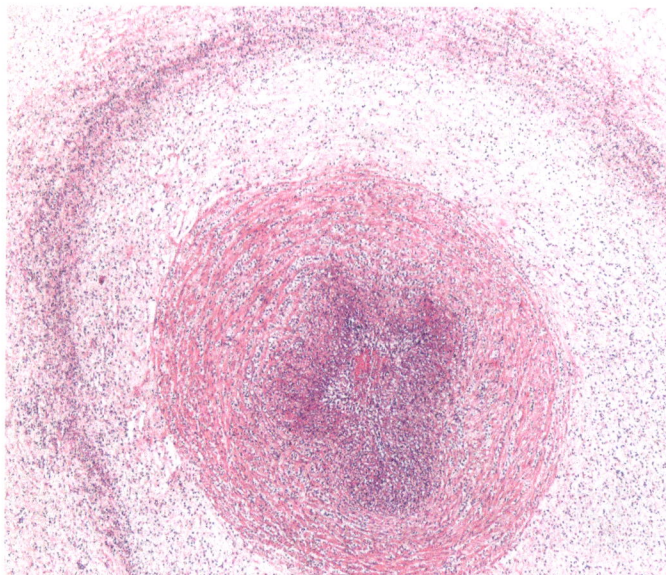

Fig. 9.10: Necrotizing funiculitis with a dense circular granulocytic omphalovasculitis. Expanded necrosis and granulocytic infiltration in the Wharton's Jelly. Placenta in GW 23 + 3. No pathogens identified.

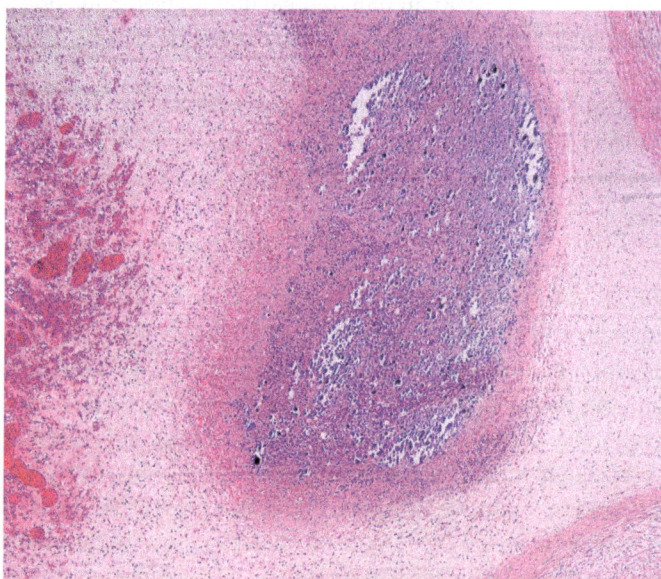

Fig. 9.11: Chronic calcifying thromboangiitis. Residual changes due to acute inflammation in the umbilical cord vessel wall and Wharton's Jelly, close to a hemangioma on the left. Placenta in GW 30 + 5. Umbilical cord prolapse and acute chorioamnionitis.

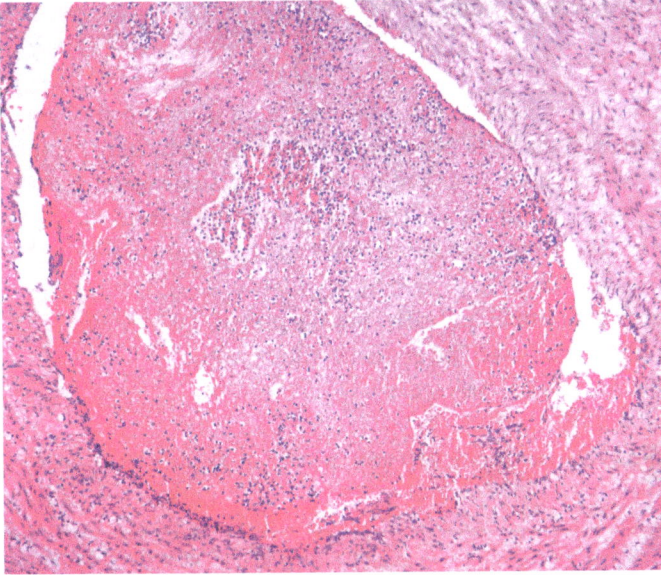

Fig. 9.12: Acute thrombovasculitis. Intraluminal thrombosis of an inflamed chorionic plate vessel in acute chorioamnionitis in GW 34. Newborn weight 2,177 g, APGAR 9-9-9.

Causes and pathogenesis

Amniotic inflammation is usually due to bacterial infection. Pathogens such as streptococcus, groups B and D, Escherichia coli, staphylococcus, bacteroides, acinetobacter and lactobacillus are well described.

Clostridium pseudomonas, listeria and candida are regional different often identified as pathogens.

Amniotic inflammation as a result of pathogens of bacterial vaginosis, such as gardnerella, mycoplasma, chlamydia, Ureaplasma urealyticum and herpes virus are more difficult to prove.

Positive pathogenic proof in the cervical smear is common [33,34], but has no significant association with amniotic infection syndrome [15,35]. On the other hand, virulent pathogens could be shown in 69.2 % of women with amniotic infection syndromes but only in 7.7 % of women without amniotic infection [36].

Direct proof of pathogens in smears from the amniotic and chorionic plate is difficult, and a negative result should not be taken as proof for a non-infectious cause of inflammation. Negative bacterial cultures, even though associated with high grade amniotic inflammation, can be caused by:

– mycoplasma,
– chlamydia trachomatis,
– ureaplasma urealyticum,
– gardnerella vaginalis,

- anaerobes (without anaerobes culture),
- viruses.

In minimal grade amniotic inflammation, a non-infectious cause should be considered.

A negative bacterial culture may be a consequence of a well-functioning immune response and amniotic inflammation does not necessarily cause neonatal disease. In high grade ascending amniotic infections, pathogens could be verified in 72% of pre-term deliveries and in 57% of term deliveries. Infection of newborns without chorioamnionitis is seen in:
- Streptococcus B cases with fulminant early onset sepsis of the newborn [7,33], 70% without a morphologically verified amniotic inflammation.
- Newborns infected in the cervical tract.

Table 9.2: Correlation of etiology and granulocytic infiltration in the chorionic plate, membranes and umbilical cord.

etiology	granulocytic infiltration in the chorionic plate, membranes or umbilical cord
infection	yes
fetal hypoxia / acidosis	yes
meconium output	yes
Blood flow decrease in the subchorionic space	yes
circulatory disturbance in the umbilical cord	yes

Predisposing factors for amniotic infection

Ascending infections with membrane rupture (70%) are more common than infection with intact membranes (30%). Amniotic rupture and loss of amniotic fluid is the most common cause of infection and may occur spontaneously before onset of labor

due to instrumentally induced labor or long duration of labor. Infection risk in PROM (Preterm Rupture of Membranes) increases with duration; in a labor of less than 6 hours duration amniotic infection was seen in 11%, whereas in labor with a duration longer than 12 hours amniotic infection was seen in 75%.

The time interval between infiltration of the inner cervical tract and chorioamnionitis, with involvement of the chorionic plate and umbilical cord, is assumed to be ca. 24 hours. It is of utmost importance to calculate the duration of amniotic infection morphologically. Predisposing factors in miscarriage and pre-term births are cervical insufficiency due to preceding vaginitis/colpitis and/or cervicitis. Cervical cerclage does not prevent amniotic infection.

Frequency of vaginal examinations before and during delivery may favor amniotic infection [37].

Rare iatrogenic avenues of infection are:
– amniocentesis and fetoscopy
– intra-amniotic infusion.

Secondary expansion of ascending amniotic infection
– Inflammation extends from the chorionic plate to the placental parenchyma. Purulent subchorionic and intervillous thromboangiitis is seen in 3–4 % of placentas with high grade amniotic inflammation at term.
– Involvement of adjacent stem villi (acute granulocytic villitis) is found in less than 1 % of placentas.
– The spread of inflammatory cells from the amnion to the marginal zone and basal plate is seen in 2 % of placentas during late pregnancy and is 10-times more common in fetal abortion, especially in terminations with marginal hematomas.

Acute purulent villitis with subepithelial microabscess formation is due to fetal hematogenous spread of pathogens into the placenta. Examples are congenital staphylococcus sepsis and listeriosis.

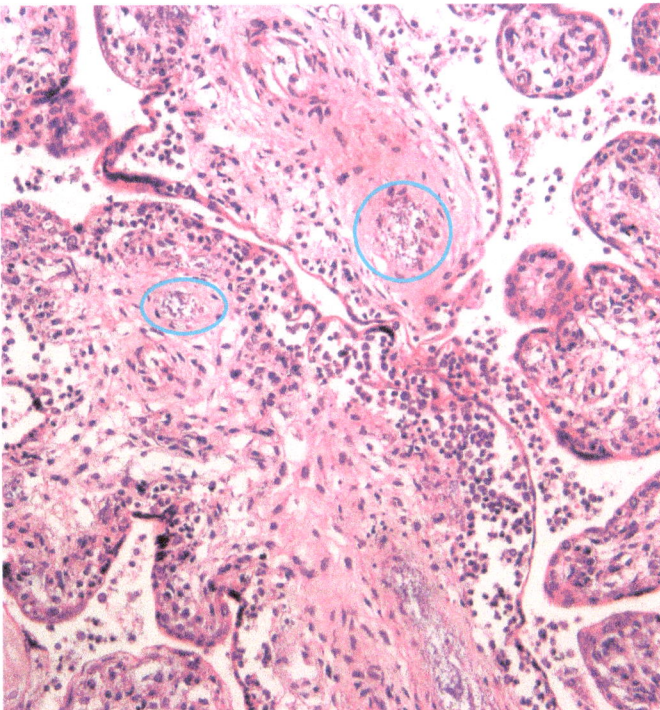

Fig. 9.13: Acute purulent villitis with intravillous subepithelial microabscesses and bacterial emboli in fetal villous vessels (circle). Late miscarriage in gestational week 21.

Clinical correlation

Clinically, "amniotic infection syndrome" is often used synonymously with "chorio-amnionitis". Clinical symptoms are:

- maternal temperature over 37.5° C,
- fetal tachycardia over 160/min,
- leukocytes over 14000/cm^3 before delivery [38],
- increasing C-reactive protein (CRP) 4–8 hours after infection.

Ascending amniotic infection is morphologically more often seen than clinically proven. Conversely, clinical symptoms correlate significantly with high grade amniotic inflammation (Table 9.3), frequency of amniotic inflammation and fetid, infectious amniotic fluid [34,39]. Positive correlation with greenish amniotic fluid and pre-acidosis in the umbilical cord artery could not be verified.

Placental findings, following pathological examination, and knowledge of clinical risk factors (fetal tachycardia, delivery duration, latency of membrane rupture, maternal temperature) improve the prognosis of newborn infections from 62.5 to 75 %.

Correlation of placental morphology and newborn infection varies between pre-term and term deliveries. Acute chorioamnionitis was found in only 3.2 % placentas delivered at term but was identified in 42.8 % of placentas delivered prior to gestational week 37. The intensity of chorioamnionitis also differed between pre-term and term deliveries.

Table 9.3: Correlation between clinical symptoms during delivery and morphological identification of ascending amniotic inflammation stage 3 [15,40].

clinical symptoms	morphological amniotic infection	
	pos (%)	neg (%)
maternal temperature > 37.5 °C and fetal tachycardia > 160/min	92	8
no temperature, no tachycardia	14	86
infectious (fetal) amniotic fluid	100	0
green amniotic fluid	40	60
clear amniotic fluid	22	78
acidotic UC blood (pH < 7.20)	30	70

Pre-term delivery

Infection may lead to preterm delivery caused by phospholipase A2 rich pathogens which become esterified and converted into:
- prostaglandin E2, causing cervical dilatation
- prostaglandin F2a, causing induction of uterine contraction.

Additionally, intradecidual macrophages and granulocytic exudates increase amniotic leukotrienes and decidual interleukins, and these may also contribute to preterm delivery [34].

Decidual mediator cytokines are also identified in amniotic fluid from normal term pregnancies [41]. TNF, interleukins 1, 6, 8 and 'neutrophilic attracting/activating peptid-1'/interleukin 8 are not produced in placental tissue or amniotic fluid. In the last trimester, before and during delivery, the cytokines increases.

During delivery cytokines promote granulocyte migration into the cervical connective tissue and this stimulates leukocytic collagenase expression and cervical maturation [42]. Furthermore, cytokines stimulate placental prostaglandin synthesis and promote labor pain. Women with PROM and premature labor pain show higher cytokine concentrations than women without premature labor pain at similar gestational age. Chorioamnionitis, associated with bacterially infected amniotic fluid, increases cytokine concentration and the highest recorded concentration was associated with a clinical amniotic infection syndrome [42]. Bacterial infection of the amniotic sac may also induce and trigger delivery due to endotoxins released by the bacteria.

Fetal consequences

The fetus can be infected via 3 different pathways:
- *infected amniotic fluid* passing into the lung and gastrointestinal tract,
- *hematogenous* spread via umbilical cord vessels,
- *transplacental-hematogenous* infection due to progression of inflammation from the intervillous space to the fetal compartment.

The typical consequences are congenital aspiration pneumonia, gastroenterocolitis, congenital meningitis, pyogenic dermatitis and blepharitis and intrauterine or intrapartum sepsis neonatorum.

Recurrence risk of amniotic infection:
- amniotic infection in the 1st pregnancy recurs in 50 % of subsequent pregnancies.
- a 1st pregnancy without infection is associated with a lack of infection in 80 % of subsequent pregnancies.

9.2 Hypoxia induced changes

Inflammatory changes caused by hypoxia and acidosis do not result in an amniotropic response in inflammatory cells [12].

To be differentiated are:

– Isolated maternal granulocytes in the subchorionic space/fibrin (minimal grade). The immediately neighbouring part of the chorionic tissue may be included (suggestion of a demarcation between maternal and fetal environment) [1].
– Greenish discoloration of the amniotic membrane and superficial chorionic plate due to meconium is seen in less than 1 hour after meconium is excreted into the amniotic fluid.
– Meconium phagocytosis of the amniotic epithelial and stromal cells.
  – Exclusively seen in amniotic cells, 2–4 hours after meconium excretion.
  – Present in stromal cells 24 hours after meconium excretion.
– Lipofuscin depositions Meconium is degraded into lipofuscin by macrophage lysosomes and is seen in the macrophages of the deep amniotic connective tissue 72 hours, at the earliest, after meconium excretion [12].
– Microthromboses in the villous capillaries indicate a microcirculatory disturbance Disseminated Intravasal Coagulation (DIC) – intrauterine shock.

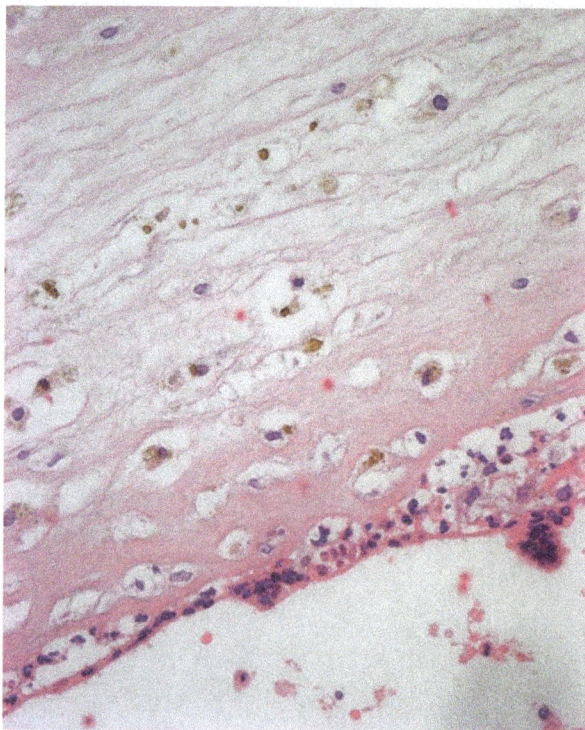

Fig. 9.14: Meconium phagocytosis of the amniotic stromal cells. Small aggregates of maternal granulocytes in the subchorionic space.

9.3 Placentitis, parenchymatous type

Characterized as an inflammatory exudate or/and subsequent tissue proliferation in the placental parenchyma. Three types are often seen in combination and should be distinguished (Fig. 9.15):
1. intervillitis (intervillositis), intervillous thrombangiitis,
2. perivillitis,
3. villitis.

Frequency
Parenchymatous placentitis is seen in 4–10 % of unselected placentas [14,43–45] and is rarely associated with maternal or fetal infection [46]. In unselected placentas, placentitis was diagnosed in 4.9 % between gestational age 28 and 42 and in 33.4 % of miscarriages.
- Intervillous thrombangiitis was seen in 0.2% of placentas, GW 28–42, and in 28.8 % of abortion material.
- Perivillitis was seen in 3.8 % of placentas, GW 28–42, and in 2.1 % of abortion material.
- Villitis was seen in 0.9 % of placentas, GW 28–42, and in 2.5 % of abortion material.

9.3.1 Intervillous thrombangiitis and intervillitis

In intervillitis, an acute and chronic variant can be differentiated:
- Acute (thrombangitis intervillosa): Perivillous fresh fibrin deposition in the intervillous space with a maternal granulocyte infiltrate and cellular and nuclear loss in the epithelium of neighbouring villi.
- Chronic (histiocytic intervillitis (intervillositis): Focal maternal mononuclear cells, mainly monocytes and a few lymphocytes, in the intervillous space.

Intervillous thrombangitis is seen in fetal abortions [2]. It appears as a fresh, granulocyte rich fibrin thrombosis in the intervillous space and is caused by maternal pathogens. Subchorionic thrombangitis is, according to some authors, included in this group.
- Pyogenic thrombi: The intervillous space is focally dilated and filled with fresh fibrin thrombi that are infiltrated by granulocytes and cell debris.
- Placental abscess: The epithelium of the surrounding villi are destroyed. Expansion into the villous stroma and destruction of villous tissue.

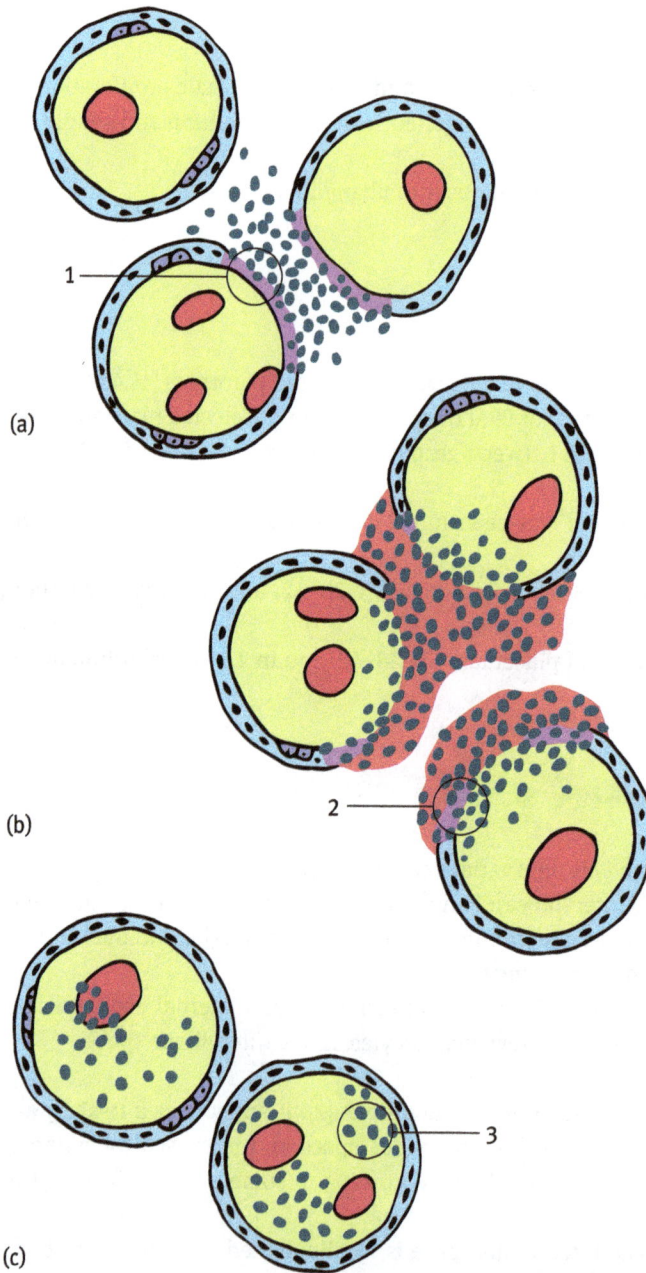

Fig. 9.15: Illustration of the 3 different types of parenchymatous type placentitis. (a) Intervillitis: (1) maternal inflammatory cells in the intervillous space and trophoblast cell destruction in the neighbouring villi; (b) perivillitis: Villous clustering with (2) maternal inflammatory cells infiltrating into perivillous fibrin, destroying trophoblast cells and infiltrating into the villous stroma; (c) villitis: fetal cellular exudate caused by (3) fetal cells leaving villous capillaries and infiltrating into the villous stroma.

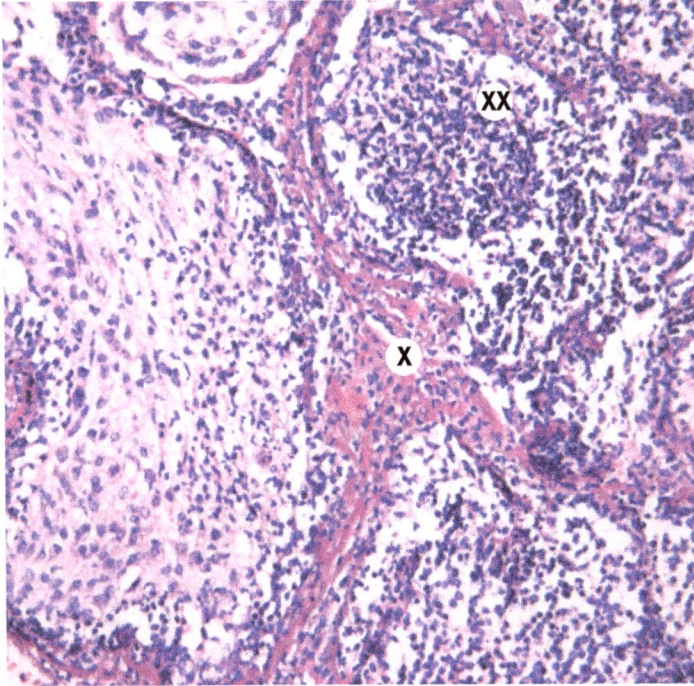

Fig. 9.16: Intervillous thrombangitis. (X) Maternal inflammatory exudate in the perivillous fibrin and expansion into neighbouring villi. Placenta abscess (XX) with focal purulent destruction of the exudate and villous tissue.

The foci are of acute character and may lead to pre-term delivery. Even though thromboangiitis intervillosum may be found in every placental region; the basal, marginal or subchorionic regions are preferentially affected.

Pathogenesis and causes

– Maternal hematogenous infection with pathogens in the intervillous space due to an extraplacental infection (tonsillitis, pyelonephritis, purulent pneumonia, florid endometritis) [47]. Intervillous thrombangiitis with microabscess formation is typically seen in listeria infection. Microabscesses located in the subchorionic space may suggest a campylobacter source of infection; however, other pathogens such as Staphylococcus aureus may cause a similar type of morphology.
– Infection continuing through the basal plate and into the intervillous space with purulent deciduitis.
– Ascending infection with
  – involvement of the placental margin with a marginal edge phlegmone,

–   chorionic placentitis spreading into the subchorionic and intervillous space; seen in more than 40 % of fetal abortions with high grade amniotic inflammation.

Clinical correlation and consequences for the fetus
–   placental affection in maternal disease and parasitemia,
–   as part of amniotic infection syndrome,
–   fetal abortion, preterm delivery,
–   fetal and prenatal sepsis.

9.3.2 Perivillitis and villitis

Definition
Perivillitis is characterized by maternal inflammatory changes that are primarily located on the villous surface, such as: epithelial necrosis, fibrin deposition and inflammatory cells.

In contrast, villitis starts primarily as a fetal cellular exudate in the villous stroma with a subsequent stromal/cell proliferation and fibrosis. Transitions between perivillitis and villitis are common.

Chronic villitis with a lymphocytic stromal infiltration and viral cellular changes may be seen in cytomegalovirus, toxoplasma and herpes simplex infections. The morphological diagnosis of viral infection is dependent on active virus replication, and this can be visualized through the use of virus specific immunostaining. However, negative cellular morphology and immunohistochemistry do not exclude a viral infection and other analytical methods, such as PCR, should be used [48].

Chronic villitis is subcategorized into the group of "villitis of unknown etiology" (VUE) if a pathogenic cause is not identifiable. A maternal immune reaction may also result in a chronic villitis [49–51].

Perivillitis: In perivillitis, the villi are clumped together by inter- and perivillous fibrin that contains inflammatory cell infiltrates. The villous epithelium appears necrotic, sub totally, and surrounded by fibrin (Fig. 9.15b). Maternal monocytes and granulocytes on the villous surface infiltrate into the villous stroma. Chronicity may be reflected in the histological findings:
–   Acute phase: epithelial necrosis, fresh fibrin depositions and numerous inflammatory cells.
–   Chronic phase: cellular connective tissue proliferation, increased collagenous fiber proliferation in the villi and small stem villous vessel obliteration.
–   Terminal phase: microinfarct like foci with complete intervillous obliteration and diffuse fibrous of the villi.

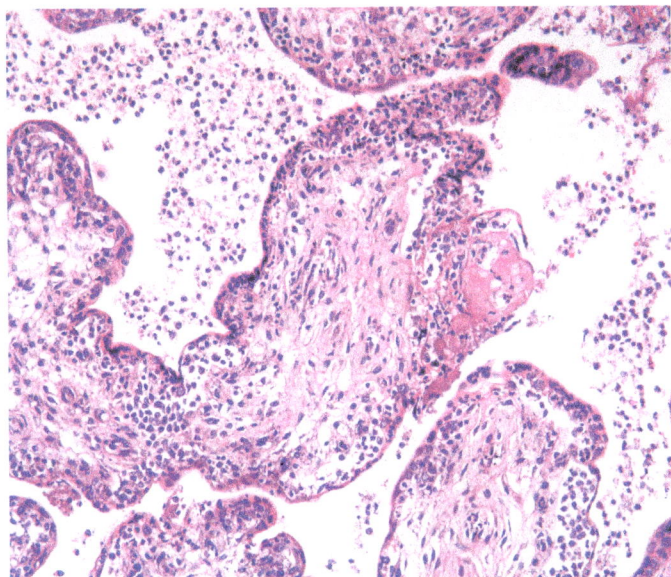

Fig. 9.17: Intervillitis, Perivillitis. Acute trophoblast epithelial necrosis, dense granulocytic infiltrate on the villous surface and infiltrating neighbouring villous stroma. Late miscarriage in GW 21.

Villitis: Villitis with a cellular infiltrate in the villous stroma can be differentiated into 6 subtypes on the basis of the inflammatory cellular component and the stromal reaction:
- acute granulocytic villitis
- lymphocytic-plasmocytic villitis.
- lymphocytic-monocytic villitis.
- necrotizing villitis.
- granulomatous villitis.
- chronic-proliferative villitis.

The different subtypes of villitis associated with chronic bacterial or viral infection display frequent repeated morphological changes (Table 9.4); however, no subtype of villitis is specific for a particular cause. Direct or indirect proof of the pathogenic agents must be acquired, and if the pathogen cannot be identified the entity of villitis of unknown etiology (VUE) should be used.

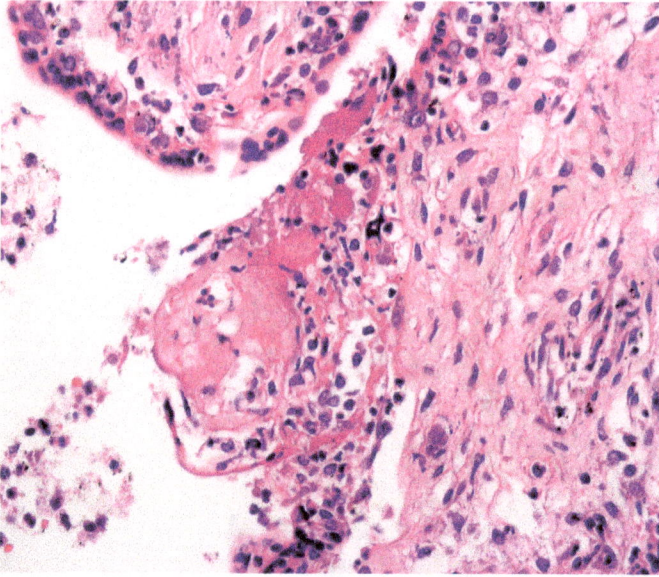

Fig. 9.18: Perivillitis (HPF). Inflammation on the villous surface and fibrin deposition.

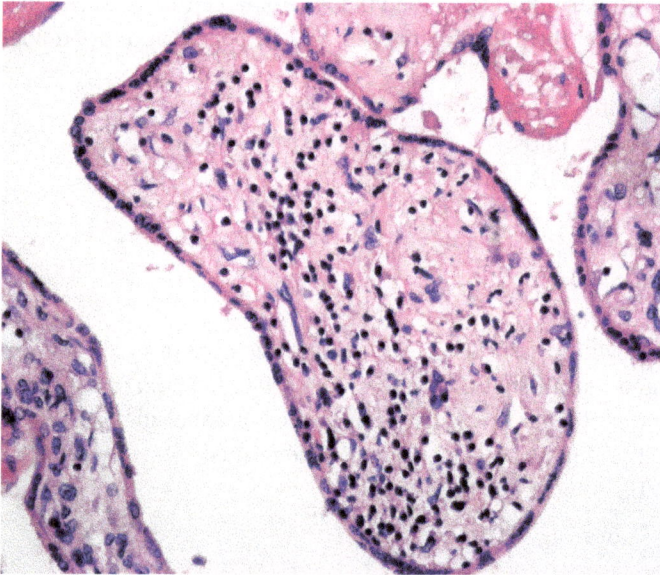

Fig. 9.19: Lymphocytic-plasmocytic villitis. Infiltration of lymphocytes and plasma cells into the villous stroma. CMV infection with IUFD in GW 24.

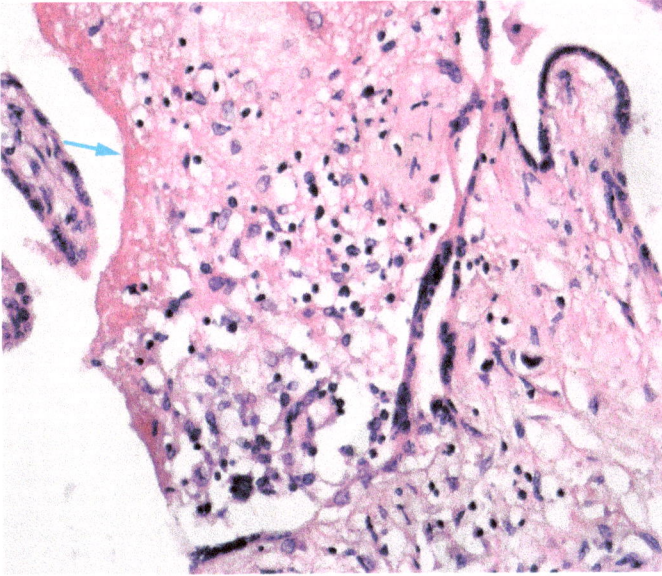

Fig. 9.20: Necrotizing villitis with stromal and chorionic epithelial necrosis (arrow) and lymphocytic infiltrates. Live birth, spontaneous delivery.

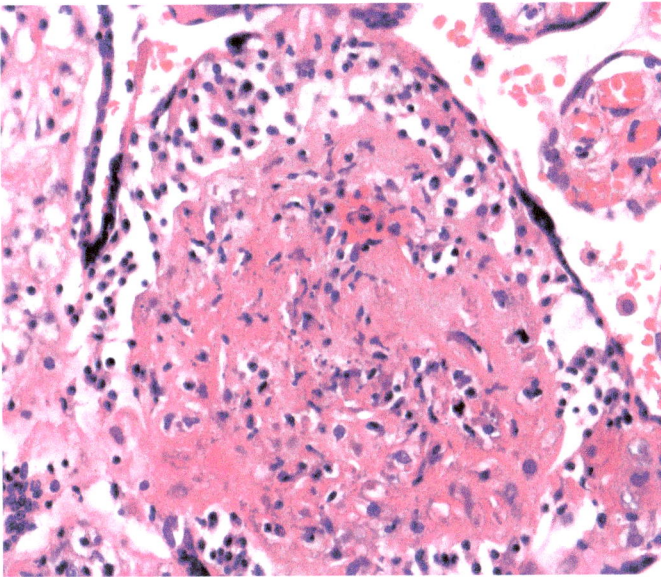

Fig. 9.21: Chronic granulomatous-like villitis with subepithelial mononuclear cell demarcation of the granuloma. (Fig. 9.22)

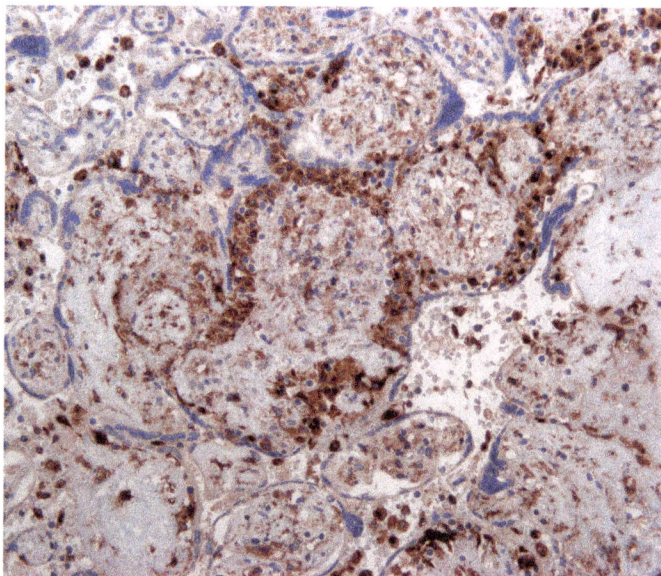

Fig. 9.22: Granulomatous-like villitis with histiocytic demarcation of the granuloma. Immunostain CD 68. (Fig. 9.21). No pathogens identified.

Other associated morphology:

- *villous maturation disorder:* Active villitis is often associated with retarded villous maturation. Chorangiosis type I may be found adjacent to chronic proliferative villitis,
- *villous stromal fibrosis* with focal hemosiderosis and/or microcalcifications is considered to represent the end stage of a primary necrotizing and/or proliferative villitis,
- *chorionic epithelial necrosis* with perivillous fibrin deposition may be due to villous inflammation in fetal-hematogenous infections with chorionic epithelial necrosis.

Table 9.4: Villitis subtypes in intrauterine infections.

granulocytic ascending villitis	listeriosis monocytogenes staphylococcus
lymphocyte-plasmocytic villitis and proliferative vasculitis	cytomegalovirus congenital syphilis
lymphocyte-monocytic villitis	rubella toxoplasma unknown etiology
necrotizing villitis associated endangiitis	cytomegalovirus varicella herpes simplex ECHO-virus Chagas disease rubella
granulomatous villitis	varicella varicella zoster tuberculosis toxoplasmosis
proliferative villitis	toxoplasmosis unknown etiology

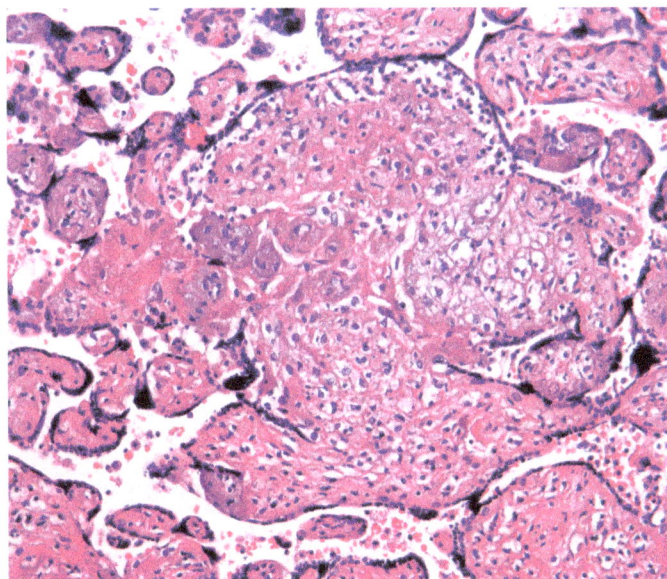

Fig. 9.23: Chronic active proliferative villitis. Villi with a stromal infiltration of mononuclear cells, a stromal cell proliferation, fibrin exudate and loss of the villous trophoblast. Emergency cesarean section due to acute fetal distress in GW 40. Fetal weight 3,410 g, APGAR 9-10. Pathogen unknown.

Pathogenesis and cause of perivillitis and villitis

Three possible causes of perivillitis and/or villitis are known:
1. infection,
2. hypoxic/toxic,
3. unknown.

1. Infectious perivillitis may follow:

– maternal-hematogenous pathogen resettlement on the villous surface (analogous to intervillous thrombangiitis),
– transdecidual affection of the placental parenchyma due to endometritis,
– amniotic inflammation with involvement of the placental margin and/or basal plate.

Perivillitis is not evident in fetal infections. An inflammatory cellular reaction and villous connective tissue proliferation may be due to a well-functioning maternal antigen-antibody immune resistance [12,44].

In contrast, infectious villitis is caused by fetal-hematogenous spread (without perivillitis) and may be associated with acute or obliterative endarteriitis of the stem villous vessels.

2. Perivillitis due to hypoxic/toxic stimuli: Hypoxia and/or other cytotoxic noxious stimuli cause chorionic epithelial injury, local hypercoagulability and secondary fibrin deposition on the villous surface. Epithelial and villous necrosis cause an acute granulocytic response, through chemotactic stimulation, and the necrotic material and fibrin depositions are removed by monocytes.

Focal loss of the chorionic epithelial immune barrier between the mother and fetus may cause localized inflammatory reactions.

Perivillitis was seen in 12.5 % of placentas with pregnancy related hypertonia/preeclampsia, was more frequently seen in women with nicotine abuse during pregnancy and is also reported in cases with systemic lupus erythematosus [52].

3. Perivillitis and villitis of unknown etiology (VUE): Groups of villi are affected and show epithelial necrosis, perivillous microfibrin deposition, lympho-histiocytic infiltrates in the stroma and intervillous space, proliferation of local tissue cells and fibrosis. The density and foci of affected villous groups vary and sometimes only the connecting villi affected. To aid correlation with clinical symptoms a two tier grading system, high and low grade, based on microscopic findings is recommended. (Table 9.5) High grade patterns seem to correlate with increased risk of FGR [53].

In cases without a verifiable viral etiology the changes are considered to be due to maternal host versus graft immune reactions [54]. Up to 60 % of perivillous maternal CD3-T-lymphocytes are identified with X-specific markers in placentas without clinical signs of maternal or fetal infection. The positive response to corticosteroid treatment supports an association between VUE and autoimmune diseases.

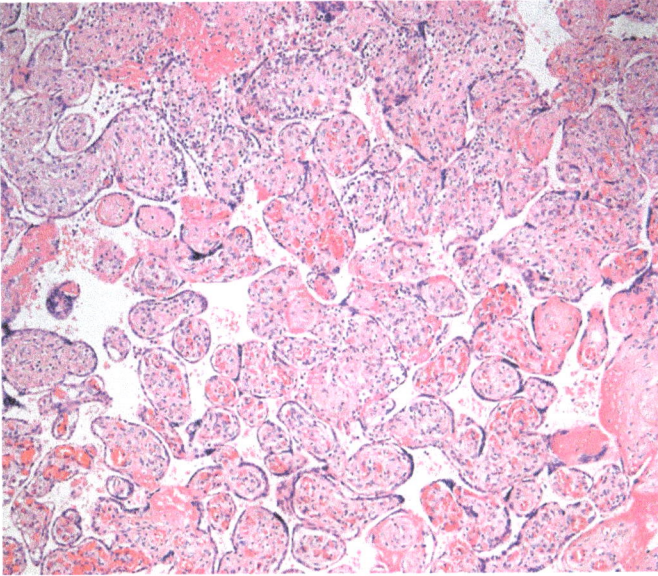

Fig. 9.24: Villitis of Unknown Etiology (VUE). Focal epithelial necrosis and perivillous fibrin deposition. Villous and intervillous lymphatic-histiocytic infiltration and a proliferative stromal reaction.

Table 9.5: Suggested grading of microscopic findings of VUE [53].

low grade VUE	high grade VUE
small clusters of 5–10 affected villi – single (focal) – multiple (multifocal)	– more than 10 villi (patchy) – all sections with more than 10 villi involved (diffuse)

Fetal consequences of perivillitis and villitis

– *Known infectious pathogen:* Generalized fetal infection in pre-term and term deliveries followed by intellectual disability and organic disease.
– *Unknown cause:* Intrauterine growth restriction (predominantly in term births), intrauterine fetal death and nonspecific increased fetal morbidity.

Recurrence risk

VUE recurrence risk is estimated to be 25%, with the grade increasing in following pregnancies, and can be associated with IUFD and FGR [55]. In contrast, recurrence of villitis of a known etiology depends on virus activity and exposure.

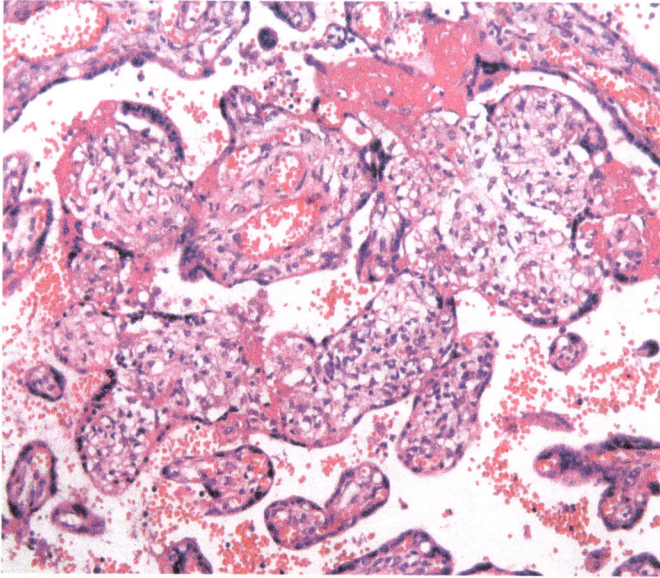

Fig 9.25: VUE. Villous group with superficial erosion of the trophoblastic epithelium and fibrin deposition. Lymphocytes and histiocytes are visible in the villi and proliferation of the villous stroma cells is seen. Cesarean section in GW 33 + 3 due of preeclampsia and FGR.

9.4 Intrauterine infection

Only a few human pathogens (rubella, herpes simplex virus, cytomegalovirus, protozoa, Toxoplasma gondii and some bacterial infections) play an important role in intrauterine infection with placental involvement [56].

9.4.1 Rubella virus

The rubella virus is a 35 nm RNA-virus and belongs to the togavirus family. After active vaccination fertile women between 15 and 40 years are immune in 85 to 93 % of cases.

Morphology
The earliest changes can be found in chorionic tissue in the late embryonic or early fetal period [57,58]:
– erosion of the chorionic epithelium with focal cellular injury and fibrin deposition
– endothelial necrosis of peripheral villous vessels
– increased number of Hofbauer cells in the villous stroma [59]
– focal stromal necrosis, cell proliferation and fibrosis in single villi

–   endangiitis in stem villous vessels with cellular necrosis, mononuclear cell infil-
    tration and, should organization occur, a myofibrocytic proliferation with vessel
    obliteration,
–   in some cases intracytoplasmic inclusions in the chorionic epithelium and decid-
    ual cells are found.

If morphological findings are identified in the 1st and 2nd trimester a viral etiology
should be investigated. Necrotic angiitis, associated with arrest of villous maturation
may be suggestive of, but not diagnostic for, viral infection. In only 50 % of therapeutic abortions following a rubella infection could a maternal infection be conclusively
demonstrated.

Verification by virus isolation/PCR from chorionic villi, amniotic fluid or blood
from the umbilical cord vein is required.

Pathogenesis
The infectious pathway is transplacental, following a maternal viremia; however, the
detailed pathogenic transmission mechanism is not completely understood.

Rubella viremia starts on day 8 post infection and persists for 5 to 7 days.

Viral infection may cause necrosis in the chorionic epithelium, the stroma and
the endothelial cells of the peripheral villi. Characteristically a lympho-monocytic villitis with arterial stem villous angiitis is seen and, if progressive, the development of
villous stromal fibrosis adjacent to affected arteries occurs.

Early arrest of villous maturation is assumed to be the result of a viral induced
anti-proliferative effect that causes inhibition of cell growth and division [18].

Rubella is a teratogen and infection between the 1st and 7th gestational week causes an embryopathy, in 55 %, that presents with eye, inner ear and cardiac malformations of varying severity (Gregg-syndrome). Between weeks 8 and 17 of gestation the
malformation rate decreases from 25 % to 8 % and infection within 4 months of gestation causes fetal growth restriction and localized organic fetopathy in 10 %.

Due to rubella vaccination cases of embryopathy have decreased to ca 1/10,000
deliveries [60].

9.4.2 Cytomegalovirus

Cytomegalovirus (CMV) is a double stranded DNA-virus from the Herpes virus family
and is the most common congenital virus infection, with an estimated infection rate
of ca. 1 % of all live births. However, the virus is only identifiable in 5–10 % of infected
children [61].

The CMV infection rate, primary or reactivated, in fertile women is ca. 45–60 %.
Approximately 0.5 % of seronegative women are primary infected and the risk to the

fetus is ca. 50 % [62]. In ca. 8 % of seropositive mothers endogenous reactivation occurs in the 2nd and 3rd trimester with an expected fetal risk of 7 %.

The progression of fetal and newborn infection may be generalized with liver and splenomegaly, or localized, and shows a preference for CNS involvement.

The prognosis of fetal intrauterine infection is adverse, with a 30 % risk of mortality.

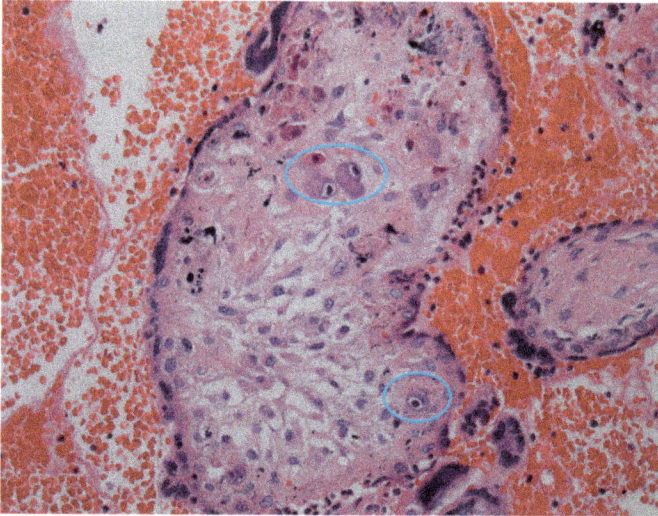

Fig. 9.26: Intranuclear CMV inclusions (owl-eye cells) in villous stroma cells (circles). Miscarriage at 18th week of gestation with previous normal pregnancy and delivery.

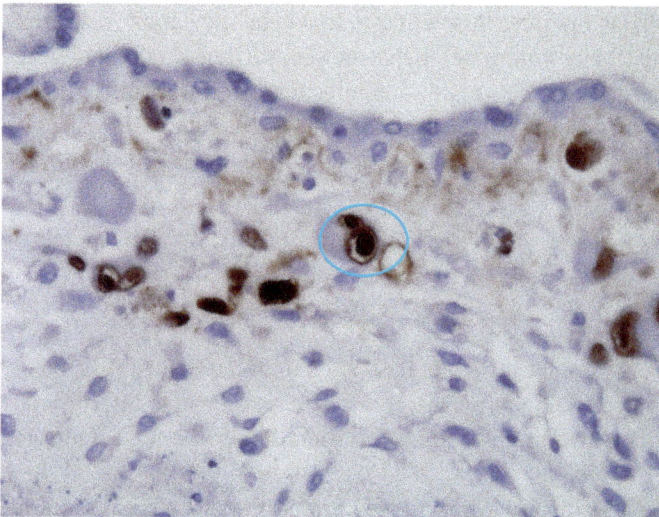

Fig. 9.27: Positive immunostaining of CMV infected cells (circle).

The virus may be identified in bodily fluids, such as urine, in tissue or in the placenta. Diagnosis is confirmed by IgM antibodies in the serum, immunostaining in tissue samples and in situ hybridization and PCR on fetal and placental tissue.

Morphology
Characteristic findings [63]:
- focal villitis with a perivascular lympho-plasmocytic infiltrate and vasculitis
- *intranuclear and intracytoplasmatic inclusions.* Diagnostic 'Owl-eye cells' are seen in 30 % of cases and are visible in the stromal and endothelial cells, but rarely in chorionic epithelial cells. Owl-eye cells have also been reported in the decidua and endometrial stroma cells [64].
- small foci of villous stromal necrosis, villous stromal fibrosis, microcalcification and siderophages,
- villous maturation disorder: Villous maturation arrest and retardation of villous maturation.

Pathogenesis
Cytomegalovirus infection is transmitted:
- intrauterine: vertically from the mother to the child by hematogenous transplacental spread
- during delivery: as the fetus passes through the infected cervical tract,
- post-delivery: by ingestion of CMV positive breast milk.

Replication of CMV occurs slowly, between 8 and 72 hours. Like other viruses, CMV may persist after an acute infection and remain in a latent stage until reactivation.

Prenatal diagnosis is possible by virus detection in cell culture, PCR of chorionic biopsies/amniocentesis/cordocentesis and CMV-specific IgM-antibodies in the fetal blood. Cytomegalovirus inclusions in placental cells are diagnostic, immunostaining.

Other examples of infection by viruses from the Herpes family which may cause congenital infections are: herpes simplex virus I and II, varicella zoster, Epstein-Barr, and rarely cytomegalovirus related human herpesvirus 6 (HHV 6) [64].

9.4.3 Herpes simplex virus infection

Primary infection with herpes simplex virus (HSV), types I and II, leads to virus persistence. In Central Europe ca. 90 % are infected with type I and 25 % with type II . Reactivation and multiplication of the virus in pregnancy affects 80–90 % of fertile women (primary infection with type I) and 20–40 % of fertile women (primary infection with type II) [61]. Secondary infection with HSV may cause abortion in the 1st and 2nd trimester. Perinatal incidence of fetal infection is ca. 1/7,500 (25 % type I and 75 %

type II). Perinatal infection may lead to generalized herpes simplex infection with encephalitis which is in lethal in 50 % of cases [65,66].

Morphology

Morphological changes due to Herpes virus infection, while rare, may be very pronounced in florid genital HSV infection:

–   necrotizing chorioamnionitis due to ascending infection with focal necrosis in the connective tissue of the chorionic plate and/or amnion. Lympho-plasmocytic and macrophage rich inflammatory infiltrate
–   intranuclear inclusions in macrophages
–   rarely villitis and necrotizing funiculitis [67].

Diagnosis of a herpes virus induced chorioamnionitis may be confirmed immunohistochemically or by in situ hybridization [68].

Pathogenesis

0.1–1 % of pregnant women suffer from a florid herpes simplex type II infection. 80 % of newborns with congenital herpes simplex infections are infected during passage through the infected genital tract at delivery. Infrequently infection occurs by hematogenous vertical transmission. The risk of infection to a child born vaginally is ca. 30–50 %, in primary infections with genital tract involvement. Reactivation of the infection at delivery is minimal with ca. 3–5 %. A generalized newborn disease has a poor prognosis. Fatality rates can be as high as 70 % and morbidity with long term sequelae, in surviving babies with CNS involvement, is greater than 50 %.

9.4.4 Varicella zoster virus

Varicella zoster is a double stranded DNA-virus and belongs to the group of herpes viruses. The incidence of a primary varicella infection (chickenpox) in pregnancy is ca. 2–7/10,000. Herpes zoster may develop after reactivation of a latent varicella virus infection, due to endogenous reinfection after primary infection, and has an incidence of 0.5–10000. Embryopathy and fetal diseases in maternal varicella are described in the 1st trimester and may cause IUFD in 30 % [61].

Morphology

Only a few cases have been described:

–   necrotizing, granulomatous villitis,
–   disseminated fibrinoid necrosis with giant cells and eosinophilic inclusions [69].

Diagnosis of a varicella induced chorioamnionitis may be confirmed by immunochemistry or in situ hybridization.

Pathogenesis
In an acute primary maternal infection the virus is transmitted hematogenously across the placenta to the fetus and 25 % of maternal infections will lead to fetal infections Maternal IgG-antibodies are capable of traversing the placenta, entering the fetal circulation and are required by the fetus, and later the developing child during the first several months after delivery, to mount an immune response. However, sufficient IgG-antibody levels are only achieved several days after primary infection and therefore the fetus is at high risk if delivery occurs within 4 days of maternal symptom onset. Only 50 % of people will display symptoms.

9.4.5 Parvovirus-B-19-infection

Human Parvovirus-B-19 is a pathogen of erythema infectiosum. This erythrovirus is an environmentally resistant single stranded DNA-virus. Since 1984 it is known to cause hydrops fetalis and intrauterine fetal death [70]. The incidence of fetal death is uncertain but frequently occurs between gestational weeks 13 and 20 with an abortion rate of 15 % [71,72]. Fetal complications are seen in each phase of pregnancy.

Morphology
– Enlarged placenta,
– characteristic triad of villous maturation arrest, focal chorangiosis, type 1 and intravascular erythroblastosis,
– intranuclear viral inclusions with glassy-pale eosinophilic chromatin in the intravascular erythroblasts, so called "lantern cells".

B19 virus particles can be shown in placentas and fetal tissue by immunostaining and in situ hybridization [73]. Prenatal diagnosis can be performed by PCR on umbilical vein blood or fetal ascites.

Pathogenesis
Virus transmission is hematogenous and virus replication occurs in fetal erythroblasts. This causes an inhibition of erythroblast differentiation with subsequent hemolysis, anemia, cardiac decompensation and generalized edema [74]. Virus affinity for erythropoietic cells is due to erythrocytic receptor P, and it is through binding to this receptor that differentiation into erythroblasts is inhibited and hemolysis occurs [75]. The effect on villous maturation arrest is unexplained. Maternal IgM-antibodies

indicate an acute infection with increased fetal risk. Viral B19 DNA can be identified in amniotic fluid and IgM-parvovirus specific antibodies can be isolated from umbilical cord blood.

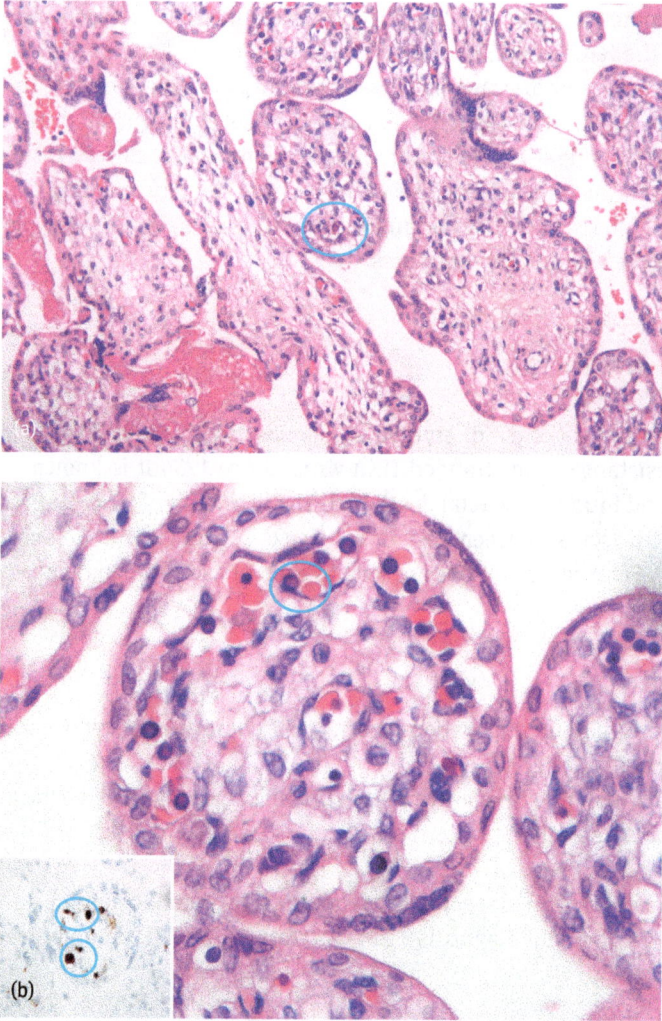

Fig. 9.28: (a) Parvovirus infection. Intranuclear inclusions in fetal erythrocytes ("lampion cells") (circle). IUFD in gestational week 24. (b) Parvovirus infection (HPF). Inlet: Positive immunostaining of parvovirus infected erythrocytes (circle).

9.4.6 ECHO Virus infection

Risk of intrauterine and perinatal infection exists if maternal viremia is present during pregnancy. Transmission is assumed to occur directly from the mother to the fetus. Histological changes in the placenta are not clearly described; however, maternal infection with ECHO virus types 27 and 33 show an acute intervillositis and villitis, epithelial and stromal necrosis and is frequently associated with proliferative villitis assumed as transplacental infections [76].

9.4.7 HIV-infection

In Europe, Africa and the USA HIV infection is related to intravenous and sexual transmission. The vertical transmission rate in Germany is ca. 19 % and between 10–15 % of children born to HIV positive mothers are infected [77]. Infection may happen in utero, during delivery and postnatally. The risk of infection is higher in vaginal deliveries than in cesarean sections.

Morphology

Histological changes in the placenta as a result of maternal HIV-infections are not well described. In a study involving 54 placentas from HIV-positive mothers, 37 showed vasculopathy of the vessels branches in the chorionic plate with:
- Endothelial cell degeneration and necrosis,
- Thickening of the tunica media with irregular type IV collagen formation in the muscle layer
- Occasional mononuclear cellular infiltrates in the subendothelium.

Vasculopathy correlates with maternal immune suppression, clinically defined as a T-lymphocyte CD4/CD8-level lower than 0.6, decreased T4-lymphocytes (CD 4) lower than 500/ml and maternal hypergammaglobulinemia with increased IgG [78].

In 33 % of the examined placentas different signs of villous immaturity were seen, and an increased incidence of amniotic infection was seen in 20 %.

In 40 % of cases of therapeutic terminations and deliveries in late pregnancy the viral antigen (p24) was identified, only in a few cells, in the placenta and the membranes [79].

P24 positive immunohistochemistry can be confirmed by PCR and in situ hybridization.

Histological changes are inconsistent, frequently minimal and in isolation are not sufficient for a definitive diagnosis.

Pathogenesis
HIV may affect all cells of the placenta and the amnion, and can subsequently enter the fetal circulation. The earliest time point for vertical transmission is gestational week 12 and viral replication has been demonstrated from gestational week 21, in lymph nodes, and from gestational week 27, in the fetal liver [80].

9.4.8 Zika virus

Zika virus is a mosquito borne Flavivirus and was first identified in monkeys in Uganda in 1947 and later in humans in 1952. Based on a literature review, the WHO has concluded that Zika virus infection during pregnancy is a cause of congenital brain abnormalities, including microcephaly, and that it is also a trigger of Guillain-Barré syndrome. Sexual transmission and other modes of transmission, such as blood transfusion, are being investigated [81].

Villitis or chorioamnionitis is not described with Zika virus infection [82].

9.4.9 Other virus infections

Single cases of villitis with small foci of necrosis and lympho-plasmocytic and plasma cell stromal infiltrates are reported in infections with Ebstein-Barr virus and Coxsackievirus A9.

Placental changes due to infection with Respiratory Syncytial Virus (RSV), a myxovirus, are not reported, likely due to a lack of viremia and diaplacental transmission [83].

Characteristic changes in the placenta due to mumps infection and hepatitis A, B and C virus infections are not known to the authors; however, several viruses are suspected to be causes for miscarriages e. g. measles, mumps, influenza and adenoviruses.

9.4.10 Intrauterine Listeriosis

Listeriosis is a ubiquitous zoonosis caused by the gram positive aerobe Listeria monocytogenes. L monocytogenes produces endotoxins and hemolytic and lipolytic enzymes. When the bacteria die a "monocytosis producing antigen" (MPA) is released and this causes granuloma formation in the tissue.

Intrauterine infection is, most frequently, sporadic. More than half of the pregnant women are primary infected but transmission to the child during birth is very low.

Perinatal mortality rates are controversial. The rate in proven listeriosis has been reported as 14 %; however, rates between 0.7 and 50 % have been described. In 28 cases the infection manifested prepartum and in 7 cases during the first days of life. The rate of Listeria infections in stillbirths is unknown [84].

Morphology

Macroscopic characteristics:
-   Irregularly distributed millimeter to 3 cm sized nodular abscesses in the placenta parenchyma. Confluent abscesses "septic infarcts" may develop. Rarely, small abscesses on the surface of the umbilical cord and membranes are described.
    Histological characteristics:
-   Acute intervillitis (intervillous thromboangiitis) with focal aggregates and bands of granulocytes, fibrin thrombosis in the intervillous space, chorionic epithelial and stromal necrosis and inter- and intravillous microabscesses (Fig. 9.16).
-   Transmission of the pathogens occurs by involvement of adjacent villi, villous vessels and the umbilical cord vein.
-   As a part of fetal sepsis the pathogens return to the placenta, i. e. fetal hematogenous involvement of the villi.
-   Intravillous pathogenic emboli, subepithelial microabscesses (Fig. 9.13).
-   Acute granulocytic and/or monocytic villitis.
-   Listerioma (granuloma) [85,86].

The pathogens are predominantly visualized by Gram stain and Dieterle-Silver stain, which highlight positive cells in the margin of necrotic areas and in cell cultures from pathogenic foci.

Pathogenesis

The source of listeria infections are pets, breeding animals, fresh products of animal origin (cheese), infected humans and healthy human carriers. Listeria bacteria are removed by the macrophage-phagocytosis system and then destroyed by parenchymal cells; however, ca. 20 % of intracellular listeria survive and multiply within a few hours. Intrauterine infection occurs due to transplacental maternal bacteremia, which leads to acute placental infection with micro- and macroabscess formation. Fetal sepsis may cause a placental reinfection with listeria emboli and the development of granulocytic monocytic villitis and intravillous listeriomas. Excretion of the pathogens by the kidneys causes a secondary amniotic fluid infection and may lead to fetal superinfection by aspiration of the infected amniotic fluid.

Additionally, a primary ascending amniotic infection can occur during delivery with subsequent fetal tracheobronchial and enteral infection.

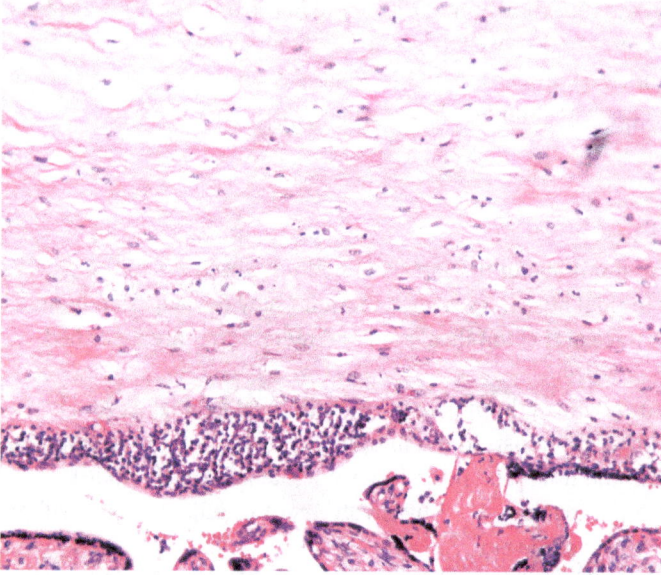

Fig. 9.29: Subchorionic phlegmonous aggregation of maternal granulocytes in the chorionic plate close to the intervillous space. Connective tissue with only a low grade infiltrate. Placenta in gestational week 22 following amniotic fluid loss in week 21 and umbilical cord prolapse.

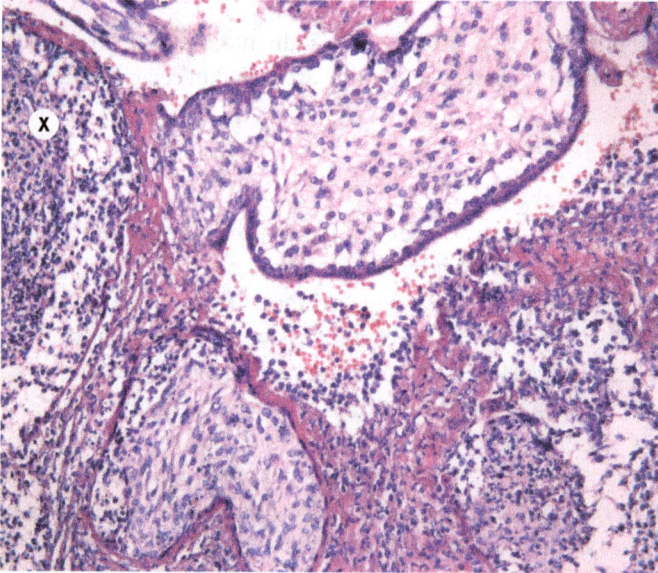

Fig. 9.30: Purulent intervillous thromboangiitis with placental abscess (X). A maternal listeriosis infection was clinically proven.

CD4 T-cell activation is necessary for development of listeria granulomas. In early stages, the granulomas are cell rich with macrophages and lymphocytes, while in later stages fibroblasts are visible in the margins of granulomas.

Primary infection occurs without antibody development.

Risk of the fetus

Fetal listeria infection can cause miscarriage, IUFD, pre-term delivery and neonatal death. As previously mentioned, perinatal death has been reported in up to 50 % of cases.

9.4.11 Congenital Toxoplasmosis

Toxoplasmosis is a chronic and cyclic zoonosis and the pathogen Toxoplasma gondii is a Gram-negative sporozoa of the Eucoccidiorida order. Two types of placental infection are described:
–   trophozoite: proliferation of the pathogen which causes tissue damage and active inflammation,
–   pathogenic cysts (terminal cysts); latent infectious stage without tissue damage [87].

The infection rate in women of fertile age is ca. 30–60 % and primary infection during pregnancies is estimated to occur in 1–6/ 1000 of women. In ca. 1/ 1000 live births a congenital toxoplasmosis is reported.

The majority of infected fetuses with manifest congenital toxoplasmosis are delivered in a post encephalitic stage with hydrocephalus. Approximately 10 % are born with florid encephalitis and only 1 % show generalized infection at delivery

Morphology

Changes in the placenta are reported in 80 % of newborns with generalized infection or florid encephalitis [88]:
–   foci of disseminated, predominantly villitis
–   focal villous stromal fibrosis with microcalcification
–   retardation of villous maturation, sometimes with maturation arrest

Villitis is usually seen as small focal lesions widespread affected villi. 3 types of villitis may be seen:
–   lymphocyte-monocytic
–   adjacent necrotizing and proliferating inflammation with vascular involvement,
–   granulomatous, infrequently seen.

Villous stromal fibrosis and maturation arrest are considered to be nonspecific tissue reactions. Stromal fibrosis may represent an end stage of proliferative villitis, with vessel involvement and villous maturation arrest, as part of a hydropic toxoplasmosis. Placental infection is confirmed through identification of the pathogen from terminal cysts in the membranes, chorionic plate, villi and umbilical cord [89].

Trophozoites in the placenta correlate with the generalized stage and florid fetal encephalitis. Terminal cysts without any inflammatory reaction may indicate a latent stage of toxoplasmosis with a fetal post-encephalitic stage at delivery [88].

Pathogens are visible on Hematoxylin-Eosin (HE) and Giemsa stains, immunofluorescence microscopy, immunohistochemistry and PCR. PCR from the amniotic fluid can be used for prenatal diagnosis [90].

Negative findings above do not exclude fetal infection.

Pathogenesis
Human transmission is diaplacental. Infection in the 2nd half of pregnancy increases the risk of generalized disease with florid signs of inflammation, whereas infections occurring earlier in pregnancy are reported to show CNS affection with post encephalic damage and Hydrocephalus.

9.4.12 Congenital Syphilis (Congenital Lues)

Congenital Syphilis is caused by Treponema pallidum. The three clinically infectious stages and the latent interval without symptoms, Lues latens, are assumed to affect the pregnancies. Serological confirmation of the pathogens leads to diagnosis and treatment [91].

Morphology
- Macrosomic placenta, some times hydrops placentae,
- villous maturation arrest/retardation, often with a cellular stroma
- endangiitis obliterans in the chorionic plate and stem villi,
- lymphocytic and plasmocytic villitis, focal stromal and chorionic epithelial necrosis [92].

Additionally, necrotizing funiculitis and necrosis of Wharton's Jelly, close to the vessels, are reported to be associated with thrombophlebitis [31].

Pathogenesis

Fetal infection is diaplacental and there is an increased risk fetal transmission in the 1st year after maternal infection. Treponema pallidum may be identified as early as gestational week 9–10 [93] and fetal manifestations of infection present in the middle fetal period. Both villitis and endangiitis are considered not to be a direct result of pathogenic infection but as consequence of an immune response to infection; such a response depends on the maturation of the fetal immune system [94].

The placenta is transmitted without reaction. Villitis and endangiitis, caused by fetal parasitemia, depend on the maturation of the fetal immune system. Villous maturation arrest and retardation indicate a late embryonic, or early fetal, villous developmental disorder without an inflammatory reaction in early pregnancy [47].

Pathogens are identified by Warthin-Starry silver stain or immunohistochemically in formalin fixed and paraffin embedded placental tissue; however, this may not be possible if the examination occurs after antibiotic treatment [95]. Diagnosis by PCR is also possible [96].

9.4.13 Congenital Tuberculosis

Placental changes due to maternal tuberculosis are only infrequently reported. Placental involvement is seen in primary tuberculosis due to hematogenous transplacental infection. Infection of the fetus can occur through infected amniotic fluid [97]. Tuberculous granulomas, with central caseating necrosis, occasionally originate from the developing primary complex in the fetal liver and hepatobiliary lymph nodes [98]. Involvement of the placenta may be due to infected deciduitis/endometritis and can be verified by histological examination of the endometrial curettage. Diagnosis often is delayed and the prognosis generally poor [99].

9.4.14 Malaria infection

Sporadic congenital infection with malaria plasmodium in central Europe is rare compared to the incidence in tropical and subtropical regions. Of the different identifiable pathogens (falciparum, vivax, ovale, malariae), Plasmodium malariae is the most globally widespread.

Morphology
- Histiocytic intervillositis with focal aggregates of mononuclear cells and macrophages, chronic histiocytic intervillositis (100),
- in ca. 20–40 % infected erythrocytes are seen, a sign of active infection [101],

- in ca. 30 % parasites may be identified and malaria pigment, fibrin covered due to cytolysis of infected erythrocytes, is seen; consistent with a chronic infection,
- in ca. 30 % exceptional pigment deposition may suggest a post infectious condition.

Identification of malaria pigment can be done under polarized light, and the parasites can be best visualized in Giemsa stained smears.

Pathogenesis

Transmission of the malaria pathogen to humans occurs via the Anopheles mosquito. The most serious malarial infections are due to Malaria tropica. Pregnancy causes a maternal immune suppression and malaria infections in this group are reported to be extremely life threatening. The frequency and type of pathogenic transmission from the mother to the fetus is, as of yet, unconfirmed, with both active transmission of the pathogen and passive transmission by infected erythrocytes suggested [26].

Identification of pathogens in the fetal circulation has not been reported as the placenta acts as an effective barrier against infection of the fetus. Congenital fetal infections have been reported in 0.2–0.4 % of maternal infections. Infected erythrocytes tend to undergo cytoadherence and this may lead to a limitation of the perfusion capacity of the placenta.

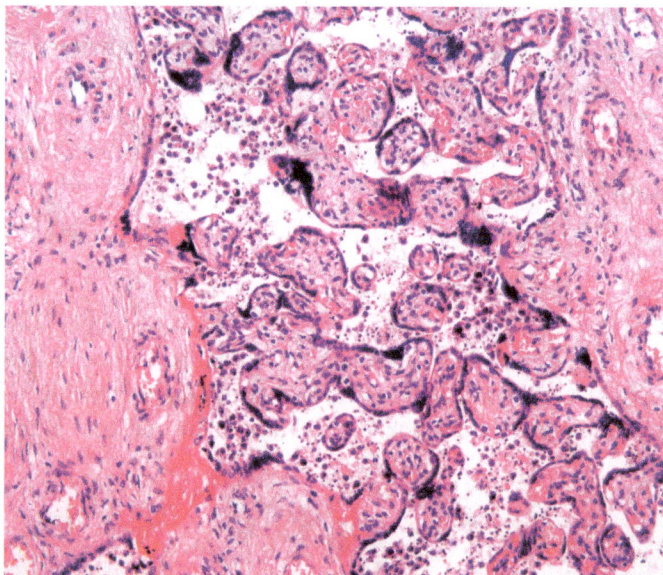

Fig. 9.31: Chronic histiocytic intervillositis. Many histiocytes (macrophages) with malaria pigment, nucleated pre-erythrocytes that are partly lytic with loss of nuclei. No pigment or parasite in the fetal villous stroma or circulation. Degenerative changes of the villous epithelium with several knots on the surface.

Fetal risk

This may cause miscarriage in early pregnancy and FGR and IUFD in late pregnancy.

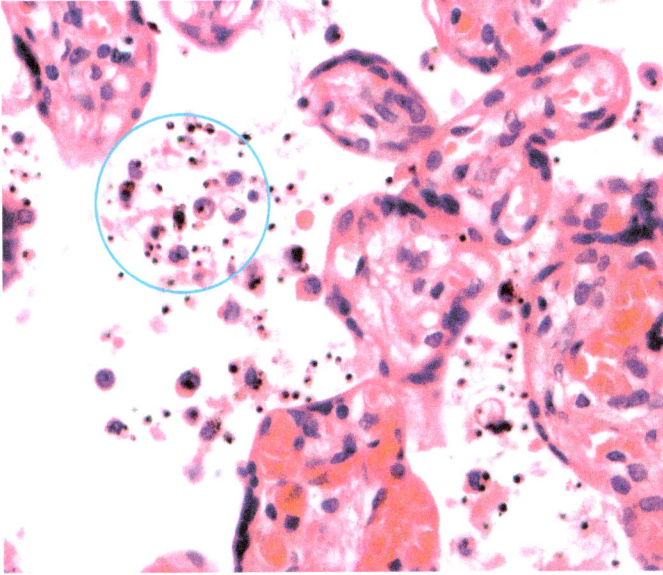

Fig. 9.32: Pigment laden macrophagocytes and lytic erythrocytes (circle).

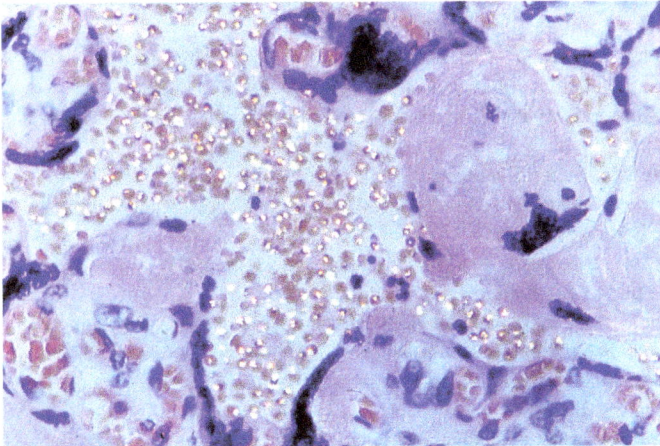

Fig. 9.33: Histiocytic intervillositis. Numerous histiocytes and macrophages in the intervillous space. Intracellular malaria pigment under polarized light. Woman from Kongo with a spontaneous delivery in gestational week 36, preceding maternal fever and intrauterine hypoxia.

References

[1] Becker V, Schiebler TH, Kubli F. Allgemeine und spezielle Pathologie der Plazenta. Die Plazenta des Menschen. Stuttgart: Thieme; 1981. p. 251–393.
[2] Benirschke K, Driscoll, SG. The pathology of the human placenta. 3 ed. Berlin: Springer; 1967.
[3] Blanc W. Pathology of the placenta, membranes and umbilical cord in bacterial, fungal and viral infections in man. In: RL N, editor. Perinatal diseases. Baltimore: Williams & Williams; 1981.
[4] Redline RW. Placental inflammation. SeminNeonatol. 2004;9(4):265–274.
[5] Redline RW. Inflammatory responses in the placenta and umbilical cord. SeminFetal Neonatal Med. 2006;11(5):296–301.
[6] Blanc WA. Pathways of fetal and early neonatal infection. Viral placentitis, bacterial and fungal chorioamnionitis. The Journal of pediatrics. 1961;59:473–496.
[7] Vogel M. Atlas der morphologischen Plazentadiagnostik. 1. ed. Berlin: Springer; 1992.
[8] Maudsley RF, Brix GA, Hinton NA, et al. Placental inflammation and infection. A prospective bacteriologic and histologic study. American journal of obstetrics and gynecology. 1966;95(5):648–659.
[9] Siddall RS. Inflammation of the amnion and chorion. Am J Obstet Gynecol. 1928;15(6):828–832.
[10] Chellam VG, Rushton DI. Chorioamnionitis and funiculitis in the placentas of 200 births weighing less than 2.5 kg. British journal of obstetrics and gynaecology. 1985;92(8):808–814.
[11] Russell P. Inflammatory lesions of the human placenta. III. The histopathology of villitis of unknown aetiology. Placenta. 1980;1(3):227–244.
[12] Altshuler G. Placental infection and inflammation. In: EVDK P, editor. Pathology of the placenta. Washington: Churchill Livingstone; 1984.
[13] Salafia CM, Weigl C, Silberman L. The prevalence and distribution of acute placental inflammation in uncomplicated term pregnancies. Obstetrics and gynecology. 1989;73(3 Pt. 1):383–389.
[14] Jimenez E, Vogel M, Hohle R, Ferszt R, Hahn H. Zum histologischen Ausbreitungsmuster entzündlicher Veränderungen der Sekundinae. In: Schnmidt E DJ, Saling E, editor. Perinatale Medizin. VIII. Stuttgart: Thieme; 1981. p. 314–315.
[15] Vogel M , Lott E, Dudenhausen JW. Korrelation zwischen morphologischem Stadium einer Amnionentzündung und klinischer Symptomatik. In: Dudenhausen JW, Saling E editor. Perinatale Medizin. X. Stuttgart: Thieme; 1984. p. 266–268.
[16] Mueller-Heubach E, Rubinstein DN, Schwarz SS. Histologic chorioamnionitis and preterm delivery in different patient populations. Obstetrics and gynecology. 1990;75(4):622–626.
[17] Guzick DS, Winn K. The association of chorioamnionitis with preterm delivery. Obstetrics and gynecology. 1985;65(1):11–16.
[18] Vogel M. Atlas der morphologischen Plazentadiagnostik. 2 ed. Berlin: Springer; 1996.
[19] Rudbeck Roge H, Henriques U. Fetal and perinatal infections. A consecutive study. Pathology, research and practice. 1992;188(1–2):135–140.
[20] Perrin EVDK. Pathology of the placenta. New York: Churchill Livingsone; 1984.
[21] Fox H. Pathology of the placenta: Saunders Elsevier; 1997.
[22] Redline RW, Faye-Petersen O, Heller D, et al. Amniotic infection syndrome: nosology and reproducibility of placental reaction patterns. PediatrDevPathol. 2003;6(5):435–448.
[23] Darby MJ, Caritis SN, Shen-Schwarz S. Placental abruption in the preterm gestation: an association with chorioamnionitis. Obstetrics and gynecology. 1989;74(1):88–92.
[24] Romero R, Espinoza J, Goncalves LF, et al. Inflammation in preterm and term labour and delivery. Semin Fetal Neonatal Med. 2006;11(5):317–326.
[25] Beck T, Bahlmann F, Weikel W. [Histology of chorioamnionitis: relations to maternal and fetal infection parameters]. Z Geburtshilfe Perinatol. 1993;197(3):129–134.

[26] Benirschke K, Burton GJ, Baergen RN. Pathology of the Human Placenta. 6 ed. Heidelberg, NY, London: Springer; 2012.

[27] Altshuler G. Pathogenesis of congenital herpesvirus infection. Case report including a description of the placenta. Am J Dis Child. 1974;127(3):427–429.

[28] Zinserling AV, Shastina GV, Melnikova VF. Changes in the fetal organs and the placenta with intrauterine mycoplasma infection. Zentralbl Allg Pathol. 1986;132(2):109–117.

[29] Madan E, Meyers MP, Amortegui AJ. Histologic manifestations of perinatal genital mycoplasmal infection. Arch Pathol Lab Med. 1989;113(5):465–469.

[30] Craver RD, Baldwin VJ. Necrotizing funisitis. Obstetrics and gynecology. 1992;79(1):64–70.

[31] Fojaco RM, Hensley GT, Moskowitz L. Congenital syphilis and necrotizing funisitis. JAMA. 1989;261(12):1788–1790.

[32] Gersell DJ, Phillips NJ, Beckerman K. Chronic chorioamnionitis: a clinicopathologic study of 17 cases. Int J Gynecol Pathol. 1991;10(3):217–229.

[33] Aquino TI, Zhang J, Kraus FT, Knefel R, Taff T. Subchorionic fibrin cultures for bacteriologic study of the placenta. Am J Clin Pathol. 1984;81(4):482–486.

[34] Romero R, Roslansky P, Oyarzun E, et al. Labor and infection. II. Bacterial endotoxin in amniotic fluid and its relationship to the onset of preterm labor. American journal of obstetrics and gynecology. 1988;158(5):1044–1049.

[35] Svensson L, Ingemarsson I, Mardh PA. Chorioamnionitis and the isolation of microorganisms from the placenta. Obstetrics and gynecology. 1986;67(3):403–409.

[36] Gibbs RS, Blanco JD. Premature rupture of the membranes. Obstetrics and gynecology. 1982;60(6):671–679.

[37] Passloer HJ. [Chorioamniotic dissociation and C-reactive protein as predictors of early premature amniotic rupture]. Z Geburtshilfe Perinatol. 1990;194(3):115–120.

[38] Muller H, Kubli F. [The amniotic infection syndrome and premature rupture of the amnion. Manifest and threatening unspecific intra-uterine infections of the last third of pregnancy (author's transl)]. Z Geburtshilfe Perinatol. 1975;179(2):77–100.

[39] Yoder PR, Gibbs RS, Blanco JD, Castaneda YS, St Clair PJ. A prospective, controlled study of maternal and perinatal outcome after intra-amniotic infection at term. American journal of obstetrics and gynecology. 1983;145(6):695–701.

[40] Martius J, Martius G. Fieber sub partu (Amnioninfektionssyndrom). Extragenitales Fieber. In Martius G, editor. Differentialdiagnose in Geburtshilfe und Gynäkologie. I. Stuttgart: Thieme; 1987. p. 94–97.

[41] Opsjon SL, Novick D, Wathen NC, et al. Soluble tumor necrosis factor receptors and soluble interleukin-6 receptor in fetal and maternal sera, coelomic and amniotic fluids in normal and pre-eclamptic pregnancies. Journal of reproductive immunology. 1995;29(2):119–134.

[42] Baergen R, Benirschke K, Ulich TR. Cytokine expression in the placenta. The role of interleukin 1 and interleukin 1 receptor antagonist expression in chorioamnionitis and parturition. Arch Pathol Lab Med. 1994;118(1):52–55.

[43] Knox WF, Fox H. Villitis of unknown aetiology: its incidence and significance in placentae from a British population. Placenta. 1984;5(5):395–402.

[44] Altshuler G, Russell P. The human placental villitides: a review of chronic intrauterine infection. Curr Top Pathol. 1975;60:64–112.

[45] Russel P. Inflammatory lesions of the human placenta I. Clinical significance of acute chorioamnionitis. Am J Diagn Gynecol Obstet. 1979;1.

[46] Altshuler G. Placentitis. Contrib Gynecol Obstet. 1982;9:113–128.

[47] Kloos K, Vogel M. Pathologie der Perinatalperiode. Stuttgart: Thieme; 1974.

[48] Turowski G, Rollag H, Roald B. Viral infection in placenta relevant cells--a morphological and immunohistochemical cell culture study. APMIS. 2015;123(1):60–64.

[49] Derricott H, Heazell AEP, Greenwood SL, Jones RL. A novel in vitro model of villitis of unknown etiology demonstrates altered placental hormone and cytokine profile. American journal of reproductive immunology (New York, NY : 1989). 2017.

[50] Redline RW. Villitis of unknown etiology: noninfectious chronic villitis in the placenta. Hum-Pathol. 2007;38(10):1439–1446.

[51] Tamblyn JA, Lissauer DM, Powell R, Cox P, Kilby MD. The immunological basis of villitis of unknown etiology – review. Placenta. 2013;34(10):846–855.

[52] Kentenich H, Schwerdtfeger R, Vogel M. [Lupus anticoagulant in pregnancy]. Geburtshilfe Frauenheilkd. 1986;46(7):467–469.

[53] Kraus FT, Redline RW, Gersell DJ, Nelson DM, Dicke JM. Placental Pathology: American Registry of Pathology Washington, DC; 2004 2004.

[54] Redline RW, Patterson P. Villitis of unknown etiology is associated with major infiltration of fetal tissue by maternal inflammatory cells. Am J Pathol. 1993;143(2):473–479.

[55] Redline RW. Villitis of unknown etiology: noninfectious chronic villitis in the placenta. Human pathology. 2007;38(10):1439–46.

[56] Müntefering H: Infektionskrankheiten des Fetus und des Neugeborenen. In: W. R, editor. Pathologie. 3. Berlin: Springer; 1984. p. 575–612.

[57] Driscoll SG, Kundsin RB, Horne HW Jr., Scott JM. Infections and first trimester losses: possible role of Mycoplasmas. Fertil Steril. 1969;20(6):1017–1019.

[58] Ornoy A, Segal S, Nishmi M, Simcha A, Polishuk WZ. Fetal and placental pathology in gestational rubella. American journal of obstetrics and gynecology. 1973;116(7):949–956.

[59] Lima MT, Machado R, Javech C, Aguilera A, Cutie E. Histopathological study of human placenta in women infected with rubella virus during pregnancy. Morphol Embryol (Bucur). 1977;23(4):257–260.

[60] Enders G, Gartner L. [Infection as a complication in early pregnancy]. Gynakologe. 1988;21(3):220–231.

[61] Enders G. [Virus and other infections in pregnancy: diagnosis and prevention. 2]. Z Geburtshilfe Perinatol. 1983;187(4):155–167.

[62] Mertens T. [Development of viral vaccines]. Immun Infekt. 1987;15(6):197–202.

[63] Benirschke K, Burton G, Baergen RN. Pathology of the human placenta. 6 ed. New York: Springer; 2012.

[64] Garcia AG, Fonseca EF, Marques RL, Lobato YY. Placental morphology in cytomegalovirus infection. Placenta. 1989;10(1):1–18.

[65] Enders G. [Viral and other infections in pregnancy: diagnosis and prevention. Rubella, cytomegalic inclusion disease, herpes simplex, varicella zoster, Epstein-Barr, measles, mumps, enteroviruses, hepatitis, toxoplasmosis, syphilis. 1]. Z Geburtshilfe Perinatol. 1983;187(3):109–116.

[66] Schneider K-T M, v. Kaisenberg C, Holzgreve W. Diagnostik und Prävention prä- und perinataler Virusinfektionen: Zytomegalie und andere Herpesviren. Steckhausen HB, editor. München: Deutsches Grünes Kreuz; 1982.

[67] Heifetz SA, Bauman M. Necrotizing funisitis and herpes simplex infection of placental and decidual tissues: study of four cases. Hum Pathol. 1994;25(7):715–722.

[68] Schwartz DA, Caldwell E. Herpes simplex virus infection of the placenta. The role of molecular pathology in the diagnosis of viral infection of placental-associated tissues. Arch Pathol Lab Med. 1991;115(11):1141–1144.

[69] Fleck M, Podlech J, Weise K, Muntefering H, Falke D. Pathogenesis of HSV-½ induced vaginitis/vulvitis of the mouse: dependence of lesions on genetic properties of the virus and analysis of pathohistology. Arch Virol. 1993;129(1–4):35–51.

[70] Knott PD, Welply GA, Anderson MJ. Serologically proved intrauterine infection with parvovirus. Br Med J (Clin Res Ed). 1984;289(6459):1660.

[71] Schwarz TF, Roggendorf M, Hottentrager B, et al. Human parvovirus B19 infection in pregnancy. Lancet. 1988;2(8610):566–567.

[72] Schwarz TF, Roggendorf M, Simader R. [Association of non-immunologically-induced hydrops fetalis with Parvovirus B19 infection]. Geburtshilfe Frauenheilkd. 1987;47(8):572–573.

[73] Burton PA, Caul EO. Fetal cell tropism of human parvovirus B19. Lancet. 1988;1(8588):767.

[74] Anand A, Gray ES, Brown T, Clewley JP, Cohen BJ. Human parvovirus infection in pregnancy and hydrops fetalis. N Engl J Med. 1987;316(4):183–186.

[75] Rodis JF, Hovick TJ Jr., Quinn DL, Rosengren SS, Tattersall P. Human parvovirus infection in pregnancy. Obstetrics and gynecology. 1988;72(5):733–738.

[76] Garcia AG, Basso NG, Fonseca ME, Outani HN. Congenital echo virus infection--morphological and virological study of fetal and placental tissue. J Pathol. 1990;160(2):123–127.

[77] Voßbeck S. HIV – Infektion und AIDSerkrankung. In: Boos R, editor. Risiken in der Schwangerschaft und kindliche Fehlbildungen. I. Spitta Balingen 2003.

[78] Jimenez E, Unger M, Vogel M, et al. [Morphologic studies of the placentas of HIV-positive mothers]. Pathologe. 1988;9(4):228–234.

[79] Backe E, Jimenez E, Unger M, et al. Demonstration of HIV-1 infected cells in human placenta by in situ hybridisation and immunostaining. J Clin Pathol. 1992;45(10):871–874.

[80] Backe E, Unger M, Jimenez E, et al. Fetal organs infected by HIV-1. AIDS. 1993;7(6):896–897.

[81] www.who.int/mediacentre/factsheets/zika/en/

[82] Rosenberg AZ, Yu W, Hill DA, Reyes CA, Schwartz DA. Placental Pathology of Zika Virus: Viral Infection of the Placenta Induces Villous Stromal Macrophage (Hofbauer Cell) Proliferation and Hyperplasia. Arch Pathol Lab Med. 2017;141(1):43–48.

[83] Müntefering H, Podlech J. Infektionskrankheiten des Embryo, des Fetus und des Neugeborenen. In: W R, editor. Pathologie. 4. 2 ed. Berlin, Heidelberg, New York: Springer; 1997. p. 461–500.

[84] Bucher HU, Nadal D, Mieth D. [Listeriosis in the newborn infant: improved prognosis due to early detection]. Monatsschr Kinderheilkd. 1989;137(6):321–325.

[85] Reiss HJ. [Pathologic anatomy of listeria infection in children]. Kinderarztl Prax. 1953:92–100.

[86] Topalovski M, Yang SS, Boonpasat Y. Listeriosis of the placenta: clinicopathologic study of seven cases. American journal of obstetrics and gynecology. 1993;169(3):616–620.

[87] Essbach H. Paidopathologie. 1 ed. Leipzig: Thieme; 1961.

[88] Vogel M. Pathologie der Spätschwangerschaft un Fetoplazentaren Einheit. In: Dietel M KG, editor. Pathologie. 3 ed. Berlin, Heidelberg: Springer; 2013. p. 543–632.

[89] Röse I. [Pathomorphology of the secundinae in congenital toxoplasmosis]. Zentralbl Allg Pathol. 1969;112(5):527–539.

[90] Hohlfeld P, Daffos F, Costa JM, et al. Prenatal diagnosis of congenital toxoplasmosis with a polymerase-chain-reaction test on amniotic fluid. The New England journal of medicine. 1994;331(11):695–699.

[91] Muller F, Lindenschmidt EG. [The problem of determining Treponema-specific IgM-antibodies with the TPHA test in primary syphilis]. Hautarzt. 1983;34(9):448–452.

[92] Walter P, Blot P, Ivanoff B. The placental lesions in congenital syphilis. A study of six cases. Virchows Arch A Pathol Anat Histol. 1982;397(3):313–326.

[93] Harter C, Benirschke K. Fetal syphilis in the first trimester. American journal of obstetrics and gynecology. 1976;124(7):705–711.

[94] Benirschke K. Syphilis-the placenta and the fetus. Am J Dis Child. 1974;128(2):142–143.

[95] Ohyama M, Itani Y, Tanaka Y, Goto A, Sasaki Y. Syphilitic placentitis: demonstration of Treponema pallidum by immunoperoxidase staining. Virchows Arch A Pathol Anat Histopathol. 1990;417(4):343–345.

[96] Genest DR, Choi-Hong SR, Tate JE, et al. Diagnosis of congenital syphilis from placental examination: comparison of histopathology, Steiner stain, and polymerase chain reaction for
Treponema pallidum DNA. Hum Pathol. 1996;27(4):366–372.

[97] Starke JR. Case 5: presentation. Pulmonary tuberculosis. Paediatr Respir Rev.
2001;2(2):196–199.

[98] Flamm H. [Another hit herto unknown virus infection of the lungs of human fetuses]. Zentralbl
Bakteriol Parasitenkd Infektionskr Hyg. 1959;176:356–357.

[99] Stahelin-Massik J, Carrel T, Duppenthaler A, Zeilinger G, Gnehm HE. Congenital tuberculosis in
a premature infant. Swiss Med Wkly. 2002;132(41–42):598–602.

[100] Nebuloni M, Pallotti F, Polizzotti G, et al. Malaria placental infection with massive chronic
intervillositis in a gravida 4 woman. Hum Pathol. 2001;32(9):1022–1023.

[101] Ismail MR, Ordi J, Menendez C, et al. Placental pathology in malaria: a histological, immunohistochemical, and quantitative study. Hum Pathol. 2000;31(1):85–93.

10 Non trophoblastic tumors

Non trophoblastic tumours may be broadly classified as:
- chorangioma/fibroma,
- teratoma,
- metastatic tumors.

10.1 Chorangioma

Definition
Chorangiomas are classified as benign expansive hamartomatous vascular tumors of the fetal placenta. 80 % of chorangiomas are less than 10 mm in size and are diagnosed as *microchorangiomas*.

Frequency
In unselected material, 136 chorangiomas were identified out of 22,439 placentas, a frequency of 0.61 % [1]. Other studies have reported a frequency between 5–7 % and a frequency of 1.4 % in monochorionic twin placentas [2,3].

Reports vary due to different examination procedures and diagnosis, such as macroscopic diagnosis (1:13000) or diagnosis on histology (5:500) [4].

Macroscopically the lesions are solitary/multiple, well circumscribed, infrequently pedunculated and up to 500 g in weight. They are positioned close to the chorionic plate and encapsulated by villous trophoblasts. The cut surface of a chorangioma is often lobule-like and multicolored, depending on the vascular and connective tissue composition of the tumor. The cut surface may also show secondary changes, such as:

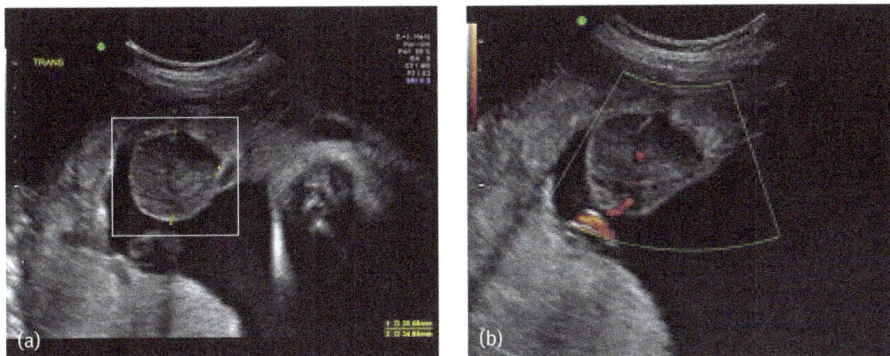

Fig. 10.1: (a) Chorangioma on ultrasound. Well circumscribed and hypoechogenic tumor with thin fibrous septa (red square). (b) Color-Doppler identifies the typical prominent blood flow within the lesion, differentiating it from a fibrous tissue tumor. (by courtesy of Prof. Dr. Braun Department for obstetrics, Charité, Germany).

https://doi.org/10.1515/9783110452600-010

necrosis, thrombosis, hemorrhage, hemosiderin deposition and calcification. Chorangiomas spread and compress adjacent parenchyma.

Microscopically there are different subtypes of chorangioma. The tumors are frequently capillary rich and larger tumors often show a greater complexity with varying cellularity and a greater heterogeneity of the reticular and fibrous stromal components. Different degrees of vascular maturation and capillary and stromal density are of no clinical relevance [5].

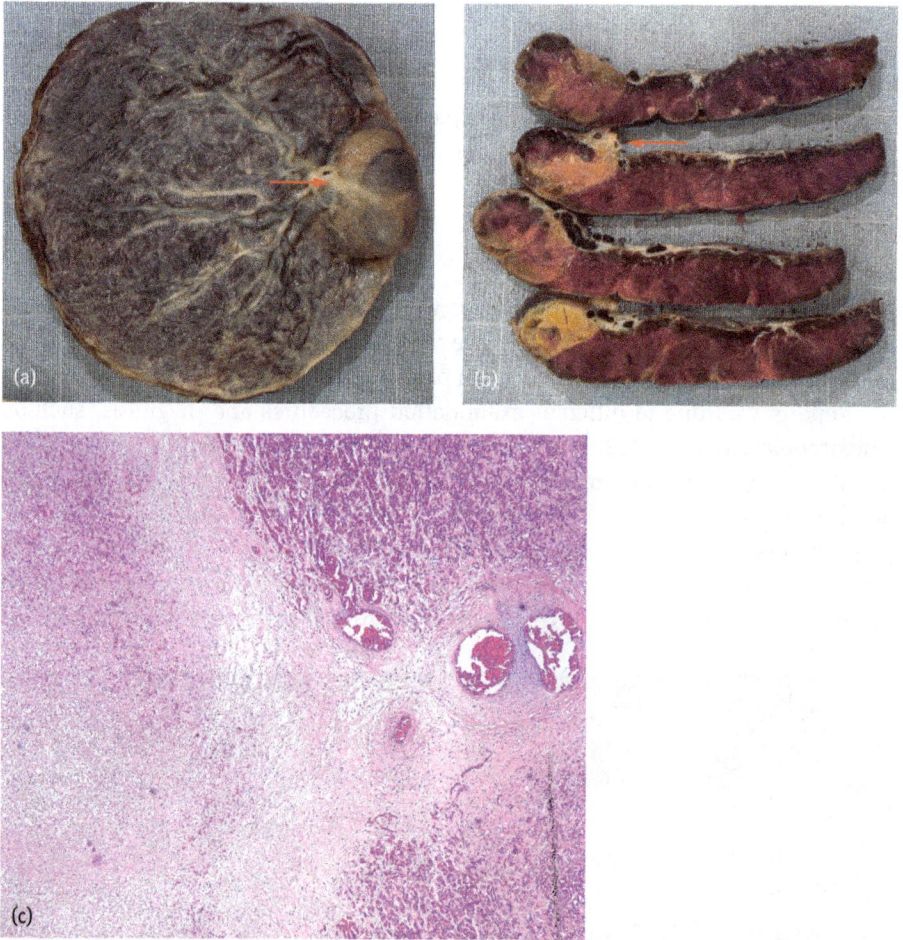

Fig. 10.2: (a) Formalin fixed placenta with a chorangioma. An encapsulated tumor measuring 3 × 2 × 2 cm that is marginally located and close to the umbilical cord insertion (arrow). Cesarean section in GW 37 + 5 on maternal indication. (b) Macroscopy of marginal chorangiomas on cut sections. The tumor has a lobular structure with a brown-red and yellow color, due to partial ischemia. Acute thrombosis in the chorionic plate vessels continued into the tumor. Umbilical cord insertion (arrow). (c) Microscopic sections of a chorangioma showing a lobular structure with capillary rich areas (right) and areas of sclerosis (left).

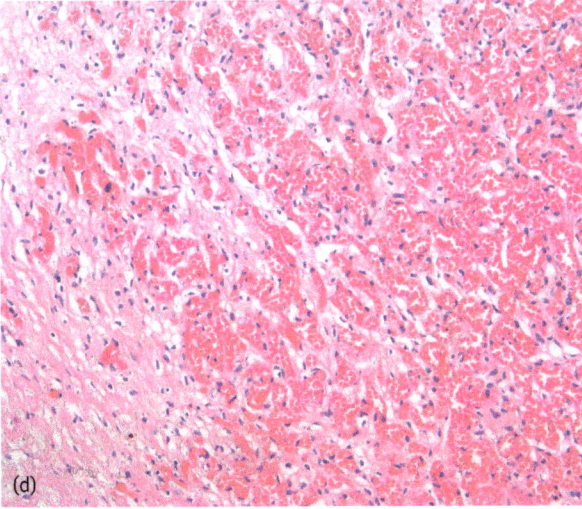

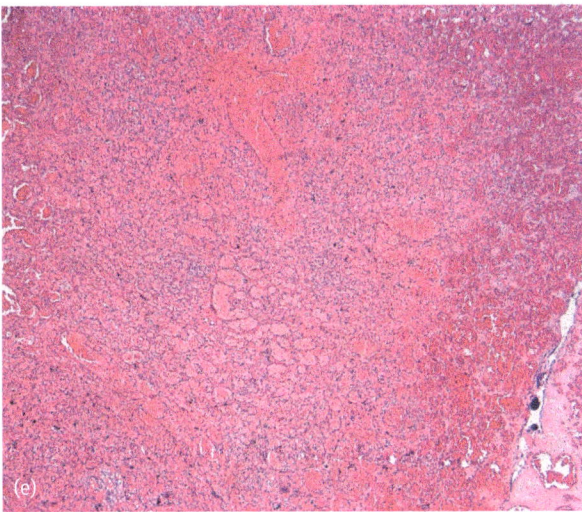

Fig. 10.2: (continued) (d) Chorangioma of the capillary type (HPF). Focal congestion and hemorrhage with partial fibrous stromal septation. (e) Chorangioma with congestion and acute hemorrhagic infarction centrally.

Extremely fiber rich tumors are classified as fibromas. Independent of the subtype 3 % of the chorangiomas (capillary, fibrous) show preserved differentiation of both the cytotrophoblast and syncytiotrophoblast and are without cellular or nuclear atypia [6].

Chorangiomatosis

Chorangiomatosis is characterized by multiple chorangiomas, a minimum of 5, with a diffuse distribution in the placenta. In contrast to chorangiomas, an increased expression of bFGF and Angiopoietin in trophoblast and endothelial cells can be identified [7].

Pathogenesis

Chorangiomas are benign hamartomatous lesions caused by maldevelopmental angiogenesis due to angioblastem disorders. The etiology is unknown and the tumor can occur without any chromosomal or cytogenetic abnormalities or may be associated with cutaneous and hepatic fetal angiomas [8].

Differential diagnosis (chorangioma)
– intermediate subacute cotyledon infarction,
– chorangiocarcinoma (rarely),
– intraplacental leiomyoma with a basal/marginal localization (rarely) [9],
– intraplacental endometrial stromal tumor [10].

Differential diagnosis (microchorangioma)
– intraplacental hepatic adenoma, these tumors are found close to the chorionic plate and are several mm in size [11],
– nodular ectopic (heterotopic) liver tissue,
– nodular adrenal heterotopia in a subchorionic stem villus [12]. Heterotopia should be differentiated from the endotheliomatous subtype of microchorangioma; however, both are without clinical meaning.

Consequences for the mother
– preeclampsia,
– polyhydramnion,
– pre-term placental abruption,
– placental insufficiency due to reduced parenchymal function.

Consequences for the fetus
– arteriovenous (AV) shunts in large tumors and fetal cardiomegaly,
– fetal anemia due to hemorrhage caused by rupture of intra-tumoral vessels,
– feto-maternal transfusion,
– hemolytic anemia due to intravascular erythrocyte destruction,
– hydrops fetalis,
– IUGR,
– IUFD.

Consequences for the newborn
– pre-term delivery,
– Kasabach-Merritt-syndrome (microthrombosis in the tumor),

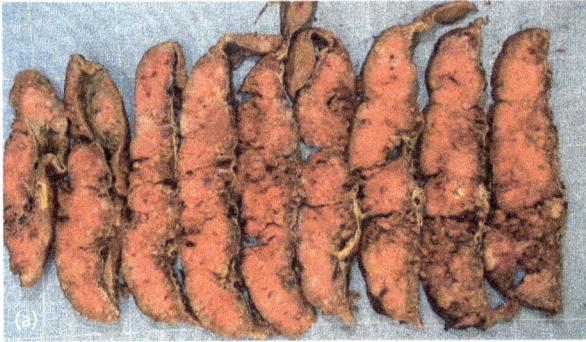

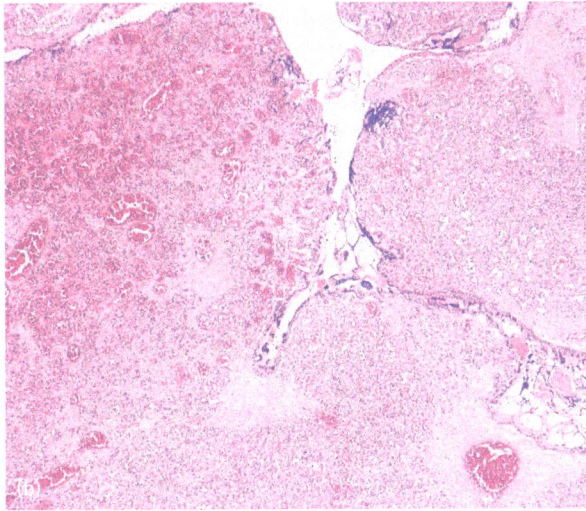

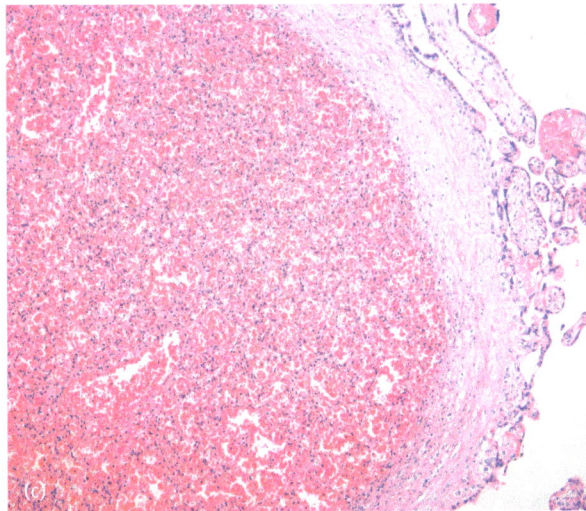

Fig. 10.3: (a) Macroscopic chorangiomatosis. Cut sections with multiple chorangiomas. Placenta in gestational week 40 + 2, net weight 627 g, fetal ascites, APGAR 2-4-7. (b) A chorangioma showing the typical lobular architecture and covered by trophoblast, mainly syncytial cells. (c) Tumor nodule of the capillary type that is separated from neighbouring villi by a broad fibrous capsule.

- hemorrhagic diathesis,
- hemolytic anemia,
- cardiomegaly,
- cardiac insufficiency,
- associated cutaneous angiomas, (without malignant potential),
- hepatic angiomas (rarely).

10.2 Teratoma

Teratomas are germ cell tumors arising from one or more of the three germ cell layers. They are rare, described infrequently in case reports, and are solid/cystic macroscopically. They are almost benign; without immature elements or malignant change in the mature elements. Teratomas may be found in the chorionic plate or in the umbilical cord.

Heterotopy of fetal tissue

Heterotopic tissue in the placenta may be identified on histology close to 2nd and 3rd order stem villi:
1. adrenal,
2. hepatic (liver tissue with portal fields, canaliculi and central vein)
   The frequency of such tissue is not adequately reported

Differential diagnosis
- fetus acardius amorphous,
- hepatic adenoma,
- teratoma (heterotopic fetal tissue is more organized)

Pathogenesis: Embryonic tissue displacement into the feto-placental circulation is considered to be the cause [12] and all three germ layers are represented (ecto, endo and mesodermal). Extraembryonic origin and monodermal teratomas are reported in cases of heterotopic hepatic adenoma [11,13]. Both should be differentiated from an endotheliomatous subtype of microchorangioma. These lesions are without any clinical significance.

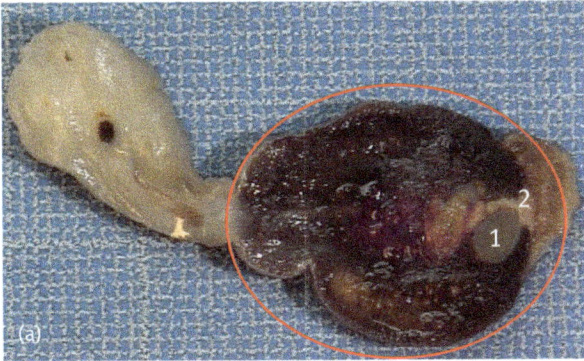

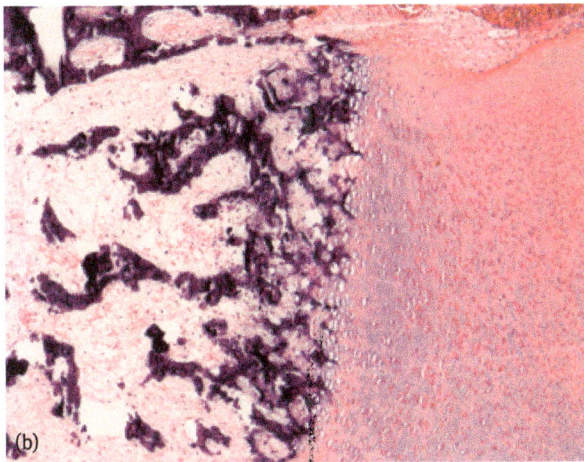

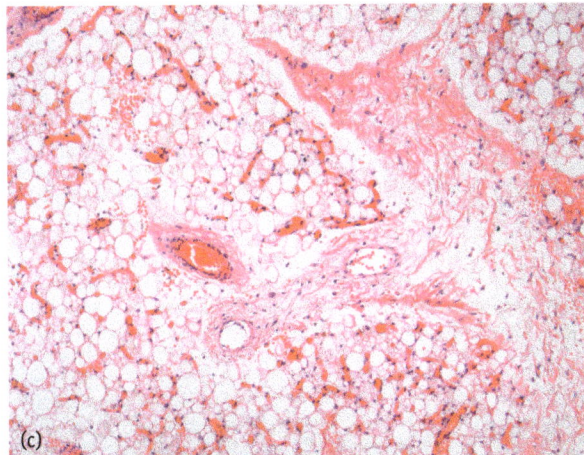

Fig. 10.4: (a) Umbilical cord teratoma (circled). Swollen umbilical cord with 2 × 1.5 × 2 cm encapsulated tumor with a dark red-brown cut surface. (1) Partly cystic areas, (2) small yellow pale fatty changes. (b) Teratoma with focal differentiation into cartilage and bone. (c) Teratoma with focal differentiation into lipid tissue. Placenta in gestational week 40.

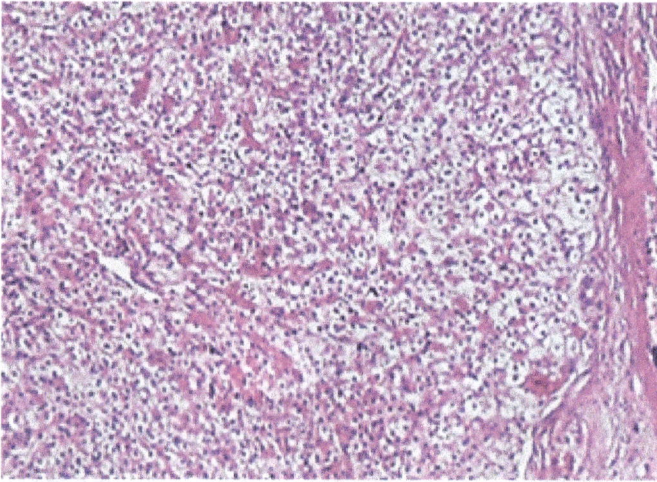

Fig. 10.5: Adrenal heterotopia with characteristic adrenocortical tissue in a stem villus.

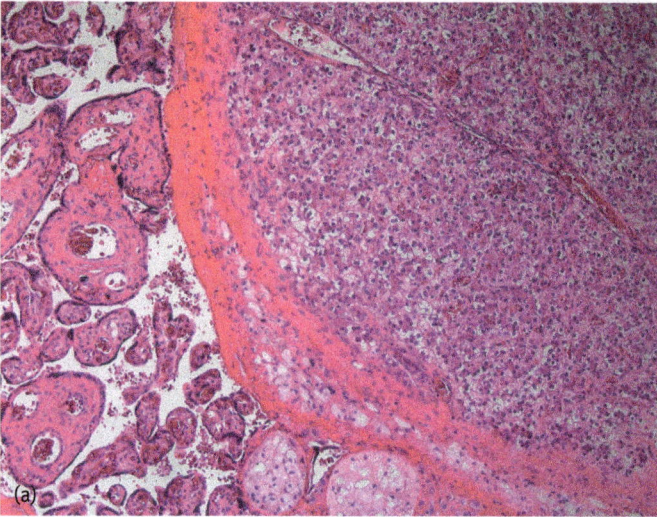

Fig. 10.6: (a) Incidental finding of ectopic liver tissue (containing a portal field, canaliculi and central vein) at an unknown gestational age (by courtesy of Dr. M. Haab, University Hospital, Institute for general and special pathology, Homburg, Saarland, Germany).

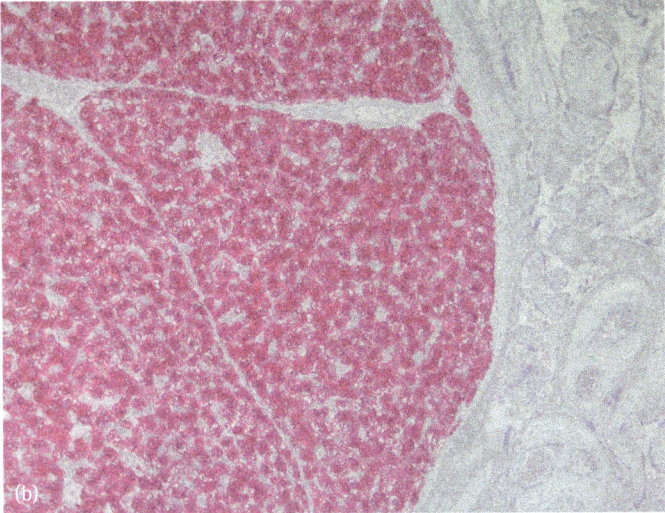

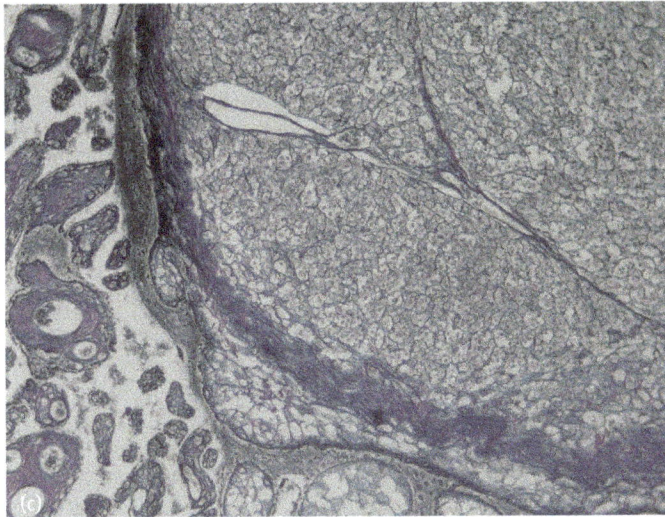

Fig. 10.6: (continued) (b) Ectopic liver tissue verified by immunohistochemistry for hepatocytes. (c) Ectopic liver tissue with architecture highlighted by reticulin staining.

10.3 Secondary tumors in the placenta

Secondary tumors in the placenta are defined as metastatic tumors originating from a primary maternal or fetal tumor.

Maternal primary tumors

Metastases from primary *maternal carcinoma* of the breast, ovary, lung, pancreas and kidneys to the intervillous space are reported [14,15]. Metastases from *malignant melanoma* have been identified in the villous stroma of the placenta, and even cases of *transplacental metastases to the fetus are reported* [13,16]. *In maternal lymphocytic leukemia* the phagocytic activity of the syncytiotrophoblast is interpreted as an immunological placental response [17]. Placental infiltration by *angioblastic sarcoma* and *Ewing sarcoma* have been reported [18,19].

Fetal primary tumors

Neuroblastomas have been reported to metastasize to the placenta and tumor cells have been identified in placental fetal capillaries; however, the etiology is not completely understood. These metastases are often associated with placental macrosomia, villous immaturity, villous stromal edema and fetal hydrops. Complications, such as decreased venous back flow due to fetal vessel tumor infiltration or long-standing venous compression by intra-abdominal tumor masses are reported [21].

Other metastases, such as *congenital leukemia* with infiltration in the fetal capillaries, *hepatoblastoma* [22] *and congenital nevus-cell-nevi melanocytes,* were seen in fetal vessels and in the stroma of stem- and intermediate villi [23].

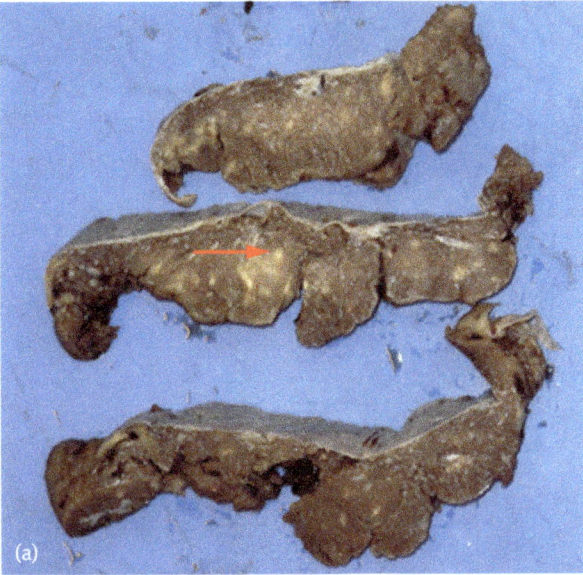

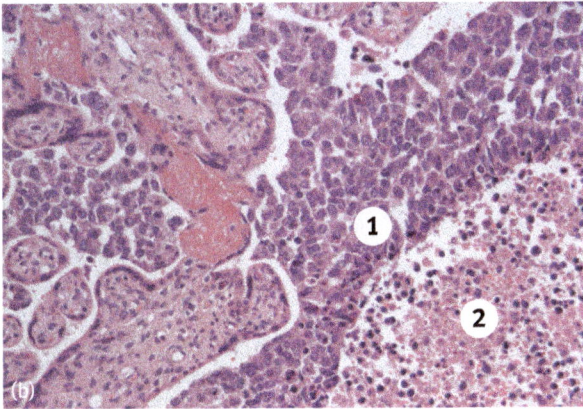

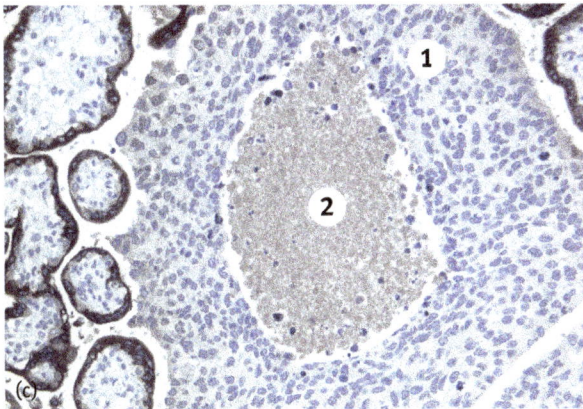

Fig. 10.7: (a) Breast cancer metastasis. Cut sections of the placenta show a pale parenchyma and small light-yellow nodular lesions focally. Placenta in gestational week 28 + 4, cesarean section on maternal indication [20]. (b) Histology of the breast cancer metastasis. Solid formation of polymorphic epithelial tumor cells in the intervillous space (1) with central necrosis (2). (c) Histology of the breast cancer metastasis. A solid formation of tumor cells (1) with central necrosis (2) is seen close to, but without evidence of infiltration in, the chorionic villi. Human chorionic gonadotropin (hCG) immunohistochemistry stains chorionic epithelium positive while the cancer metastasis is negative.

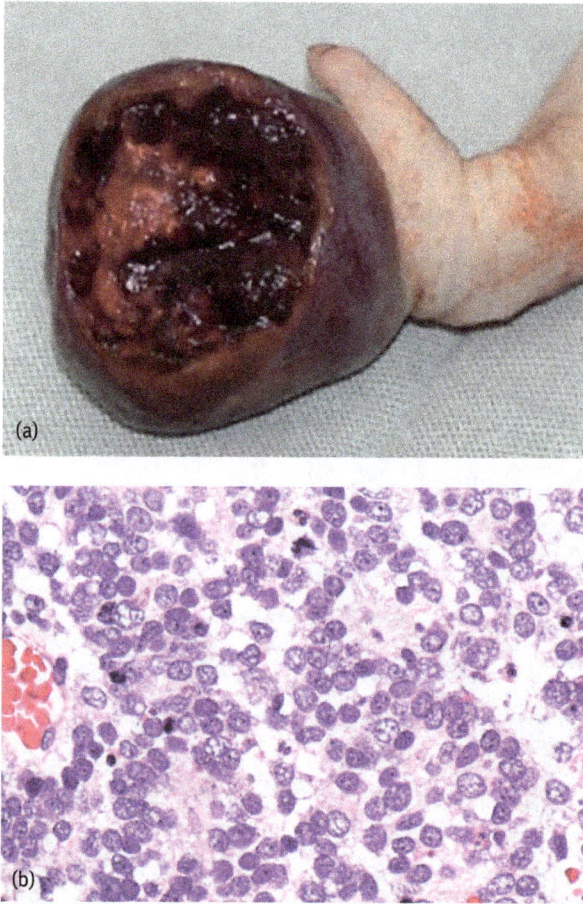

Fig. 10.8: (a) Fetal soft tissue sarcoma of the left hand of a neonate. The infant died 116 days after birth. Large dark-red and vascular tumor with excessive tumor necrosis. (by courtesy of Prof. Dr. Ratschek, Pathological Department, University Hospital Graz, Austria) [23]. (b) Undifferentiated tumor. Cells with round nuclei, granular chromatin and small nucleoli.

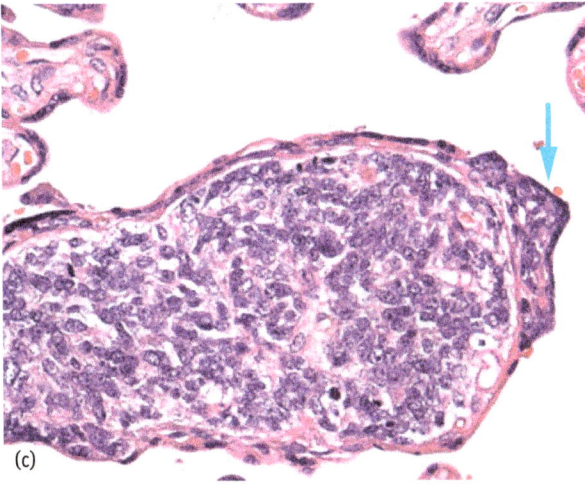

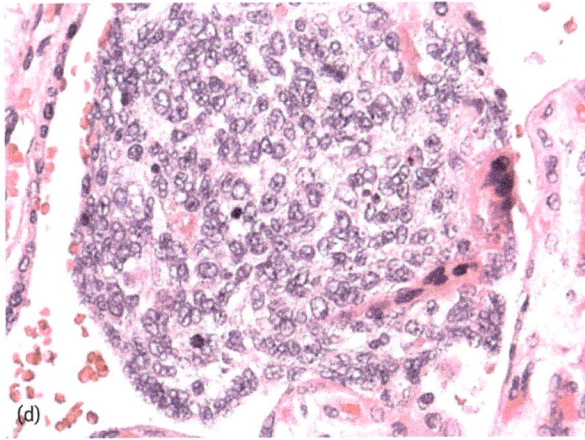

Fig. 10.8: (continued) (c) Intraplacental metastasis. Villus containing a solid sheet of tumour cells and a villous trophoblast with a small focus of infiltrating tumor cells (arrow). (d) Tumor cells infiltrating into the maternal intervillous space.

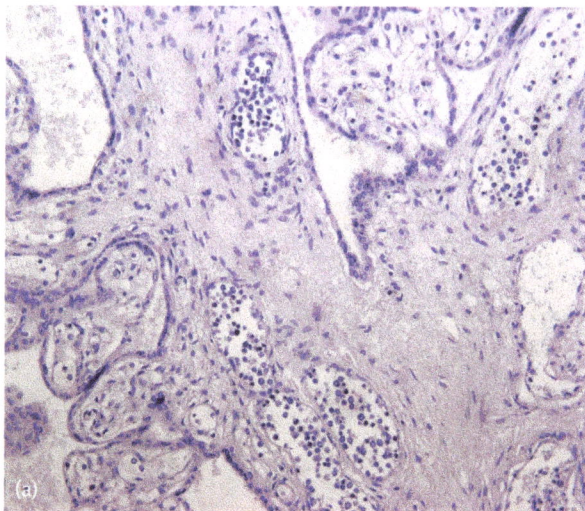

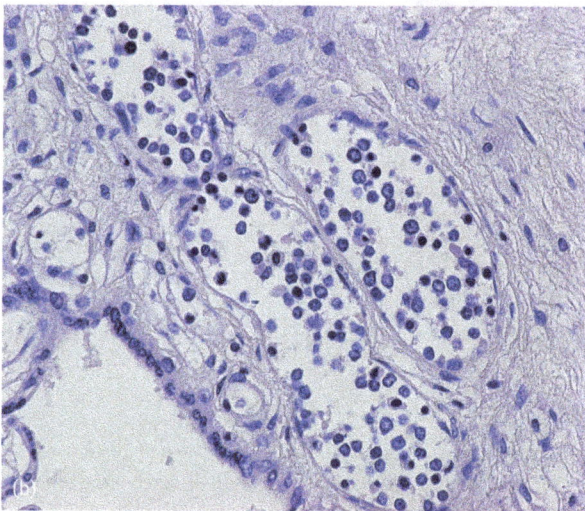

Fig. 10.9: (a) Congenital acute myeloblastic leukemia. Stem villus vessels with intraluminal atypical, blast-like fetal blood cells of varying size. Spontaneous delivery in GW 36 with fetal anemia and perinatal death at 8 days of age. (b) Congenital acute myeloblastic leukemia (HPF).

References

[1]   Guschmann M, Henrich W, Entezami M, Dudenhausen JW. Chorioangioma--new insights into a well-known problem. I. Results of a clinical and morphological study of 136 cases. J Perinat Med. 2003;31(2):163–169.

[2]   Altshuler G. Chorangiosis. An important placental sign of neonatal morbidity and mortality. Arch Pathol Lab Med. 1984;108(1):71–74.

[3]   Ogino S, Redline RW. Villous capillary lesions of the placenta: distinctions between chorangioma, chorangiomatosis, and chorangiosis. Hum Pathol. 2000;31(8):945–954.

[4]   Fox H. Haemangiomata of the placenta. J Clin Pathol. 1966;19(2):133–137.

[5]   Becker V, Schiebler TH, Kubli F. Allgemeine und spezielle Pathologie der Plazenta. Die Plazenta des Menschen. Stuttgart: Thieme; 1981. p. 251–393.

[6]   Vogel M. Atlas der morphologischen Plazentadiagnostik. 2 ed. Berlin: Springer; 1996.

[7]   Guschmann M. [Growth factors and apoptosis rate in an unusual chorangioma]. Pathologe. 2002;23(5):389–391.

[8]   Manzke H, Mau G. [Correlation of obstetrical and clinical data with nevi flammei in the newborn (author's transl)]. Monatsschr Kinderheilkd. 1975;123(3):124–127.

[9]   Ernst LM, Hui P, Parkash V. Intraplacental smooth muscle tumor: a case report. Int J Gynecol Pathol. 2001;20(3):284–288.

[10] Karpf EF, Poetsch B, Langner C, Nogales FF, Regauer S. Endometrial stromal nodule embedded into term placenta. APMIS. 2007;115(11):1302–1305.

[11] Dargent JL, Verdebout JM, Barlow P, et al. Hepatocellular adenoma of the placenta: report of a case associated with maternal bicornuate uterus and fetal renal dysplasia. Histopathology. 2000;37(3):287–289.

[12] Guschmann M, Vogel M, Urban M. Adrenal tissue in the placenta: a heterotopia caused by migration and embolism? Placenta. 2000;21(4):427–431.

[13] Benirschke K, Burton G, Baergen RN. Pathology of the human placenta. 6 ed. New York: Springer; 2012.

[14] De Carolis S, Garofalo S, Degennaro VA, et al. Placental and infant metastasis of maternal melanoma: a new case. J Obstet Gynaecol. 2015;35(4):417–418.

[15] Potter JF, Schoeneman M. Metastasis of maternal cancer to the placenta and fetus. Cancer. 1970;25(2):380–388.

[16] Brodsky I, Baren M, Kahn SB, Lewis G Jr., Tellem M. Metastatic Malignant Melanoma from Mother to Fetus. Cancer. 1965;18:1048–1054.

[17] Wang T, Hamann W, Hartge R. Structural aspects of a placenta from a case of maternal acute lymphatic leukaemia. Placenta. 1983;4(2):185–195.

[18] Frick R, Rummel H, Heberling D, Schmidt WO. [Placental metastases from a maternal angioblastic sarcoma of the vagina (author's transl)]. Geburtshilfe Frauenheilkd. 1977;37(3):216–220.

[19] Greenberg P, Collins JD, Voet RL, Jariwala L. Ewing's sarcoma metastatic to placenta. Placenta. 1982;3(2):191–196.

[20] Froehlich K, Stensheim H, Markert UR, Turowski G. Breast carcinoma in pregnancy with spheroid-like placental metastases-a case report. APMIS. 2018;126(5):448–452.

[21] Smith CR, Chan HS, deSa DJ. Placental involvement in congenital neuroblastoma. J Clin Pathol. 1981;34(7):785–789.

[22] Robinson HB Jr., Bolande RP. Case 3. Fetal hepatoblastoma with placental metastases. Pediatr Pathol. 1985;4(1–2):163–167.

[23] Reif P, Hofer N, Kolovetsiou-Kreiner V, Benedicic C, Ratschek M. Metastasis of an undifferentiated fetal soft tissue sarcoma to the maternal compartment of the placenta: maternal aspects, pathology findings and review of the literature on fetal malignancies with placenta metastases. Histopathology. 2014;65(6):933–942.

11 Pathology of the placenta in early pregnancy

Definition

Abortion may be defined as a spontaneous or induced pre-term termination of a non-viable gestational product in the first half of gestation (up to week 20) or, if accurate dating is not possible, a gestational product less than 500 g in weight:

- spontaneous abortion
- therapeutic abortion: Artificial (medical or instrumental) pre-term limitation of pregnancy on medical, ethical or social indications
- forensic abortion: Termination of a pregnancy occurring in a jurisdiction with laws prohibiting such terminations [1].

Classification

1. Early loss of pregnancy: loss of products of conception before, during or shortly after implantation. The pregnancy perishes in ca. 50 % in the first 3 weeks after fertilization; ca. 20 % before implantation, 10 % during implantation and 20 % during the first two weeks after implantation [2].

2. Embryonic abortion: loss of products of conception between Gestational Week (GW) 5–14. The critical developmental embryonic stage, with a high susceptibility to noxious insults, finishes in week 8 (Gestational Week 10) and formal organogenesis is completed in week 12 (Gestational Week 14)

The majority of developmental embryonic disorders result in spontaneous abortion. Embryonic abortion should be subclassified into:

- early abortion: Abortions until Gestational Week 8 p. c. (gestational week 10).
- late abortion: Abortions occurring after Gestational Week 10 (1).

Implanted embryos have an abortion rate of ca. 15 %, of which 90 % are spontaneous abortions before gestational week 14. Similar pregnancy loss is observed in IVF treatment [3].

3. Fetal abortion: a termination of pregnancy from gestational week 15 onwards with a fetus less than 500 g in weight (lawful in Germany) [4].

Both spontaneous and therapeutic abortions, from Gestational Week 15 onward, are of a different etiology than embryonic abortions and, therefore the procedure of fetal autopsy and placental examination is different [5].

11.1 Early embryonic loss of pregnancy

Early embryonic abortion may be diagnosed by β-HCG and β-Glycoprotein (SP1) levels. It frequently presents as delayed menstrual bleeding and is defined as a pre-clinical abortion [6].

https://doi.org/10.1515/9783110452600-011

Morphology

The gestational sac is a few millimeters in diameter and shows, if identifiable, decidualized mucosa.

Extrauterine pregnancy should be considered when menstrual bleeding is not documented.

Pathogenesis

- chromosomal aberration (monosomy and trisomy),
- hormonal dysregulation,
- implantation disorder: inadequately developed endometrium (such as pre-term decidualization)
- defective endometrial estrogen deficiency(due to mechanical and toxic factors hampering implantation) [7],
- disorder of maternal immune tolerance [8], by maternal immune system deficiency.

11.2 Embryonic abortion

Definition

Loss of products of conception between gestational week 5 and 14.

Pathogenesis

- Chromosomal aberrations (monosomy, trisomy et al)
- hormonal dysregulation,
- local implantation disorders,
- feto-maternal immune disorder,
- maternal disease,
- environmental factors,
- infection

11.2.1 Examination of abortion material

In many cases morphological examination alone does not explain the cause of abortion and supplementary investigations, such as: cytogenetics, molecular biology, immunology, biochemistry, microbiology and virology may be required.

Macroscopy

Abortion material includes the gestational sac, decidua and blood clots. The gestational sac may be preserved, but it is often ruptured or fragmented. Careful examination of the material is paramount, and to easily distinguish chorionic villi from decidua it is recommend to perform the examination with the material submerged in water as the chorionic villi will float and enfold.

The embryo should be examined separately and macroscopic photography is strongly advised.

If genetic investigations are necessary the tissue to be examined (chorionic, amniotic or even embryonic tissue) should be stored in an antibiotic containing medium.

Macroscopic essential findings:
- total weight and weight of the gestational sac and embryo,
- maximum diameter in mm of the gestational sac (both open and closed),
- amniotic cavity and yolk sac,
- length and diameter of the umbilical cord,
- embryonic length in mm and macroscopic characteristics.

Maldeveloped embryos are classified according to the grade of developmental disorder (Table. 11.1).

Table 11.1: Categorization of the morphological disorganization of the embryo into GD 1–4.

GD	embryonic growth disorganization
1	missing embryo, empty gestational sac
2	nodule like embryo, up to 4 mm length, with no retinal pigment and no differentiated caudal and cranial poles
3	cylindrical embryo, from 4 to 10 mm length, with partial retinal pigment and partially differentiated caudal and cranial poles
4	embryo longer than 10 mm with profound malformation and partially differentiated caudal and cranial poles. Extremity stubs may be present

GD = embryonic growth disorganization [9].

Embryonic disorganization may be further classified according to the following:
- embryo with local defect
- autolytic embryo: the criteria mentioned above are less useful in this situation,
- umbilical cord rudiment with missing embryo: caused by complete resorption [10].

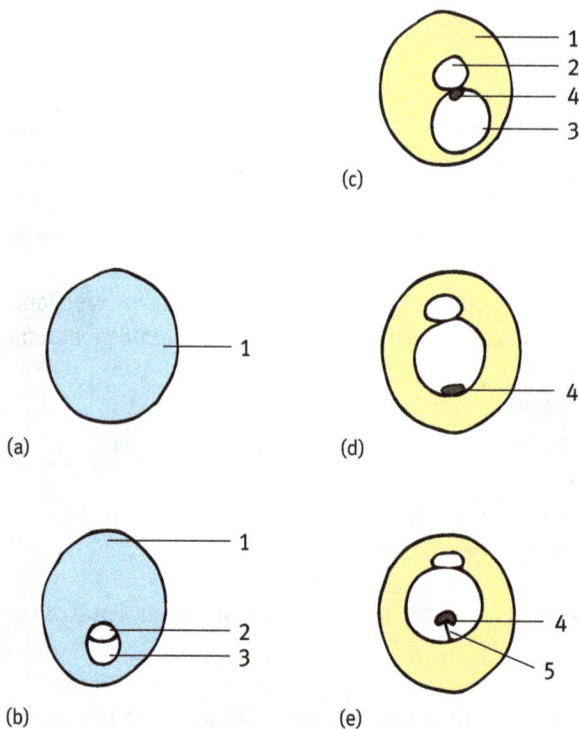

Fig. 11.1: Illustration. Embryonic growth disorganization subtypes GD 1–4 (Table 11.1): (a) GD 1: (1) empty gestational sac ; (b) GD 1: (1) gestational sac; (2) yolk sac; (3) amniotic sac; (c) GD 2: (4) nodular embryo; (d) GD 3: (4) cylindrical embryo; (e) GD 4: (4) profound malformed; (5) umbilical cord.

Abortion material up to GW 8 (age determination by CRL (crown-rump-length)/SSL (Scheitel-Steiß-Länge) or size of the gestational sac), shows findings of:
– a whole and empty gestational sac in 13 %,
– a torn gestational sac without umbilical cord, yolk sac and amnion in 23 %,
– a torn gestational sac with umbilical cord, yolk sac and amnion in 25 %,
– an embryo in 25 % [11,12].

50 % of early abortions are considered complete (containing both an embryo and a gestational sac), and 50 % are incomplete [13]:
– *complete* products of conception (50 %):
  – GD embryo 24 %,
  – normal embryo 10 %,
  – embryo with focal defect 8 %,
  – fragmented, degenerative or malformed embryo 8 %.
– incomplete (50 %):
  – open or fragmented 38 %,
  – decidua only 12 %.

Cut sections: The gestational sac should be opened and cut in serially in sagittal sections, with chorionic plate (Fig. 11.2). Products of conception with a gestational sac diameter less 30 mm should be completely embedded.

Cut sections from the decidua and umbilical cord should also be embedded.

Morphology

Histological examination should include the chorionic villi and (also presumptive) chorionic plate. The umbilical cord vessel branches, seen in longitudinally oriented connective tissue close to the chorionic plate vessels, should be distinguished from capillaries in the suprachorionic loose mesenchyme. Stem and peripheral chorionic villi should be distinguished.

Stem villi are characterized by the infiltration of branching chorionic plate vessels in the villous axis and early paravascular differentiation of collagenous fibers. Evidence of allantois vessels in the chorionic plate and stem villi are evident after embryonic implantation. Even if the embryo is not macroscopically visible, developmental age and developmental disorders may be evaluated.

Peripheral villi represent an important differentiation of the chorionic epithelium and they, as well as, the quality of villous stroma and the differentiation of autochthone capillaries should be assessed.

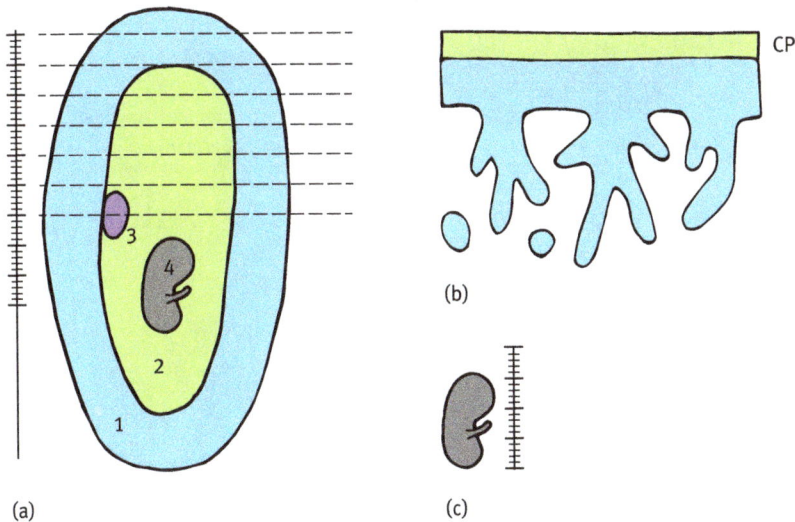

Fig. 11.2: Illustration. Recommended macroscopic sectioning for histological examination: (1) amniotic sac; (2) chorionic sac; (3) yolk sac; (4) embryo; (a) serial cut sections of the gestational sac; (b) chorion frondosum, chorionic plate (CP); (c) embryonic examination should be done separately (4).

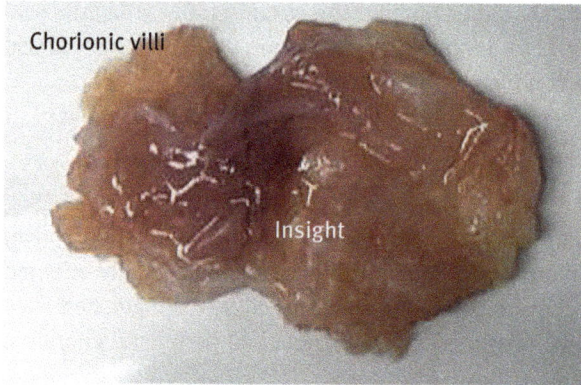

Fig. 11.3: Normal open gestational sac in gestational week 7, after formalin fixation. View insight

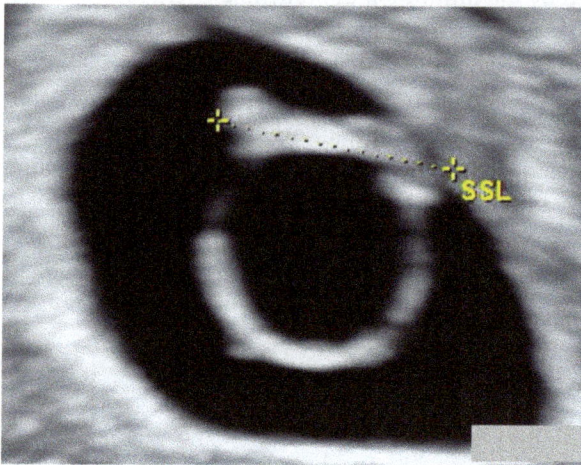

Fig. 11.4: Ultrasound. Normal pregnancy in Gestational Week 6. Measurements show the CRL / SSL (by courtesy of Prof Brückmann, office for prenatal diagnostics in Erfurt, Germany).

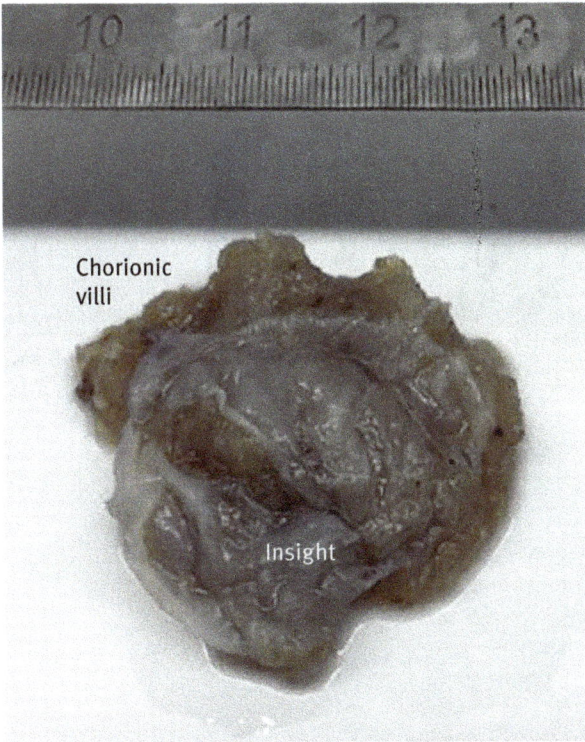

Fig. 11.5: Formalin fixed gestational sac in GW 8. Open and without embryo (by courtesy PD. Dr. Tennstedt-Schenk, Mühlhausen, Germany).

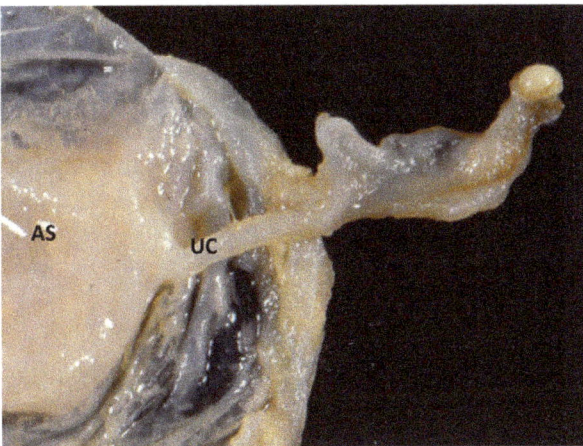

Fig. 11.6: Embryonic growth disorganization, GD 2, with a nodule like embryo: amniotic sac (AS), umbilical Cord (UC) [39].

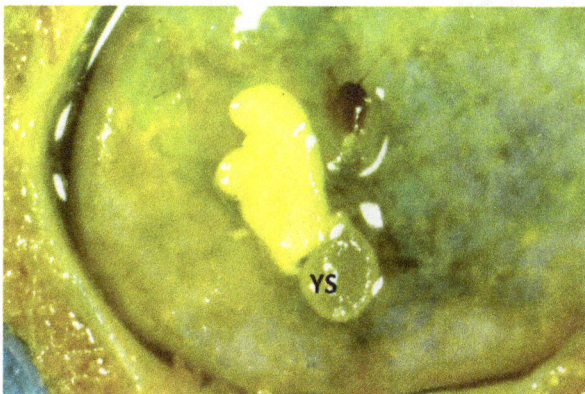

Fig. 11.7: Embryonic Growth Disorganization, GD4: yolk sac (YS) [39].

11.3 Special pathology in embryonic abortions

- Villous developmental disorders,
- villous changes due to chromosomal abnormalities
- villous maturation disorders,
- circulatory disturbance,
- implantation disorder,
- inflammation,
- villous retention,
- rudiments of implantation.

Placental developmental disorders, villous maturation disorders, circulatory disturbance and implantation pathology are most often seen in spontaneous abortions during the 1st trimester. Inflammation of the chorionic tissue is an infrequent finding.

11.3.1 Villous developmental disorders

Definition

Villous developmental disorders are defined as primary developmental disorders of the villous trophoblast and the extraembryonic mesenchyme. They are examples of non-molar "villous trophoblastic diseases" and are seen in more than 55 % of spontaneous embryonic abortions up to gestational week 12 [14]. If villous developmental disorders are sufficiently diffuse the gestational product is unable to develop. The embryo may be absent or may show global or multiple areas of localized growth disorganization (GD). In approximately 60 % of cases chromosomal abnormalities could be shown.

Morphological classification
1. blighted ovum (Windmole), anembryonic pregnancy,
2. embryonic mole with malformed embryo,
3. unclassifiable, frequently in cases of prolonged retention.

Morphological anembryonic and embryonic moles are frequently referred to as hydropic abortions in the literature, partly associated with polysomal chromosomal abnormalities [15,16].

Both, "Windmole" and "Embryonic mole" are not included in the WHO classification of villous "Gestational Trophoblastic Diseases" (GTD), which lists (see Table 12.1):
– partial hydatidiform mole,
– complete hydatidiform mole,
– invasive mole

Instead, the WHO defines abnormal (non-molar) villous developmental disorders as villous lesions which may mimic a partial hydatidiform mole (PHM) clinically and histologically [17].

Macroscopy is diagnostic for both anembryonic (Windmole) and embryonic mole, with microscopic examination only a supplement to the diagnostic process. In 15 % of the cases the findings are equivocal and such cases are considered unclassifiable.

11.3.1.1 Blighted ovum (Windmole)

Definition: A non-molar villous developmental disorder with a hypoplastic villous trophoblast and without an embryo.

Macroscopy: The amniotic sac is empty (anembryonic) and without evidence of early resorption. (GD 1)

Morphology:
– Chorionic plate without visible fetal vessel branches (from the connecting stalk or umbilical cord) in the chorionic plate,
– no stem villi,
– predominantly irregular villous diameters,
– smooth villous surface,
– flattened, irregular single- and double-layered villous epithelium that can be nuclear free,
– few nuclear sprouts (hypoplastic villous epithelium),
– loosely meshed stroma with hydropic, mucoid and occasionally fibrous degeneration,
– Rare endothelial tubes and/or small autochthone capillaries.

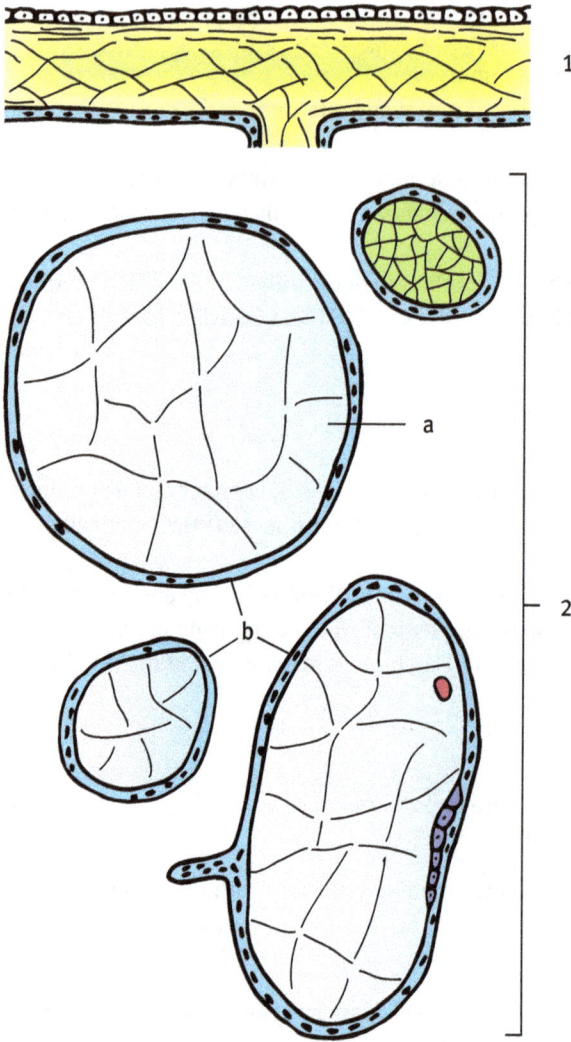

Fig. 11.8: Illustration. Blighted ovum (anembryonic pregnancy): (1) corionic plate without fetal vessels; (2) villi; (a) stroma mainly mucoid / hydropic, rarely fibrous; (b) hypoplastic and flattened villous trophoblast.

Pathogenesis: Developmental disorder with loss of embryonic conception before embryonic-placental circulation occurs. The critical phase of termination is considered to be late in the 3rd developmental week; the late secondary villous and early tertiary villous developmental period. In 60 % of anembryonic pregnancies karyotyping identified chromosomal abnormalities, mainly autosomal trisomy and tetrasomy. Risk factors in cases of non-chromosomal disorders are shown in Table 11.3.

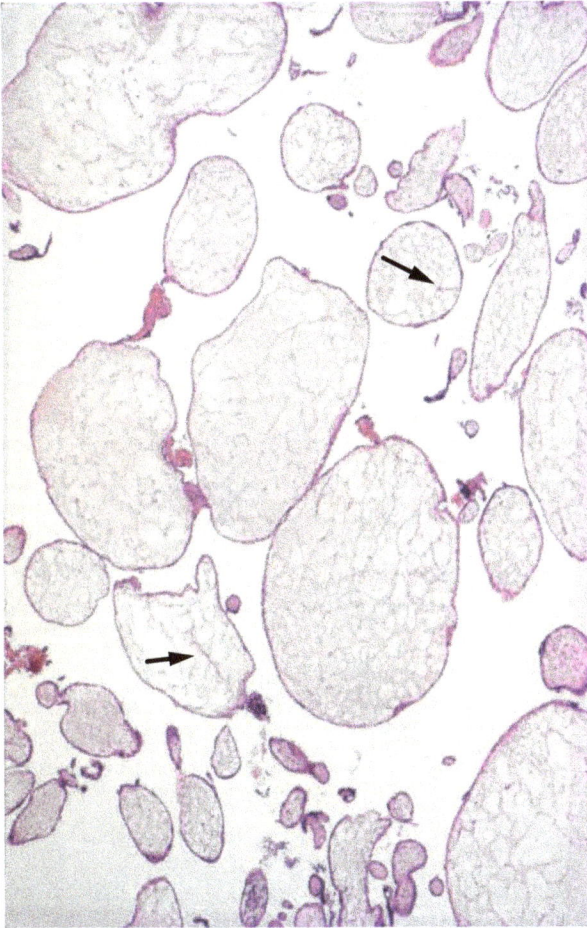

Fig. 11.9: Blighted ovum in GW 8. Enlarged villi without stem villi, mucoid and hydropic stroma with small capillaries (arrows), fibrous stroma in small villi and a hypoplastic villous trophoblast with a flattened single- and double-layered epithelium with areas lacking nuclei.

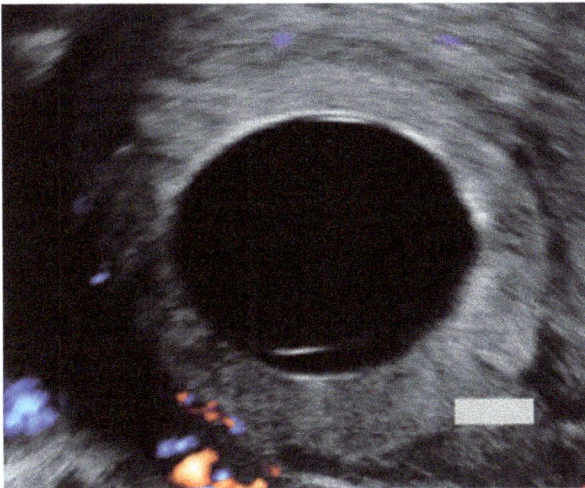

Fig. 11.10: Ultrasound. Blighted ovum (Windmole) in gestational week 6 (by courtesy of Prof Brückmann, office for prenatal diagnostics in Erfurt, Germany).

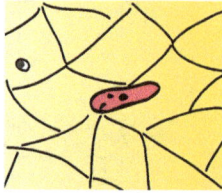

(1)

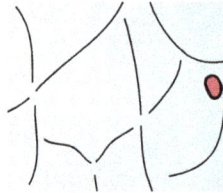

(4)

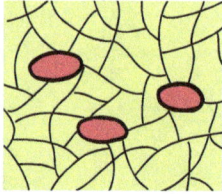

(2)

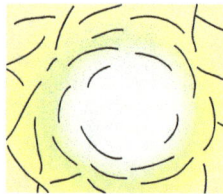

(5)

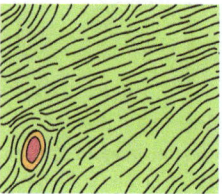

(3)

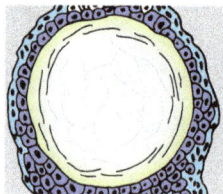

(6)

Fig. 11.11: Illustration. Stroma types in embryonic abortions. (1) Embryonic, (2) reticular, (3) fibrous, (4) hydropic/mucoid, (5) mole-like, (6) villous bulla.

11.3.1.2 Embryonic mole

Definition: A villous developmental disorder with a dysplastic villous trophoblast and a global growth disorganization of the embryo (GD malformation).

Macroscopy: Embryo with global GD malformation (GD 2–4) /a residual umbilical cord.

Morphology:
- Chorionic plate vessels with thin and primitive walls,
- stem villi with abortive vessels in the villous axis and few capillaries,
- peripheral villi of varying diameter, with partly indented surfaces,
- irregular single- and double-layered villous epithelium with nuclear sprouts,
- dysplastic villous trophoblast with single migrating villous trophoblast cells (intermediate type) in the stroma,
- dysplastic villous trophoblast with solid or small and cystic endovillous trophoblast cell clusters,

- variation in the villous stroma; dense embryonic, hydropic or partly mole-like, degenerated, reticular, fibrous ('multicolored stroma picture'),
- few capillaries with rare nucleated erythrocytes.

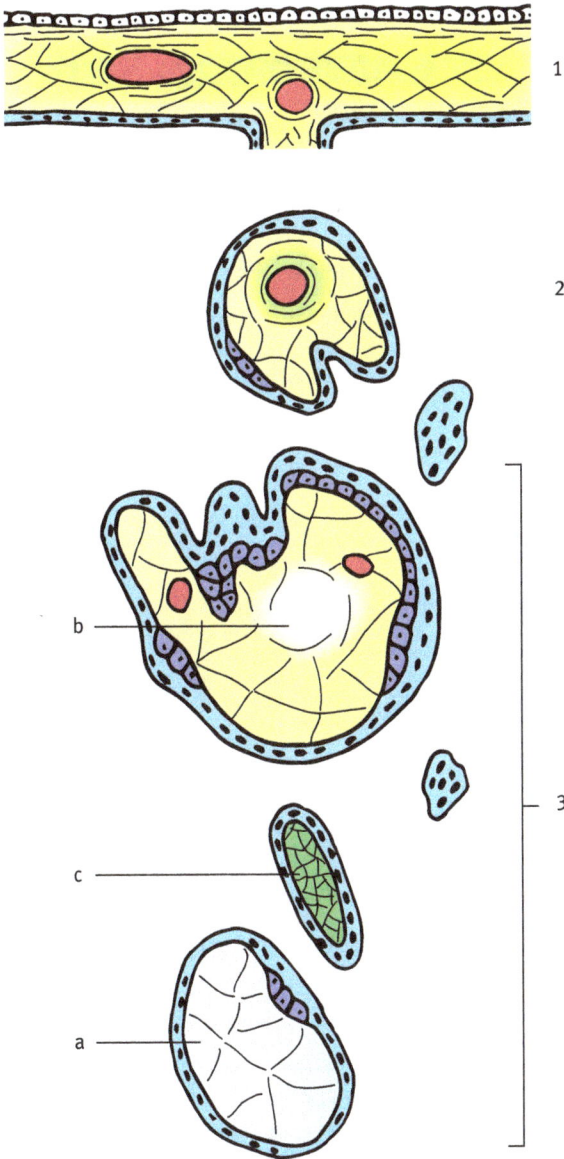

Fig. 11.12: Illustration. Embryonic mole. (1) Chorionic plate, (2) Stem villi, (3) Peripheral villi with (a) hydropic / mucoid stroma, (b) mole-like stroma and (c) fibrous stroma.

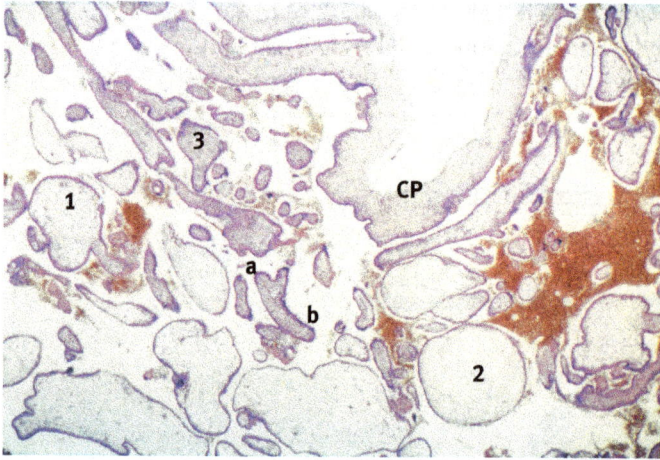

Fig. 11.13: Embryonic mole in gestational week 9 with a "multicolored stroma" picture (MPF). Chorionic plate (CP) with villi of various diameter showing a partly embryonic stroma (1); hydropic stroma (2); fibrous stroma and a (3) prominent single- (a) and double-layered (b) villous trophoblast.

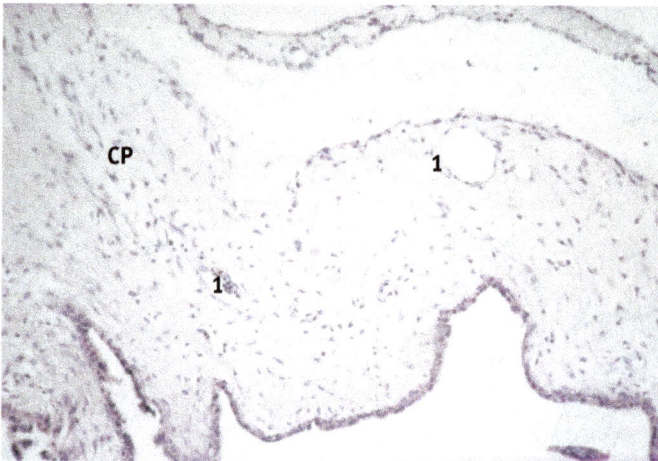

Fig. 11.14: Embryonic mole in Gestational Week 11. Chorionic plate (CP) with hypoplastic fetal vessel branches (1) (by courtesy PD. Dr. Tennstedt-Schenk, Mühlhausen, Germany).

Pathogenesis: Developmental disorders with a preserved embryo and embryonic-placental vessels. The critical phase for termination occurs early in developmental week 4. In embryonic moles, more often than in anembryonic pregnancies, aneuploidy due to non-disjunction is identified by karyotyping. Chromosomal abnormalities such as trisomy and x-monosomy have been identified in these cases (Table 11.2).

Relative frequency of classifiable placental developmental disorders:
- blighted ovum 28%
- embryonic mole in 55 %
- partial hydatidiform mole (PHM) in 14.5 %,
- complete hydatidiform mole CHM) in 2.5 % [18]

Differential Diagnosis
- Regular villous development (Ch. 1)
- Arrest of villous maturation (Ch. 8)
- Partial mole/early complete mole (Ch. 12)
- Retention changes ("missed abortion") (Ch. 11.3.7)

11.3.2 Villous changes/phenotype in chromosomal aberrations

Comparisons between histological findings in early embryonic abortions and cytogenetic controls show that early embryonic abortions are more frequently associated with villous developmental disorders due to chromosomal abnormalities. Clinically they are classified as abortive products or missed abortions between Gestational Weeks 5 and 14.

Table 11.2: Histological and cytogenetic findings in spontaneous abortion between Gestational Weeks 5 and 14.

histological findings	number of cases	cytogenetic karyotype			
		normal (n)	%	aberrant (n)	%
anembryonic(Windmole)/embryonic mole	260	71	27.3	189	72.7
PHM	59	3	5.1	56	94.9
CHM	7	7	100	0	
villous maturation arrest, hypoplasia of fetal vessels	68	40	58.8	28	41.2
circulatory disturbance	33	26	78.8	7	21.2
implantation disorders	8	8	100.0	0	
retention, unclassified	75	33	44.0	42	56.0
normal development	102	87	85.2	15	14.8

Karyotyping of early embryonic abortions identified, in order of decreasing frequency, the following numerical chromosomal abnormalities: trisomy, triploidy, XO monosomy, tetraploidy and rarely structural anomalies.

While morphological examination may suggest a chromosomal abnormality, as some histological characteristics are more often seen in early embryonic abortions than in normal euploid controls, a single finding is rarely pathognomonic.

Table 11.3: Characteristic changes in abortion material due to chromosome abnormalities between GW 5 and 14. A combination of histological findings is required for diagnosis. Isolated findings are insufficient [19]. *Chi²-Test after Yates; + = p < 0,05, ++ = p < 0.01

diagnostic characteristics of abortion with chromosomal aberration	significance in opposite to abortion *with normal karyotype
chorionic plate	
– allantois vessel hypoplasia (capillary)	+
stem villi	
– lack of vessel development	+
– absent or partial development of villi	+ +
peripheral villi	
– irregular and reduced branching	+
– large diameter	+ +
– multicoloured stroma picture	+
– hydropic and molar	+ +
– hydropic and fibrous	+ +
– lack of capillaries	+
chorionic epithelium	
– irregular, single- and dual-layered with migration of trophoblast cells	+ + +
– hyperplasia of syncytiotrophoblast	+ +
– epithelial invagination / endovillous microcysts	+ +

The diagnosis of chromosomal abnormalities on histology alone is controversial. Diagnosis of abortion, with aneuploidy, on chorionic villus histology alone is in 50 % to 55 % accurate. In a prospective study of abortion material, using comparative histological and cytogenetic examinations, chromosomal abnormalities were correctly diagnosed in 60 % of cases by histology alone. In a subsequent examination, non-blinded to cytogenetic results, the diagnoses rate increased to 75 %; however, even ca 20 % of abortions with a normal karyotype were diagnosed as having villous developmental disorders. This occurred if the gestational sac was sufficiently damaged at a very early stage to cause an abortion. Suspicion of a chromosomal abnormality on morphology needs to be reported promptly to allow for clinical discussion and parental counseling [20].

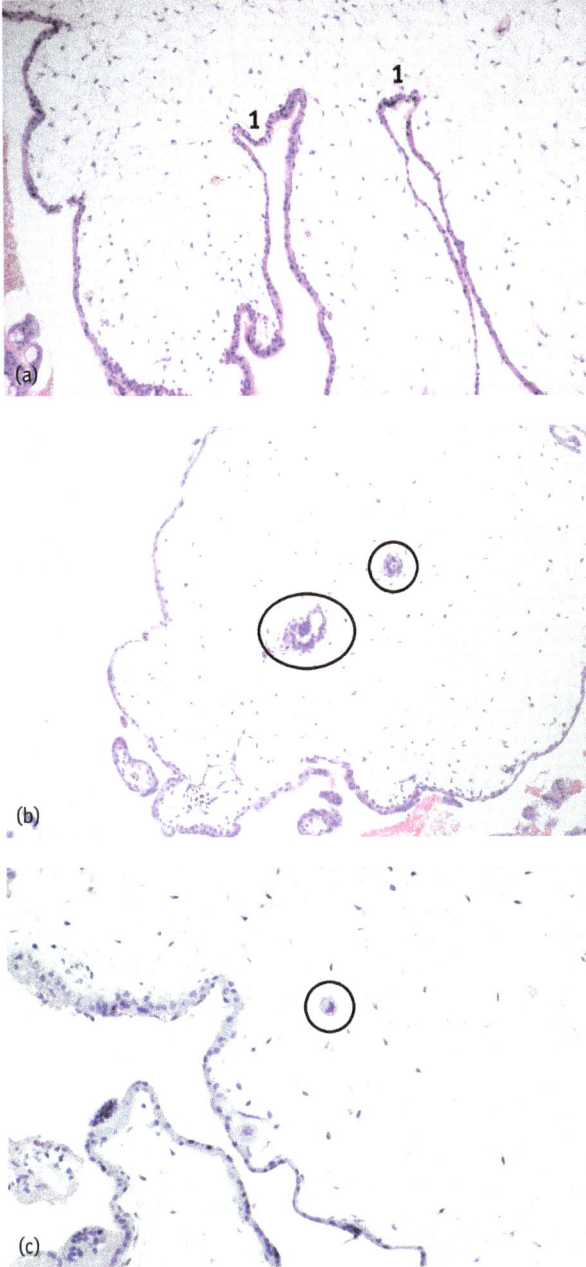

Fig. 11.15: (a) Trisomy 16. Endovillous trophoblastic invagination (1). (b) Trisomy 16. Microcystic trophoblastic inclusions (circled). (c) Trisomy 16. Endovillous intermediate trophoblast cell migration in the stroma (circled). [39]

Risk factors in spontaneous abortion with a normal karyotype

Retrospectively the following risk factors were identified in the maternal history:
- maternal age greater than 30 years
- nicotine use; greater than 20 cigarettes a day before and during pregnancy
- hormonal contraceptive use up to the beginning of pregnancy
- irregular cycle
- history of two or more miscarriages
- history of abortion immediately prior to pregnancy
- maternal obesity, BMI > 40
- maternal disease, such as: diabetes mellitus, chronic hypertension, systemic lupus erythematosus

11.3.3 Villous maturation disorders (Ch. 8)

Villous maturation disorders are identified in many abortions with embryo-lethal developmental disorders with a normal placental formation. Villous maturation disorders affect normal villous development and the formation of the stem and peripheral villi. The embryo may be: normal, malformed, have focal defects, may be better developed than in an embryonic mole, may demonstrate maldevelopment of different grades or be autolytic. Villous maturation disorders are the 2nd most prevalent of the villous developmental disorders during the 1st trimester. Villous maturation disorders were seen in 6 % of abortions and in more than 11 % of spontaneous abortions. Villous maturation disorders that are focal and occur before gestational week 10 are challenging to diagnose.

The most significant villous maturation disorders are:
- arrest of villous maturation
- chorangiosis type I.

Arrest of villous maturation

Morphology:
- umbilical vessel branches in the chorionic plate,
- homogeneous connective tissue in the chorionic plate,
- thin walled vessels in the stem villi with paravascular loose fibres and a very small tunica media,
- deficient villous branching resulting in groups of large and medium sized villi,
- flat single-layered and adjacent dual-layered villous trophoblast with reduced cytotrophoblastic cells,
- embryonic stroma with few capillaries.

Arrest of villous maturation is more frequently focal rather than diffuse. Identification of vessels in the chorion and stem villi is most important distinguishing factor between an embryonic mole and anembryonic pregnancy (blighted ovum) (Table 11.4). Stem villous vessels are often hypoplastic with poorly developed media.

Table 11.4: Differential diagnosis of blighted ovum, embryonic mole and arrest of villous maturation.

	anembryonic pregnancy (blighted ovum)	embryonic mole	arrest of villous maturation
embryo	missing	global malformation	normal embryo, localized defect
chorionic plate			
– umbilical vessel branches	missing	few and hypoplastic vessel walls	hypoplastic vessels
– suprachorionic capillaries	missing/very seldom	few	varying
– stem villi			
– axial vessels	missing	abortive, rudimentary	present, thin vessel wall
– axial paravascular fiber rings		sparse, irregular	loose fibres
villous diameter	predominantly large	irregular and large	large-/medium sized
chorionic surface	smooth	irregular, invaginations	smooth
villous chorionic epithelium	smooth, mainly single-, or adjacent double-layered, partly nuclear free (villous trophoblast hypoplasia)	single/double-layered, endovillous trophoblast cell migration, small cell clusters (villous trophoblast dysplasia)	flat, single/ > double-layered
nuclear sprouts	few	frequent, many	some
trophoblast islands	few	frequent/partial fibrinoid degeneration	some
villous stroma	loose and cell poor. Hydropic/mucoid, partly molar like, rarely fibrous	varying, side by side embryonic, hydropic/ molar like, cell rich, reticular, fibrous	embryonic – hydropic/ reticular
villous capillaries	seldom	few	few

Pathogenesis: The majority of spontaneous abortions with maturation arrest show a normal karyotype. In approximately 40 % chromosomal abnormalities, such as trisomy 13, 18 and 21, and rarely Monosomy X, are identified.

Maternal risk factors:
- implantation disorders,
- long term use of contraception until the beginning pregnancy,
- diabetes mellitus,
- obesity,
- maternal thyroid dysfunction.

Chorangiosis

An infrequently reported villous maturation disorder in embryonic pregnancy that is characterized by excessive vessel proliferation in a few/many villi (Ch. 8).

11.3.4 Circulatory disturbance

Acute circulatory disturbance

This is seen as fresh intervillous hemorrhage or thrombosis in
- prostaglandin induced abortions and is often associated with hemorrhage and thrombosis of the same age in the decidua. Villous changes are limited to loose stromal edema, or hydropic swelling, and fresh hypoxic cytoplasmic degeneration of the trophoblast cells.
- Intradecidual hematoma may be seen in the transition between the embryonic and fetal periods due to preterm rejection of the gestational product.
- Formally, genetic spontaneous abortion are caused by intradecidual bleeding with splintering of the adhesion zone in the implantation bed. Implantation disorders and decidual vasculopathy, in the late embryonic period, in chronic maternal hypertonia may be causative, but often the etiology remains unknown.

Chronic circulatory disturbance

This is seen as mesh-like, massive fibrin depositions that enclose villous groups of variable sizes. The villi in these enclosed groups show regressive changes with eosinophilic cytoplasmic degeneration of the syncytiotrophoblast, trophoblast nuclei with pyknosis and/or karyorrhexis, stromal edema and fibrosis obliteration of villous capillaries and fine granular microcalcification in the stroma.

In the final stage of the circulatory disturbance the villi become necrotic and are visible as ghost villi.

In contrast to retention grade 3 circulatory disturbances are always local findings.

Frequency:
- spontaneous abortion in 10.4 %
- interruptio in 1,6 %

Pathogenesis and cause: the cause of the majority of abortions with a circulatory disturbance remains unknown.

Important pathogenetic factors are:
- Partial abruption of a superficially implanted gestational sac, especially in early abortions before GW 10.
- Lack of trophoblast cell invasion into the spiral arteries is reported; however, in abortions invasion was regularly seen.
- Stenosis of the intradecidual spiral arteries is rarely seen in abortions towards the end of the embryonic period (after GW10). In a few cases it has been associated with maternal diseases, such as chronic hypertension or diabetes mellitus with vascular involvement.
- Acute atherosis and wall necrosis may be associated with a perivascular lympho-monocytic infiltrate, possibly indicating that a maternal immune response is associated with, but not causative of abortion.

11.3.5 Implantation disorder

Defective or absent implantation as a cause of early pregnancy loss is well known [15]. In ca. 10 % of missed abortions it is diagnosed morphologically as an implantation disorder, often of the implantation bed.

Findings indicating implantation disorders
- endometrial hypoplasia,
- hypoplasia of the gestational sac,
- placenta membranacea of early pregnancy.

Endometrial hypoplasia
Irregular shedding of endometrium with abortive signs of secretion may cause superficial implantation of the blastocyst and pregnancy loss. Endometrial curettage shows localized groups of trophoblast cells and fibrinoid matrix on the superficial mucosa of the endometrium.

Gestational sac hypoplasia
The gestational sac is too small and is primarily localized within the superficial mucosa of the endometrium.

Macroscopy: the gestational sac measures less than 10 mm in diameter and is often partly opened. The embryo is infrequently seen.

Morphology: the implantation depth is shallow, often cup-shaped with surrounding hemorrhage. Subchorionic and intrauterine hemorrhage with villous disruption is seen. The chorionic plate is thin and contains single capillaries. Villi show reduced branching. The anchoring villi and trophoblast columns are rare or completely absent, indicating a failure of the trophoblast to invade.

Consequences: deficient trophoblastic invasion and expansion results in hemorrhage early pregnancy loss before GW 10.

Placenta membranacea of the late embryonic period

Macroscopy: flat gestational sac. The gestational sac often shows subtotal hemorrhage. The embryo is most often dead /autolytic and partly resorbed.

Morphology: the slender chorionic plate shows rudimentary collapsed vessels. The villi often have a slender diameter and show regressive changes: perivillous microfibrin depositions, acute intervillous hemorrhage and hemorrhagic necrosis. Only a few trophoblast columns are present at the base of the stem villi and within the decidua band-like granulocytic infiltrates and hemorrhage may be seen.

Consequences: placenta membranacea is primarily found in maldevelopment of the uterus and in acquired uterine anomalies. It results a superficial undefined villous growth and pregnancy loss frequently occurs after GW 10.

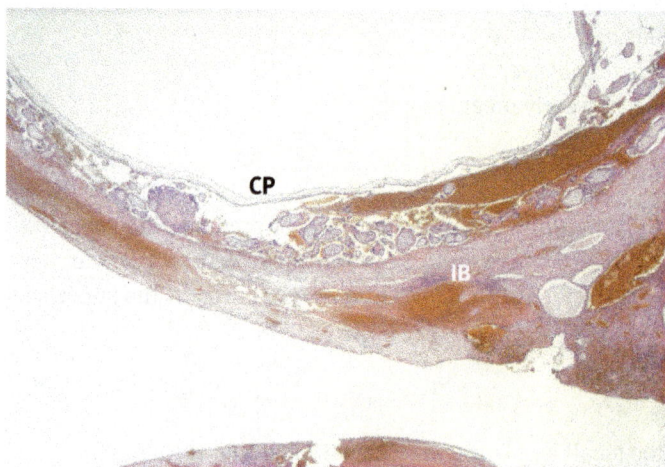

Fig. 11.16: Placenta membranacea. Chorionic plate (CP). Flat placental parenchyma and rare trophoblast columns with extensive and acute subchorionic, intervillous and intradecidual hemorrhage in the implantation bed (IB) [39].

Pathogenesis and cause Implantation damages
Successful implantation of the blastocyst depends on the quality of the gestational product as well as the condition of the maternal mucosa. A suboptimally receptive implantation bed predisposes towards deficient implantation and subsequent expulsion, with additional post zygotic damage, of the embryo.

Implantation damage may be caused by implantation disorders due to:
– exogenous hormonal dysregulation due to ovulation inhibitors with variable loss of mucosal hormone receptors and lack of decidualization [7],
– corpus luteum insufficiency with different grades of disharmonized retarded maturation of the endometrium with underdeveloped glands and stroma,
– uterus maldevelopment of any type,
– without correlation to chromosome or hormone dysregulation [21].

Habitual abortions:
– the most frequent cause is the congenital malformation uterus subseptus. This results in implantation displacement and a malperfused septum [22],
– acquired uterine changes causing localized endometrial circulatory disturbances (adhesions [synechia] and myomas) [22],
– in most cases a causative morphological finding is not identified.

11.3.6 Inflammation

Inflammation of the amniotic type in gestational week 12, possibly due to ascending infection, is reported. Iatrogenic inflammation, post chorionic biopsy, is also rare.

Maternal infection and transplacental infection with bacteria, protozoa and viruses are reported as causes of abortion [23]. Hematogenous infection may lead to embryonic resorption and abortion; however, morphological proof is first seen in late abortions.

Aside from the direct pathogenic effect of maternal infection; increased temperature, circulating toxins or metabolic disorders due to infection may also lead/contribute to abortion [23].

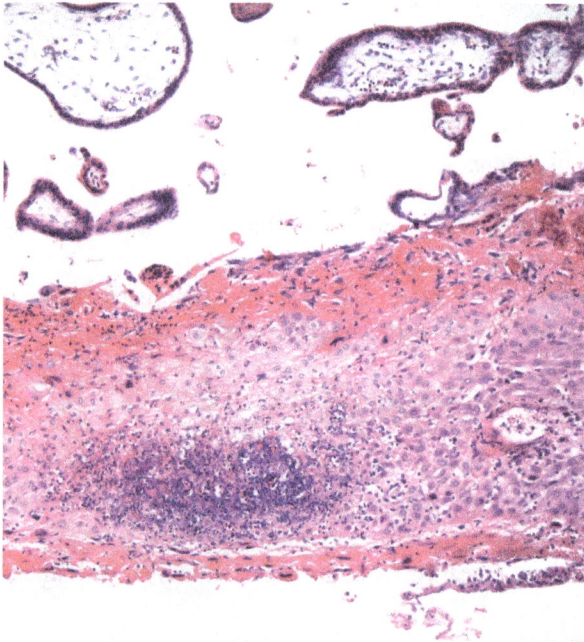

Fig. 11.17: inflammation in the implantation bed.

11.3.7 Villous retention

Several days to weeks may pass between the arrest of chorionic development, embryonic death and the expulsion of pregnancy products. Secondary changes known as retention phenomena depend on the grade of the primary developmental disorder and the duration of retention (Table 11.5).

The earliest changes (stage I) include a more prominent eosinophilic cytoplasm of the syncytium and syncytial knots. Later on the nuclei become hyperchromatic, pyknotic and karyorrhectic. Villi without vessels tend to undergo an earlier and more intensive hydropic and mucoid stromal degeneration. In contrast, villi with vessels and a developed embryonic placental circulatory system tend to undergo condensation of the stroma with stromal cell enrichment and increased collagenous fiber development.

With progressive retention the changes progress from discrete findings in the chorionic epithelium and stroma to villous destruction, epithelial necrosis, loss of capillaries, fibrinoid intervillous obliteration (microfibrin and fibrinoid type), fetal vessel luminal collapse and fibrotic vessel occlusion.

Table 11.5: Signs of retention in abortion.

retention stage	I (< 1 week)	II (several weeks)	III (several weeks, "missed abortion")
chorionic epithelium	eosinophilic syncytium, increased syncytial knots	nuclear pyknosis and karyorrhexis in syncytium and nuclear knots	epithelial loss
		perivillous fibrin / fibri-noid	increased perivillous fibrin / fibrinoid
		loss of cytotrophoblast	fibrous obliteration of the intervillous space
villous stroma	low grade condensation of the ground substance	hydropic mucoid degen-eration	mucoid or hyaline trans-formation
		increased fibers	fibrosis
		collagenous fiber swell-ing	cell loss
connective tissue cells	nuclear pyknosis	cellular enrichment	cellular loss
		abundant nuclear pyknosis	
vessels	acute luminal collapse	endothelial loss	endothelial loss
		luminal collapse	luminal occlusion of the capillaries and fetal vessels
		fibrosis of stem villous vessel walls	diffuse luminal oblitera-tion of vessels

Missed abortion

The term is not universally defined and can refer to:

- abortion with intrauterine fetal death 6 weeks prior to expulsion of gestational products.
- sonographically: a dead embryo without cardiac activity.
- morphologically: retention phenomena stage III.

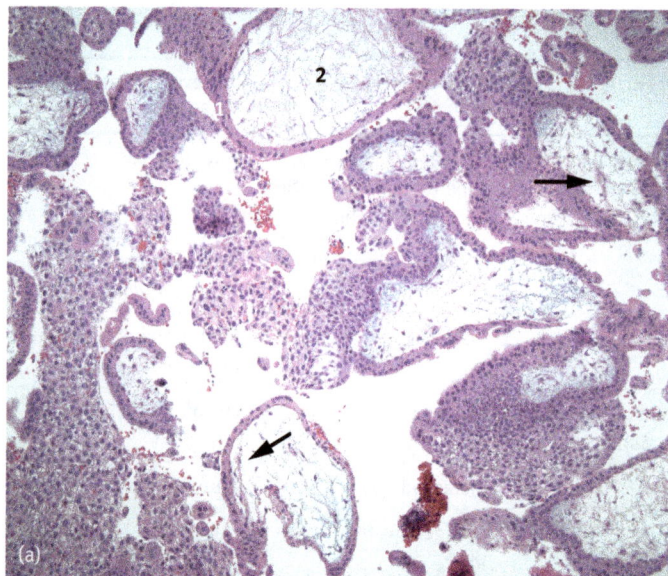

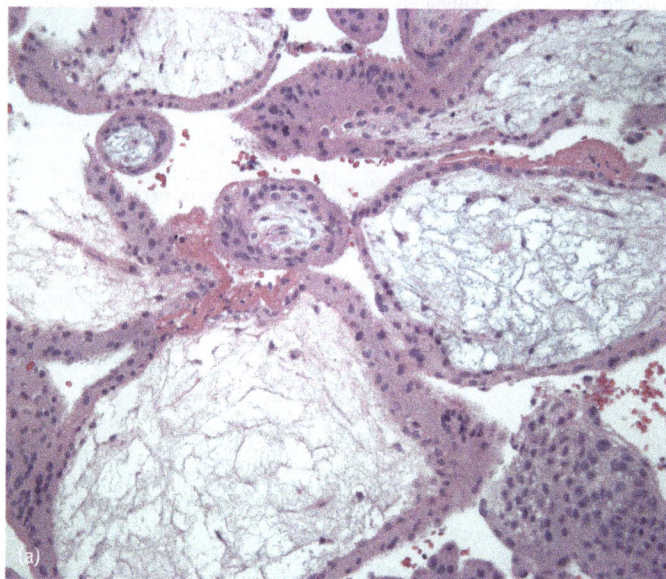

Fig. 11.18: (a) Retention stage I/II (MPF). (1) Eosinophilic chorionic epithelium, (2) mucoid villous stroma with nuclear pyknosis, (arrows) Collapsed vessel lumen. (b) Retention stage I/II (HPF).

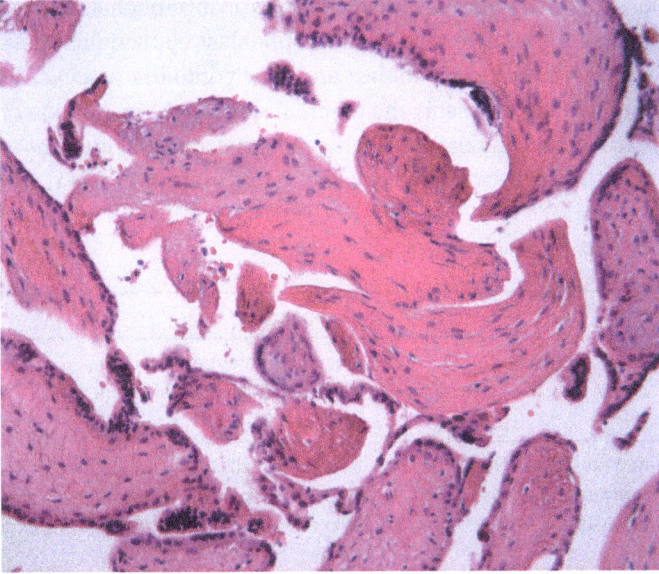

Retention stage III. Villi with loss of epithelium and endothelium, fibrous stroma.

11.3.8 Rudiments of an intrauterine implantation

Histological changes indicating a pre-existing pregnancy:
– chorionic tissue,
– intradecidual trophoblast cells,
– superficial decidua, hyaline plaques,
– placental bed nodule (Ch. 12)

11.4 Implantation bed (placental bed) in early pregnancy

Development of the chorionic villi enables differentiation between the villous and non-villous trophoblast due to their localization and differentiation (Table 11.6).

1. Villous trophoblast:
– chorionic epithelium, syncytial sprouts,
– cyto-, intermediate-, syncytiotrophoblast.

2. Extravillous trophoblast:
– implantation/placental bed, trophoblast columns, septa, islands, chorion leve,
– cyto-, Intermediate-, syncytiotrophoblast.

The stem cell of the villous and extravillous trophoblast is the cytotrophoblast (Langhans cell) and it functions as the reserve pool of the trophoblast epithelium. These cells differentiate into the intermediate trophoblast and finally into the syncytiotrophoblast. The syncytiotrophoblast represents the terminal stage of differentiation of the cytotrophoblast, and it acts as a border between the maternal and fetal portions of the placenta, facilitating exchange between the two circulatory systems (Table 11.6).

Table 11.6: Trophoblast. Differentiation and morphology.

differentiation		morphology
cytotrophoblast	undifferentiated stem cell	small undifferentiated cells Increased nuclear-cytoplasmic ratio IHC: CK+, PLAP+
intermediate trophoblast	intermediate differentiation between cytotrophoblast and syncytiotrophoblast	polyhedral cells, clear amphophilic cytoplasm, hyperchromatic nuclei, partly giant cell-like. IHC: CK+, HPL+, β-HCG(+), PLAP+
syncytio-trophoblast	terminally differentiated cell	cell syncytium, differentiated cells irregular nuclei, giant cells, microvilli IHC: CK+, β-HCG+

In the implantation/placental bed cytotrophoblast the stem cells are part of the trophoblast columns and remain adjacent to the basal membrane. They are mitotically active and divide steadily and asymmetrically. The post mitotic daughter cells are passively dispersed from the basal layer and the solid cellular formation of stem cells. These cells lose their mitotic ability and differentiate into cells with invasive characteristics, the extravillous intermediate trophoblast.

The cells invade the decidua as invasive interstitial trophoblasts and the wall of the spiral arteries as invasive endovascular trophoblasts (Fig. 11.20) They cause a loss of contractile and elastic vessel wall elements and result in fibrinoid transformation of the vessel wall. These changes result in widened vessel lumina and decreased vascular resistance and are responsible for the formation of a low resistance circulation [24].

In contrast to malignant tumor growth, the proliferation and invasion of the EV Tr is strictly controlled and limited. The cells lose their capability for invasion within days and normally do not invade the deeper uterine wall. Invasion depth is normally less than 1 cm, which means that the inner $\frac{1}{3}$ of the muscle layer, close to the uterine cavity, is not exceeded [37].

intervillosum

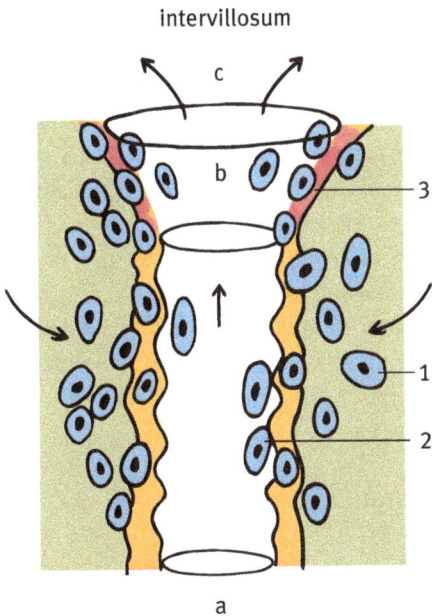

Fig. 11.20: Illustration. Interstitial and endovascular trophoblast invasion: (1) invasive interstitial EvTr cells, (2) endovascular migration of EvTr cells, (3) fibrinoid transformation of the vessel wall, (a) normal lumen of the artery, (b) transformation zone of the vessel wall, (c) large opening to the intervillous space.

The loss of the cells invasive capability is considered as:
- a result of trophoblast polyploidization,
- syncytial cell fusion with giant cell formation,
- and apoptosis.

These factors lead to a cessation of cell growth after abortion or delivery, assuming that the trophoblast columns are completely expelled. The polyploid giant cell intermediate trophoblast is identifiable in the implantation/placental bed for months, even years, following pregnancy and demonstrates no evidence of mitotic activity or invasion (Ch. 12).

Histology of the implantation bed in the 1st trimester shows a zonal organization:

- *Zone I: mainly daughter cells* arising from the *stem cell reserve pool.* The tight and closely packed cell group becomes less densely packed as the cells move further from the basal layer. In the embryonic period, this zone can demonstrate a relatively high amount of Ki-67 positive cells. The cells show a progressive lightening of the cytoplasm and eventually invade the adjacent decidua.
- *Zone II:* adjacent to zone I and containing *large polygonal trophoblast* cells embedded in a *fibrinoid-matrix.* The cells are dispersed throughout fibrinoid, but demonstrate no invasive capabilities at this stage. Some cells contain giant nuclei with anisonucleosis and hyperchromasia; both caused by polyploidization of the

trophoblast. Spindle-like cells of the interstitial invasive trophoblast can be identified in this zone.

– *Zone III*: a cell rich zone with *EV TRbL cells* (cytokeratin, CK 18, positive) is present between the maternal decidua cells, fibroblasts, large granular endometrial lymphocytes and macrophages. Trophoblast cells are found individually and may appear as a fish cord like formation. Additionally, deeper in the decidua *multinucleated trophoblast giant cells* are seen. These originate through fusion of the spindle-like invasive trophoblast cells and contain many, partly indistinct, nuclei and scant cytoplasm. The *spindle cells become apoptotic.*

– *Zone IV*: in the decidual-myometrial limitation zone *the giant cells become more numerous* and are seen between adjacent fibers of the myometrium. Multiple cells, giant cells and separation of muscle fibers by the trophoblast cells (without necrosis) point to 'exaggerated placental site reaction' (Ch. 12).

Limitation of the invasive capabilities of the extravillous intermediate trophoblast is achieved through:

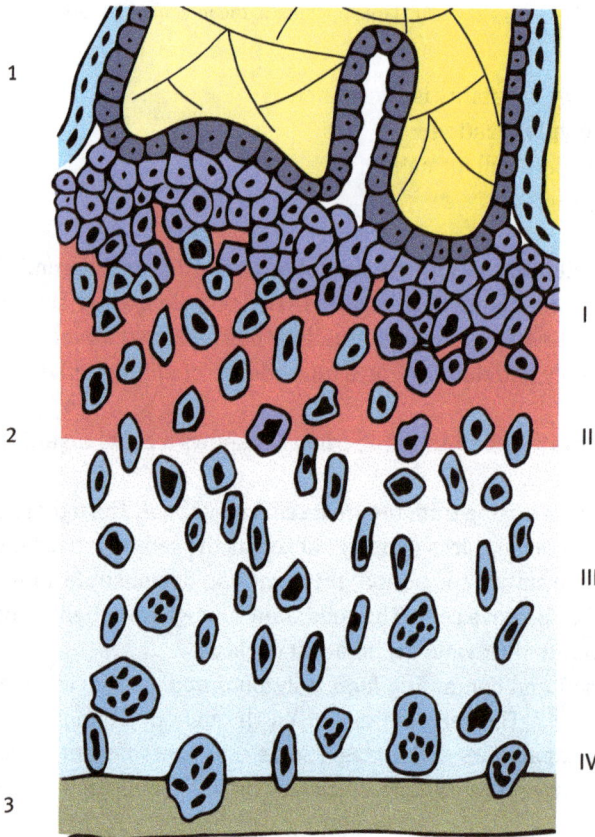

Fig. 11.21: Illustration. Zonal organization of the placental bed in early pregnancy: (1) anchoring villus with solid trophoblastic columns; (2) implantation bed, decidua; (3) transition to myometrium. Zone I: proliferation of the EvTr; Zone II: fibrinoid-matrix containing large polygonal EvTr; Zone III: invasion by interstitial trophoblasts, many spindle-like EvTr cells; Zone IV: decidual-myometrial transition area with trophoblast giant cells [38; modified].

- duration of the cell cycle of the cytotrophoblast
- polyploidization
- syncytial cell fusion
- apoptosis
- control by decidua cells and maternal macrophages
- invasion depth of 1 cm

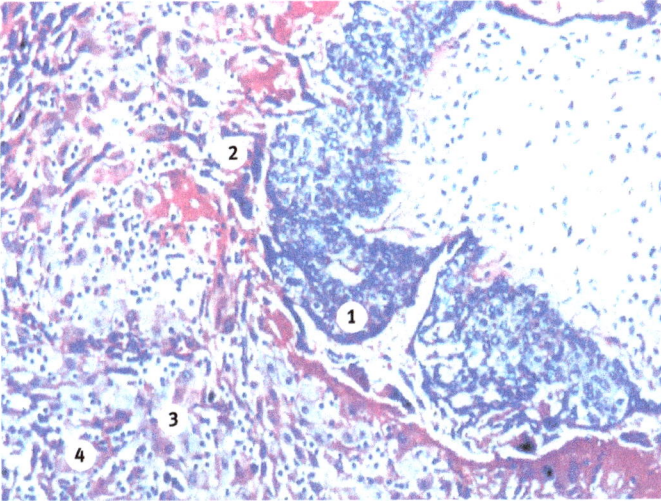

Fig. 11.22: Implantation/placental bed in gestational week 13. Anchoring villi with embryonic stroma: (1) basophilic cytotrophoblast with daughter cells, (2) small fibrinoid matrix zone, (3) interstitial invasive spindle like trophoblast cells, (4) fish-cord-like formation.

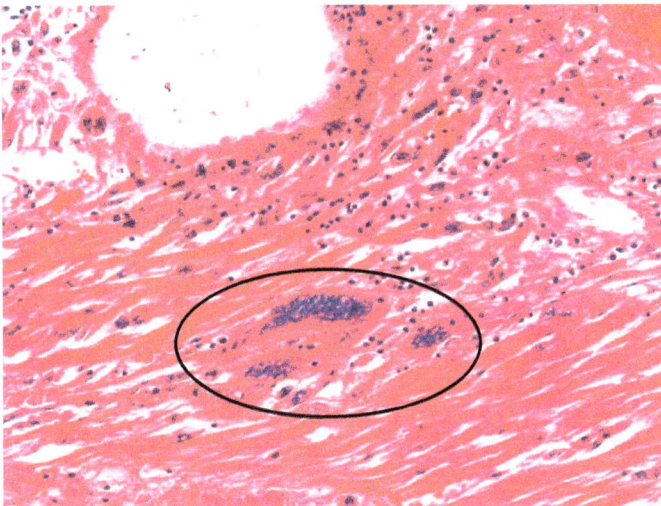

Fig. 11.23: Multinucleated giant cells in the myometrium (circle).

The invasiveness of the trophoblast cell is regulated by decidua cells and maternal macrophages. Two mechanisms are well known:

– secretion of TNF-α by maternal macrophages which binds to the trophoblastic TNF-receptor,

– secretion of Indoleamine 2,3 Dioxygenase (IDO) which induces in the trophoblast cell an apoptotic cascade [25].

11.5 Fetal (late) abortion

Spontaneous fetal abortion occurred in 5 % of all pregnancies until the 1990s and occurred after implantation as clinical abortions [26]. Induced terminations in the following years reduced statistically the incidence of spontaneous abortions (legally in Germany: fetal weight/ < 500 g). The vast majority of abortions for lethal malformations and syndromic diseases are induced terminations.

The most frequent cause of fetal abortions is amniotic infection and it is associated in ca. 30 % with pre-term placental abruption of a normally positioned placenta.

Table 11.7: Fetal spontaneous abortion (≤ GW 15; < 500 g, n = 356), from 1993 to 1994) [27].

cause of fetal death	n	(%)
amniotic infection – of those with premature abruption	172 (51)	48.3
general infection	6	1.7
lethal umbilical cord complication	32	9.0
acute circulatory disturbance (premature abruption, infarct greater than 20 %)	25	7.0
implantation disorder with acute circulatory disturbance	9	2.5
chronic infarction of the placenta	8	2.2
endangiopathia obliterans /villous fibrosis	23	6.5
twin pregnancy – FFTS (feto-fetal transfusion syndrome) – concordant twin death (of FFTS) – discordant twin death (of FFTS)	26 (10) (12) (4)	7.3
lethal malformation / syndrome	30	8.5
hydrops universalis	14	3.9
unknown	11	3.1

Frequent placental changes in fetal abortion are (Table 11.7):
–   inflammation
–   umbilical cord complication
–   maternal vascular malperfusion
–   fetal vascular malperfusion
–   implantation disorders
–   villous maturation disorders
–   mesenchymal placental dysplasia,
–   chromosome aberrations in fetal and neonatal death
–   hydrops universalis.

11.5.1 Inflammation

Inflammatory reaction in the amnion, umbilical cord and/or placenta is the most frequent finding in fetal abortions and is caused, predominantly, by an ascending amniotic infection.

Inflammation of amniotic type with granulocyte exudates in the amnion, chorionic plate and/or umbilical cord was seen in 67 % of spontaneous abortions, but only in 5 % of induced abortions; regardless of stage or grade of inflammation.

High grade amniotic infection was seen as causative of 45.3 % of spontaneous pregnancy losses. Additional findings of maternal inflammatory reactions, such as chorioamnionitis, and fetal reactions, such as chorionic plate vasculitis, omphalovasculitis and funiculitis, suggest an inflammatory cause of abortion and that the findings are not merely secondary changes.

A secondary inflammatory reaction is seen in the basal placenta with intrauterine fetal death with signs of retention as *"morphallactic demarcation"* and in fetal abortions with intrauterine fetal death of a twin in a multiple pregnancy [28].

Amniotic inflammation caused by ascending infection is most frequently seen in:
–   cervix insufficiency,
–   premature membrane abruption,
–   rarely after diagnostic amniocentesis; less than 4 days after the procedure and occurs in ca. 1:1000.

Pathogenic causes
See Ch. 9.

11.5.2 Umbilical cord complication (see also Ch. 3)

Lethal umbilical cord complications are found in 9 % of autopsies of fetal sponta-neous abortions (Table 11.7).
- *Umbilical cord strangulation:* entanglement, one or more, of fetal extremities and/or torso by the umbilical cord with strangulation signs, fetal death and re-tention lasting several days to weeks.
- *Strangulation due to amniotic bands* (amnion rupture sequence or amniotic defor-mity adhesion mutilation, ADAM-complex). In abortions with a fetal weight less than 500 g weight this was seen in 1:70 fetal and placental autopsies.
- *Umbilical cord stricture:* most frequently seen close to umbilical ring or umbilical cord insertion on the placental chorionic plate, infrequently the middle portion of the umbilical cord may be involved. Close to the stricture Wharton's Jelly is reduced, or missing entirely, and this is classified as a segmental thin-cord com-plex. Histologically the umbilical cord vessel wall is thinned, the vessel lumina is compressed but not obliterated, and the surrounding tissue shows fibrosis. The neighbouring Wharton's Jelly shows edema while other parts of the umbilical cord are of normal or increased diameter. The cord stricture is considered to be the cause of death/abortion if the stricture reduces the umbilical cord diameter to less than a few millimeters.
- *Acute infrafunicular bleeding with vessel congestion* (Ch. 3).

11.5.3 Maternal circulatory disturbance (see Ch. 7)

The majority of intraplacental *acute circulatory disturbances* show small focal chang-es, affecting less than 20 % by volume of the placenta. Acute circulatory disturbances above 20 %, seen as large hemorrhagic infarcts, intraplacental hematomas or acute thrombosis, were seen in 9.5 % of fetal spontaneous abortions, in less than 3 % of placental abruptions.
- *Acute and chronic circulatory disturbances* show an increased association with placental implantation disorders; such as placenta circumvallata, membranacea partialis and placental displacements.
- *Chronic circulatory disturbances* with macroscopic large mesh-like infarcts and massive infarcts (chronic infarcted placenta) were seen in less than 3 % of spon-taneous abortions; however, small foci can be seen in nearly 50 %. Chronic cir-culatory disturbances affecting more than 10 % of the placental volume were not identified. Macroscopic chronic vascular disturbances were histologically con-firmed by increased inter- and perivillous microfibrin deposition. Additionally, chronic circulatory disturbance was more frequently associated with villous stro-mal fibrosis (45 %) and Endangiopathia obliterans (42 %).

- 85 % of placental *abruption due to prostaglandin induction* showed acute, large basal hematomas and intradecidual hemorrhage.

11.5.4 Fetal circulatory disturbance

- *Endangiopathia obliterans:* in spontaneous abortions endangiopathia obliterans was seen in 16 % of high grade fetal vascular malperfusion, but was only causative for fetal death in 6.5 % of cases. In cases of low grade malperfusion it caused death in less than 5 % of cases.
- Endangiopathy was associated with villous stromal fibrosis in 52 % of cases; however, *villous stromal fibrosis* of grade 2 and 3 was seen without any evidence of endangiopathy.
- Endangiopathy is caused by fetal placental malperfusion with endothelial cell damage due to *hypoxidosis* and subsequent fibromyocyte proliferations extending from the vessel wall causing septation and obliteration of the lumen. The fetus often is growth restricted.
- *Endangiitis obliterans* with cellular exudates and vessel wall necrosis was seen in less than 2 % of spontaneous abortions and 4 % of induced abortions. Not infrequently an associated lympho-monocytic villitis, with partial microcalcifications, is found.
- Pathogens such as rubella virus are associated with malperfusion and can be identified by PCR of chorionic villi, amniotic fluid and umbilical cord blood. Rubella infection in the middle fetal period causes placental changes as well as fetal organ damage, such as: congenital hepatitis, myocarditis, inner ear damage and ocular lens damage.
- *Collapse sclerosis* is a secondary event related to the complete loss of vessel perfusion and is the most important differential diagnosis.

11.5.5 Implantation disorders

The significance of placenta membranacea, extrachorialis circumvallate and placental displacements in the fetal period:
- *Placenta membranacea* is found in both the early and late fetal period and is caused by a shallow implantation depth of the trophoblast. Recurrent circulatory disturbances in the intervillous space are a common finding in this condition. Villi may show regressive changes, especially in the epithelium, and the stroma contains increased collagenous fibers and a deficiency of fetal vessels. These changes result in fetal growth restriction. It may be associated with ascending amniotic infection.

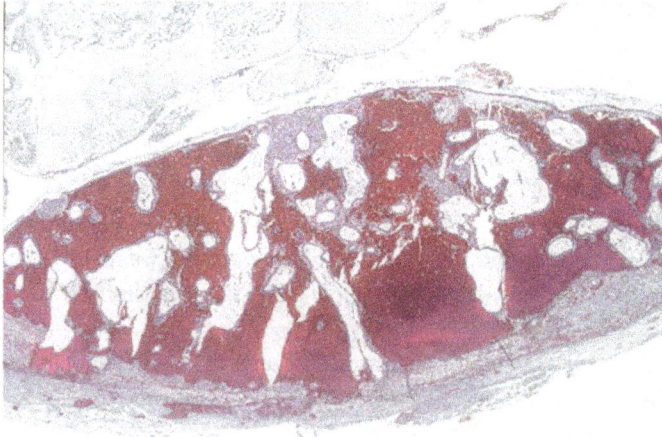

Fig. 11.24: Massive intervillous bleeding, distension and rupture of the villous syncytium (spontaneus abortion 9. SSW) [39].

–   *Placenta extrachorialis circumvallata* occurs 2–3 times more often in fetal abortion than in late pregnancy. It has an increased risk of partial premature placental abruption and placental marginal bleeding.
–   *Placental displacement,* such as low lying placenta or *placenta previa,* before gestational week 28 only infrequently causes bleeding, death and expulsion of the fetus.

11.5.6 Villous maturation disorders (Ch. 8)

Villous maturation disorders are seen in 50–75 % of aborted placenta and vary according to the grade and extent of the disorder. They may be classified into 3 main groups:
–   arrest of villous maturation
–   deficiency of intermediate villi,
–   pre-term/accelerated villous maturation,
–   (rarely, it may also present as chorangiosis type 1).

Arrest of villous maturation
Villous maturation arrest is seen in more than 50 % of spontaneous abortions. Cervical insufficiency was especially associated with low grade villous maturation arrest and ascending amniotic infection. The pathogenesis is unknown.

Arrest of villous maturation with large paw like villi was seen in ca. 14 % of abortions and in nearly 30 % of placental abruptions.

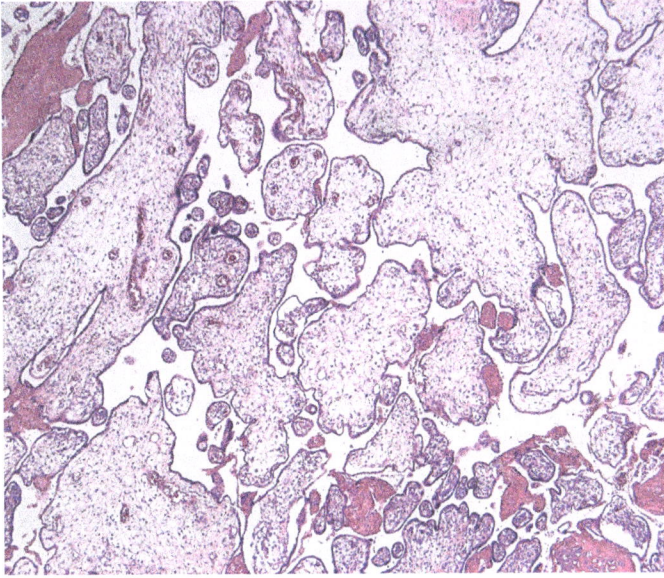

Fig. 11.25: Paw-like villi in Trisomy 21.

Characteristics of paw like villi
- large diameter stem villi,
- extremely irregular villi with the irregularity continuing into the short intermediate villi,
- hypoplastic and thin walled stem villous vessels,
- embryonic and loose reticular villous stroma,
- irregular and flat single- and double-layered villous trophoblast, often with invaginations and endovillous trophoblast inclusions.

Frequency
- An increased number of paw like villi may be seen in spontaneous abortions, terminations and in syndromes, such as autosomal Trisomy and XO-Monosomy (ca. 65 %). In placentas from fetuses with local malformation, especially of the central nervous system, paw like villi can be found distributed among villi showing various stages of maturity that are independent of gestational age.
- In placentas from fetuses without malformation paw like villi were found in less than 2 % specimens.

The *pathogenetic consequences* of villous maturation arrest for the fetal outcome is not completely understood. Generalized stromal edema (hydrops placenta) is often associated with fetal hydrops, as hydrops universalis, and is a cause of spontaneous fetal abortion (Ch. 11.5.9).

Deficiency of intermediate villi

An early onset maturation disorder of the early fetal period with a deficiency of the intermediate villi and densely packed stem and terminal villi. Stenotic decidual vasculopathy in the pre-placental vascular bed is an important pathogenetic factor.

Associated maternal diseases:
- chronic hypertension,
- chronic nephropathy
- diabetic angiopathy
- collagenosis
- systemic lupus erythematosus.

Consequences

A numerical deficiency of the intermediate villi causes a reduction in fetal vessel volume and an associated limitation of fetal perfusion capacity. Due of the interdependent nature of the fetal and maternal blood flow within the circulatory units, the total intervillous circulation and placental perfusion capacity is affected, and this causes an early fetal growth restriction before gestational week 20.

Intermediate villous deficiency may be interpreted as extreme type of:

Pre-term accelerated villous maturation

Pre-term accelerated villous maturation was seen in 28.6 % of placentas from spontaneous abortion but the grade was 2–3 in less than 18 %. In contrast to intermediate villous deficiency, pre-term maturation was predominantly seen in placentas after the 20th gestational week and was associated with villous stroma fibrosis.

The origin of preterm/accelerated villous maturation in early and middle pregnancy is assumed to be due to the same pathogenetic factors as in late pregnancy; a compensatory stimulation of villous maturation in placental hypoplasia, implantation disorders and chronically decreased uteroplacental perfusion. Preterm accelerated villous maturation is also seen in ca. 50 % of twin pregnancies.

Chorangiosis type 1

Chorangiosis type 1 was seen in 2.9 % and was high grade in 1.7 %.

The etiology is unknown. Some cases are associated with generalized edema and fetal hydrops. Vessel proliferation in the placenta may cause a chronically increased fetal cardiac output and result in cardiac insufficiency. In cases of cardiomegaly and chorangiosis type 1 it is difficult to distinguish between a cardiac and a chorangiosis cause of edema. Chorangiosis type 1 and hydrops fetalis may be associated with immunological or non-immunological hemolytic anemia.

11.5.7 Mesenchymal placental dysplasia

Mesenchymal placental dysplasia is a villous developmental disorder associated with placentomegaly, stem villous bullae, stromal hypoplasia, and partial capillary hyperplasia (chorangiosis).

Macroscopy
- enlarged placenta (more than 1.000 g)
- varicosis and aneurysms of the large chorionic and subchorionic stem villous vessels

Morphology
- stem villous bullae of varying size,
- hypoplastic stem villi vessels with slender tunica media and very loose perivascular contractile cell and fiber sheath (Ch. 1)
- irregular villi with a fibroblast rich and partly mucoid/pseudocystic loose stroma,
- focal chorangiosis Typ I,
- no hyperplasia of villous trophoblast,
- secondary vessel changes; acute intraplacental hemorrhage, thrombi and calcification.

Facultative:
- accelerated villous maturation,
- endangiopathy obliterans.

Changes are often in combination [29].

Pathogenesis
The pathogenesis is unknown. Newborns may be clinically normal or show growth restriction. Rarely fetal abortion or intrauterine fetal death occurs in late pregnancy [30].

Cytogenetics
Chromosomal analysis shows no abnormalities. There is a well known association with Beckwith-Wiedemann-syndrome and/or an isolated omphalocele and up to 50 % of the fetuses/newborns are affected [31]. A possible explanation of mesenchymal dysplasia without fetal disease may be that Beckwith-Wiedemann-syndrome (11p15-) is limited to the placenta.

Differential diagnosis

A partial hydatidiform mole may be suspected on ultrasound but placental dysplasia does not have any trophoblastic hyperplasia histologically, triploidy is not identified cytogenetically and some fetuses do not demonstrate any symptoms. Stem bullae may present in other conditions, such as Turner-syndrome and Trisomy 18, but these show single, not multiple, bulla. An absence of bullae provides a significant diagnostic challenge in differentiate mesenchymal placental dysplasia from large focal chorangiosis type I or chorangiomatosis.

11.5.8 Chromosome abnormalities in fetal and neonatal disease

Spontaneous abortions are mainly caused by chromosomal abnormalities prior to gestational week 12. In the 2nd trimester, fetal and neonatal death due to numeric chromosome abnormalities and gonosomal aneuploidy decreases as the pregnancy proceeds towards term; however, ca. 20 % of spontaneous fetal abortions due to trisomy are registered in the 2nd trimester, which continues as peri- and postnatal mortality due to Trisomy 13, 18, 21 and XO-Monosomy [32].

In fetal abortions the combinations of placental findings and fetal injury that are suggestive of chromosomal disorders are rare: Patau, Edwards, Down and Turner syndrome (bilateral hydropic neck).

Trisomy 13 (Patau syndrome)

Macroscopy
- placental hypoplasia (weight < 10th percentile),
- solitary umbilical cord artery (50 %).

Morphology
- arrest of villous maturation with paw-like villi (70 %),
- occasionally mole-like stromal degeneration.

Trisomy 18 (Edwards syndrome)

Macroscopy
- placental hypoplasia; small and low weight (70 %),
- solitary umbilical cord artery (20 %).

Morphology
- villous maturation arrest with paw-like villi (66 %),
- rarely stem villous bullae,
- varying cell poor / cell rich fibrous stroma (66 %),
- endovillous trophoblast cell clusters (60 %),

- accelerated villous maturation,
- thromboangiitis obliterans.

Trisomy 21 (Down syndrome)

Macroscopy
- placental hypoplasia (66 %),
- solitary umbilical cord artery (30 %),
- hydrops universalis (10 %).

Morphology
- villous maturation arrest with paw-like villi (70 %),
- hydropic degenerated stroma,
- mainly embryonic stroma and few endovillous trophoblast cell clusters (70 %),
- normal findings seen in ca. 15 %.

Paw-like villi and hydrops universalis were more often seen in spontaneous fetal abortions with Trisomy 21 than in terminations (73 %:53 %) and (13 %:7 %) respectively. Spontaneous abortions also more frequently show chronic circulatory disturbances with villous stromal fibrosis (27 %:2 %) and pathologically increased microfibrin depositions, grades 2 and 3, (40 %:10.5 %). Subtle findings of paw-like villi were seen in less than 4 % of placentas from live births with trisomy 21 [33].

XO-Monosomy (Turner syndrome)

Macroscopy
- placental growth restriction (50 %),
- hypoplasia of the umbilical cord vessels and branches on the chorionic plate.

Morphology
- few Paw-like villi (70 %),
- partly hydropic or mole-like stroma,
- varying villous diameter,
- pencil-like fibrous villi.

Triploidy syndrome

Macroscopy
- placental growth restriction (50 %) and placental overgrowth (30 %),
- irregular disseminated villous bullae.

Morphology
- side by side villi with large and very small diameters,
- stem villous bullae with different sizes,
- paw-like villi with 'fjord like' exophytic hyperplasia of the syncytiotrophoblast; in combination with endovillous invagination and trophoblast buds,
- frequent endovillous trophoblast cell clusters,
- irregular reticular, hydropic and fibrous stroma, rare capillaries.

Growth restricted placentas, villous stromal fibrosis and pre-term or normal villous maturation according to gestational age, are more frequently seen in fetal abortions with triploidy than in embryonic and early fetal abortion. Additional chromosomes are often of maternal origin [34].

Confined placental mosaic
A postzygotic chromosome disorder with different sets of chromosomes in the placenta and fetus, for example mosaic-trisomy:
- postzygotic chromosome disorder due to separation in the outer trophoblast shell or inner cell mass of the morula (blastocystic epiblast).
  Three different types:
- trisomy in the cytotrophoblast/ – Diploidy in the villous stroma (embryo)
- trisomy in the villous stroma/- Diploidy in the cytotrophoblast.
- trisomy in the cytotrophoblast and villous stroma/ Diploidy in the embryo.

Intrauterine growth restriction and intrauterine fetal death is seen especially in the 3rd trimester [35].

11.5.9 Hydrops universalis (fetalis and placentae)

Definition and pathogenesis
Hydrops universalis is an increased extravascular fluid content due to disturbance of fluid exchange between intra and extravillous (interstitial) compartment. In disturbed balance, of the hydrostatical pressure (in vitium cordis):

Table 11.8: Pathogenesis of Hydrops universalis.

oncotic pressure	congenital nephrotic syndrome
capillary permeability	hypoxia, anemia, infection
lymph drainage	jugular lymphatic obstruction sequence

Table 11.9: Causes and relative frequency of non-immunologic hydrops fetalis [36].

cause	frequency in %
complex cardiac malformation, cardiomegaly, cardiac insufficiency, cardiac tumor	20–76
arrhythmia (AV-Block)	15
chromosome abnormality (trisomy 18, 21, XO-Monosomy)	14–18
malformation syndromes: polysplenia-S, skeletal dysplasia, Pena-Shokeir	10
chronic twin to twin transfusion syndrome	10
intrauterine infection (CMV, parvovirus B19, toxoplasmosis, varicella)	ca. 4
monozygotic α-thalassemia	ca. 57 in south-east Asia

Causes
- *immunological hemolytic Hydrops (IH-hydrops)* in Rh -incompatibility and ABO-incompatibiliy,
- *non immunologic Hydrops (NIH-hydrops).*

Non-immunologic hydrops is more frequent than immunologic hemolytic hydrops.

Other causes
- gastrointestinal malformations (atresia, malrotation),
- adenomatoid cystic lung malformation,
- teratoma sacralis, placental chorangioma, chorangiomatosis,
- umbilical cord vein thrombosis,

Maternal causes: diabetes, anemia, hypoalbuminemia.

A special case occurs in monochorionic twin placentas with vessel anastomoses (Ch. 13) and feto-fetal transfusion-syndrome. The acceptor fetus may show Hydrops fetalis due to intrauterine cardiac insufficiency. It may also, albeit rarely, be found in the donor twin due to decreased albumin and total protein concentration.

In approximately 1 in every 10 cases of congenital hydrops no etiology is identified, despite autopsy of the fetus, examination of the placenta and relevant clinical data:
- idiopathic Hydrops universalis

Macroscopy
Hydrops placentae presents as a macrosomic, heavy and pale placenta. Cut surfaces are moist and show edematous swollen contours of the villi/villous tree.

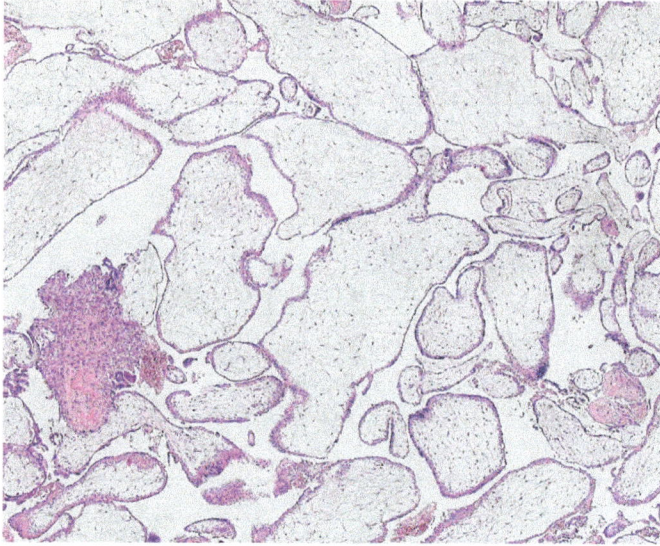

Fig. 11.26: Hydrops placentae. Edematous increased villous diameter, invisible fetal vessels and flattened trophoblast. Induced abortion in Gestational Week 19.

Morphology

- frequent villous maturation arrest,
- hydropic, bullae-like villous stroma,
- displaced stroma cells,
- compressed capillary lumen,
- flattened villous trophoblast.

Facultative changes

- capillary hyperplasia (chorangiosis) in a single villi or villous groups,
- intravascular erythroblastosis, seen in chronic anemia or viral infection as a sign of compensatory increased erythropoiesis.

References

[1] Vogel M. Pathologie der Schwangerschaft. In: Blümcke S. editor. Pathologie Berlin, New York: W de Gruyter 1995; 789–815.
[2] Höpker WW. Missbildungen. Berlin: Thieme; 1984.
[3] Bar-Ami S, Seibel MM, Pierce KE, Zilberstein M. Preimplantation genetic diagnosis for a couple with recurrent pregnancy loss and triploidy. Birth Defects Research Part A: Clinical and Molecular Teratology. 2003;67(11):946–950.
[4] Rushton DI. The classification and mechanisms of spontaneous abortion. Perspectives in pediatric pathology. 1984;8(3):269–287.

[5]   Tennstedt C, Vogel M. [Autopsy of the fetus. Proposed investigatory strategy as a decision aid in the autopsy of fetues with special conditions]. Der Pathologe. 2000;21(5):383–387.
[6]   Edwards RG. Causes of early embryonic loss in human pregnancy. Human reproduction (Oxford, England). 1986;1(3):185–198.
[7]   Dallenbach C, Sterzik K, Dallenbach-Hellweg G. [Histologic endometrial findings in patients on the day of planned embryo transfer]. Geburtshilfe Frauenheilkd. 1987;47(9):623–629.
[8]   Donat H, Fritzsche C, Morenz J. [Incidence and significance of humoral antibodies in females with recurrent spontaneous abortions]. Zentralbl Gynakol. 1989;111(12):811–815.
[9]   Poland BJ, Miller JR, Harris M, Livingston J. Spontaneous abortion. A study of 1,961 women and their conceptuses. Acta Obstet Gynecol Scand Suppl. 1981;102:1–32.
[10] Vogel M. Pathologie der Schwangerschaft, der Plazenta und des Neugeborenen. In: W R, editor. Pathologie. 3. Berlin: Springer; 1984. p. 510ff.
[11] Fantel AG, Shepard TH, Vadheim-Roth C, Stephens TD, Coleman C. Embryonic and fetal pheno-types. In: Porter IH HE, editor. Human embryonic and fetal death. New York: Academic Press; 1980. p. 71–87.
[12] Streeter GL. Development horizons in human embryos. In: Washington Clo, editor. Embryology. Reprint II. Washington DC, 1951.
[13] Kalousek DK, Lau AE. Pathology of spontanous abortion. In: Dimmick JE, Kalousek DK, editor. Developmental Pathology of the Embryo and Fetus. Philadelphia: Lippincott; 1992. p. 55–82.
[14] Vogel M, Horn LC. [Gestational trophoblastic disease, Villous gestational trophoblastic di-sease]. Pathologe. 2004;25(4):269–279.
[15] Baergen RN. Manual of Pathology of the Human Placenta. 2 ed. New York: Springer; 2011.
[16] Kraus FT, Redline RW, Gersell DJ, Nelson DM, Dicke JM. Placental Pathology: American Registry of Pathology Washington, DC; 2004.
[17] Buza N, Hui P. Partial hydatidiform mole: histologic parameters in correlation with DNA genoty-ping. Int J Gynecol Pathol. 2013;32(3):307–315.
[18] Kurman RJ, Carcangiu ML, Herrington CS, Young RH. Gestational Trophoblastic Disease in WHO Classification of Tumours of Female Reproductive Organs. 4th ed: IACR Press; 2014.
[19] Seeger-Held A, Vogel M, Minguillon C. Significance and discriminant analysis of histomor-phological characteristics in embryonal abortions with and without chromosomal aberrations. Pathol Microbiol (Basel). 1992; 25.
[20] Vogel M. Atlas der morphologischen Plazentadiagnostik. 2 ed. Berlin: Springer; 1996.
[21] Byskov AG HP. Embryology of mammarian gonads and ducts. In: Knobil E NI, editor. The physio-logy reproduction. New York: Raven; 1988. p. 265.
[22] Campo RL, Schlosser HW. [Congenital and acquired organ changes of the uterus and habitual abortion]. Gynakologe. 1988;21(3):237–244.
[23] Enders G, Gartner L. [Infection as a complication in early pregnancy]. Gynakologe. 1988;21(3):220–231.
[24] Benirschke K, Burton G, Baergen RN. Pathology of the human placenta. 6 ed. New York: Springer; 2012.
[25] Reister F, Frank HG, Kingdom JC, et al. Macrophage-induced apoptosis limits endovascular tro-phoblast invasion in the uterine wall of preeclamptic women. Lab Invest. 2001;81(8):1143–1152.
[26] Shapiro S, Bross D. Risk factors for fetal death in studies of vital statistics data: interference and limitations. In: PorterJH HE, editor. Human embryonic and fetal death. London: Academic press; 1980.
[27] Tennstedt-Schenk C, Vogel M. Pathologie der Fetalperiode. In: Remmele W, editor. Pathologie. Berlin, Heidelberg: Springer; 2013. p. 661–725.
[28] Becker V, Schiebler TH, Kubli F. Allgemeine und spezielle Pathologie der Plazenta. Die Plazenta des Menschen. Stuttgart: Thieme; 1981. p. 251–393.

[29] Gibson BR, Muir-Padilla J, Champeaux A, Suarez ES. Mesenchymal dysplasia of the placenta. Placenta. 2004;25(7):671–672.

[30] Jauniaux E, Nicolaides KH, Hustin J. Perinatal features associated with placental mesenchymal dysplasia. Placenta. 1997;18(8):701–706.

[31] Lage JM. Placentomegaly with massive hydrops of placental stem villi, diploid DNA content, and fetal omphaloceles: possible association with Beckwith-Wiedemann syndrome. Hum Pathol. 1991;22(6):591–597.

[32] Hook EB. Spontaneous deaths of fetuses with chromosomal abnormalities diagnosed prenatally. The New England journal of medicine. 1978;299(19):1036–1038.

[33] Vogel M. Atlas der morphologischen Plazentadiagnostik. 1. ed. Berlin: Springer; 1992.

[34] Kalousek DK. Confined placental mosaicism and intrauterine development. Pediatr Pathol. 1990;10(1–2):69–77.

[35] Kalousek DK, Barrett I. Confined placental mosaicism and stillbirth. Pediatric pathology. 1994;14(1):151–159.

[36] Boos R. Non-immunologischer Hydrops fetalis (NIHF). In: Boos R. editor. Risiken in der Schwangerschaft und kindliche Fehlbildungen. 2. Balingen: Spitta; 2000.

[37] Kaufmann P. Control of normal trophoblast invasion in the human. In: Hauptmann S, Dietel M. editors. Surgical of Pathology update; Berlin ABW Wissenschaft: 2001;161–165.

[38] Kertschanska S. Trophoblast invasion intubular compared to normal intrauterine pregnancy. In: Hauptmann S, Dietel M. editors. Surgical of Pathology update; Berlin ABW Wissenschaft: 2001;165–168.

[39] Vogel M. Pathologie der Frühschwangerschaft. Frühschwangerschaft und Abort. In: Dietel M, Klöppel G editors. Pathologie; Springer Berlin Heidelberg, 2013; 519–541.

12 Gestational trophoblastic disease

Lars-Christian Horn

12.1 Definition of Gestational Trophoblastic Disease

The term gestational trophoblastic disease (GTD) is used by both the World Health Organisation (WHO) and the International Federation of Gynecology and Obstetrics (FIGO) classification systems to describe a variety of diseases, including benign, tumor-like and highly malignant lesions of trophoblastic differentiation. GTDs represent a clinically and histopathologically heterogeneous group of diseases and are mostly associated with a history of pregnancy (Fig. 12.1).

A common feature of all GTDs is abnormal growth of different cell types of the placental trophoblast, sometimes associated with villous dysmaturity. GTD classification, according to the WHO is summarized in Table 12.1. PHM, CHM and IHM are classified as villous GTDs, all other lesions are considered as non-villous GTD.

The diagnostic terms of an-embryonic mole (German "Windmole") and embryonic mole (see Ch. 11) do not exist within the WHO-classification system. Instead, the WHO defines abnormal (non-molar) villous lesions as villous lesions which may mimic a partial hydatidiform mole (PHM) clinically and histopathologically [1]. Some may be associated with genetic alterations (predominantly trisomies [2]) harbouring the same low-risk of persistent GTD as any other morphologically unremarkable non-molar conception. Because of their malignant or potential malignant behaviour, CC, PSTT and ETT may be summarized under the term gestational trophoblastic neoplasia (GTN).

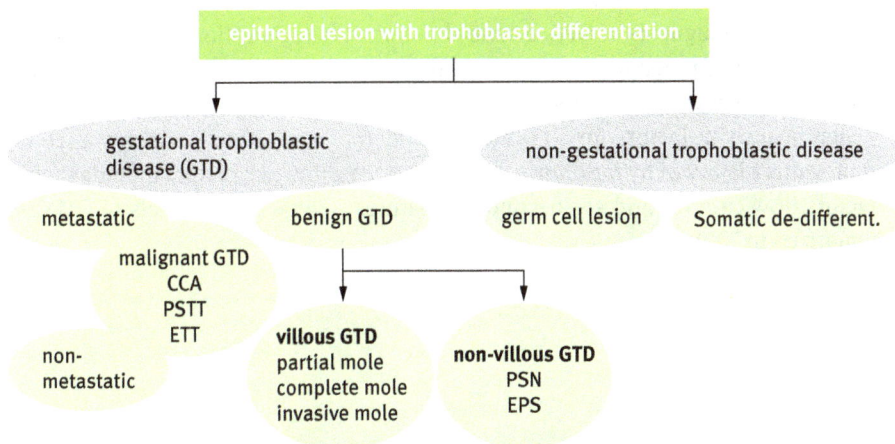

Fig. 12.1: Classification of epithelial lesions of the female genital tract representing trophoblastic differentiation (for details see text, [136]).

https://doi.org/10.1515/9783110452600-012

Table 12.1: Classification of Gestational Trophoblastic Disease (GTD).

1) villous GTD	
Partial Hydatidiform Mole (PHM)	ICD-O: 9103/0
Complete Hydatidiform Mole (CHM)	ICD-O: 9100/0
Invasive Mole (IM)	ICD-O: 9100/1
2) Non-villous GTD	
Chorioncarcinoma (CC)	ICD-O: 9100/3
Placental Site Trophoblastic Tumor (PSTT)	ICD-O: 9104/1
Epitheloid Trophoblastic Tumor (ETT)	
Placental Site Nodule (PSN)	
Exaggerated Placental Site (EPS)	SNOMED 79420

12.2 Incidence of GTD

The prevalence of GTD varies markedly by country but there is a well documented high incidence in south-eastern Asia [3–6]. This increased incidence rate persists in migrants from this area who show the same high incidence as their counterparts still living in Asia and show a 1.95-higher risk for GTD than a Non – Asian population [6]. Reports from South Korea show a decrease of molar pregnancies from 4.4/1.000 births in the Sixties to 1.6/1.000 in the Nineties [7]. The SEER-database reported a decrease of choriocarcinoma within the United States [8] while the incidence of GTD increased in the Netherlands between 1995 and 2008 [9] with a subsequent stabilisation after that period [10]. The initial increase may be a result of improved diagnostic clinical methods for the diagnosis of GTD, a central nationwide registration processes, an increased number of pregnancies in women and a previous history of > 40 years of age and an increase of women with Asian ethnicity within the country [9].

Significant risk factors for GTD include maternal age < 20 and > 40 years [11–13] and previous history of hydatidiform mole [11,14]. Possible risk factors include dietetic factors (low carotin) and socioeconomic features [11,14]. General facts of GTD are summarized in Table 12.2.

Table 12.2: General Facts Gestational Trophoblastic Disease (GTD.)

Definition
– wide range of clinical presentation ranging from benign to highly malignant
– different cytogenetic background; the majority of molar disease androgenetically based
– failure of normal trophoblastic differentiation, sometimes associated with trophoblastic hyperplasia
– the majority of GTD is associated with pregnancy
– time interval between most recent pregnancy and GTD ranges between days and up to more than 20 years
– tumor marker for the majority of GTD: b-HCG
– GTN = Gestational Trophoblastic Neoplasia according to the FIGO definition: persistency or rise of HCG-values and /or histologically proofed choriocarcinoma
– persistent GTD: patients with persistency or rise of HCG-values
– GTT = Gestational Trophoblastic Tumor
  – may be used in all cases which are associated with tumor development
  – may be used for choriocarcinoma, PSTT and ETT

Incidence
– molar pregnancy occurs in about 1:500–1.000 pregnancies in Europe and North America
– choriocarcinoma 1:40.000–50.000 pregnancies
– within Asian population 3-fold higher incidence
– PSTT, EPS, PSN an ETT are very rare diseases

Age distribution and risk factors
– majority of cases are premenopausal
– molar pregnancy may be occur in women > 50 years-of-age
– GTD associated with intermediate trophoblast (PSTT and ETT) may occur postmenopausal
– women < 21 and > 35/40 years-of-age with higher incidence of GTD
– the only well accepted risk factors are age and previous history of GTD
– familial clustering of complete mole may occur and may associated with alterations of the NLRP-7-gene locus at 19q13.3–13.4 as well as for KH3C3L and PADI6 for complete and of MEI1 for partial hydatidiform moles

12.3 Pathology of GTD

12.3.1 Partial hydatidiform mole (PHM)

The majority of PHM is of androgenetic origin, representing a triploid chromosomal composition [16], mostly 69, XXX (Fig. 12.2). Rare cases are tetraploid [17].

Clinically: The majority of patients present with vaginal bleeding by missed/incomplete abortion and are less likely to have symptoms and signs similar to those seen in complete mole, especially in first trimester pregnancy (120). Serum HCG may be elevated, but is less than 10 % of what is seen in patients with complete moles with values > 100.000 IU/ml [11,19].

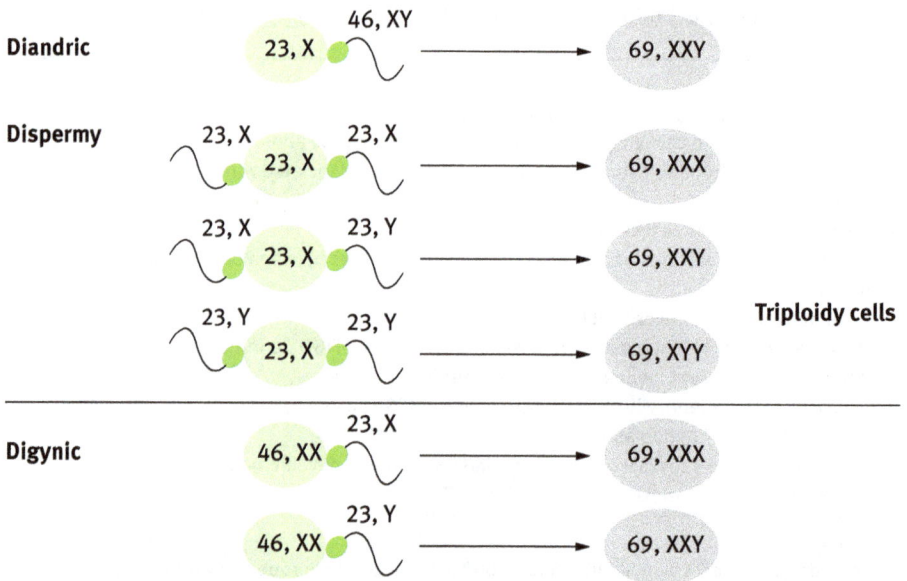

Fig. 12.2: Genetic background of partial hydatidiform mole [16,18].

Macroscopically: The evacuated material during dilatation and curettage (D & C) may be voluminous. If PHM occurs in the second or rarely third trimester, the placenta may be enlarged with some cystic changes. In a significant number of cases, the embryo/fetus or embryo/fetal tissue can be identified.

Morphologically: PHM is characterized by [1,20–22] Fig. 12.3; Fig. 12.4:
- two intermixed populations of placental villi (normal-sized, but fibrotic villi and enlarged hydropic villi), sometimes with central cistern formation (which is not so pronounced as in CHM),
- within the villous stroma, trophoblastic inclusions are often present, however these are not specific for PHM and may also be seen in trisomic abortions [23],
- chorionic villi appear often irregular and scalloping, a "fjord-like" pattern,
- villous trophoblast of the enlarged villi often shows focal, multifocal syncytial proliferation while polar or lateral proliferation [13,22],
- blood vessels containing fetal red blood cells may be present and embryonal/fetal tissue can be seen.
- blood vessels represent sometimes an angulated shape

An *early-PHM* may occur [24,138] and is comprised of enlarged villi with some hydropic stromal alterations but with small cystic transformation, trophoblastic inclusions and poorly developed trophoblastic hyperplasia may be present.

Immunohistochemically: p57-staining is preserved in PHM (see below).

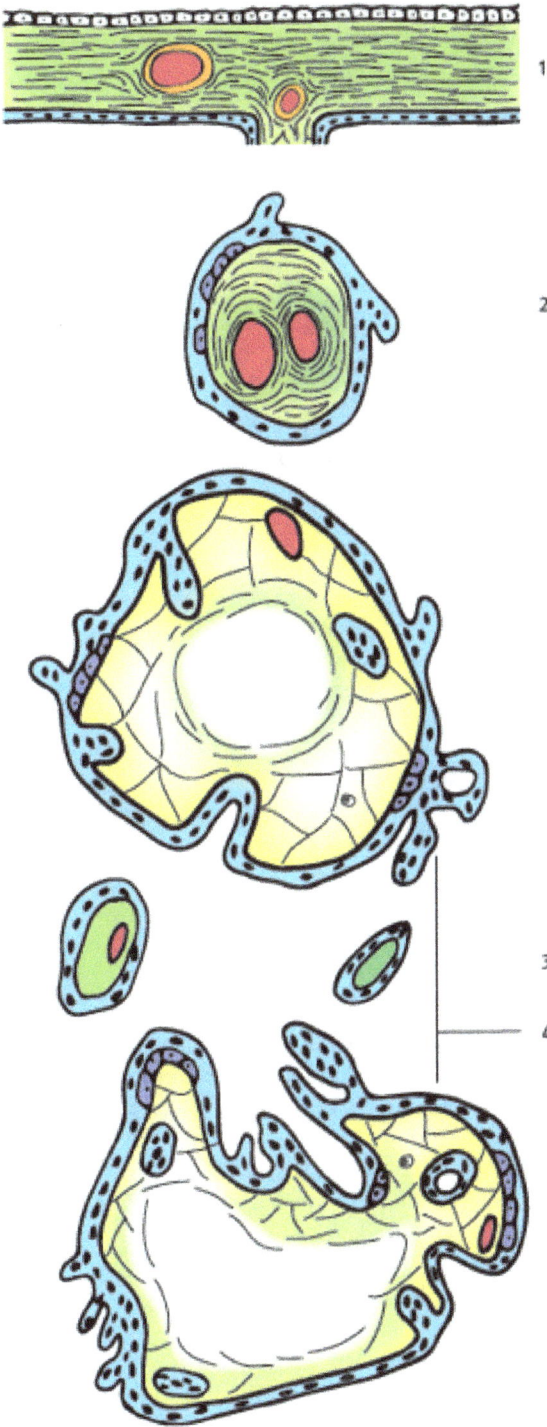

Fig. 12.3: Partial hydatidiform mole. Schematic presentation of the histological criteria for partial hydatidiform mole: (1) chorionic plate representing fetal vessels; (2) stem villi with normal appearance; (3, 4) presence of two distinct populations of chorionic villi: enlarged hydropic villi, sometimes associated with central cysts, mixed with normal appearing villi.

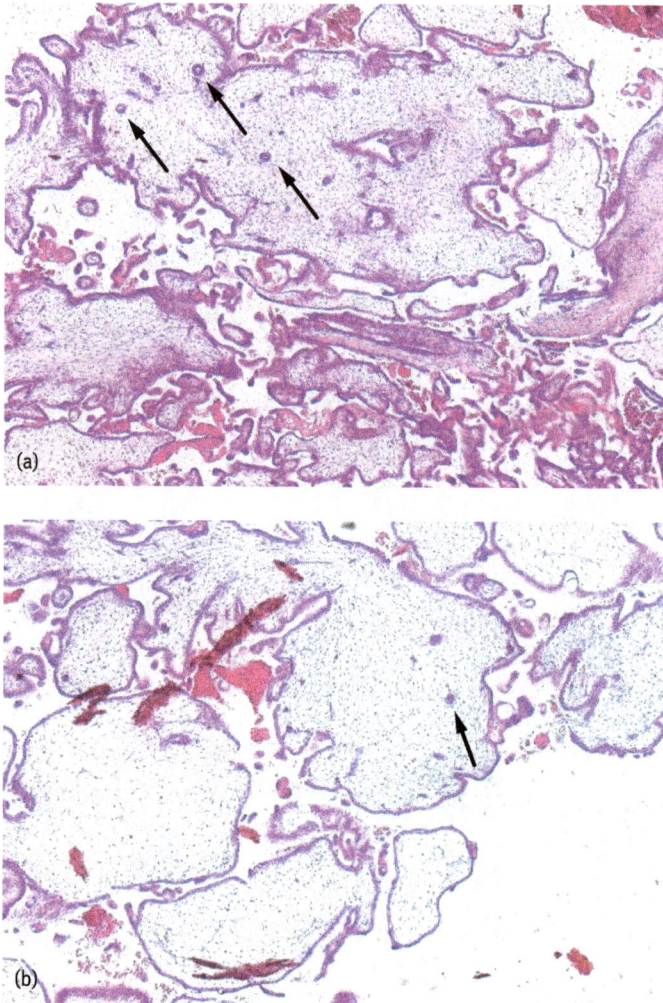

Fig. 12.4: Partial hydatidiform mole (a) mixture of enlarged and normal sized villi and intravillous trophoblastic inclusions (arrows), (b) hydropic and enlarged villi with intravillous trophoblastic inclusions.

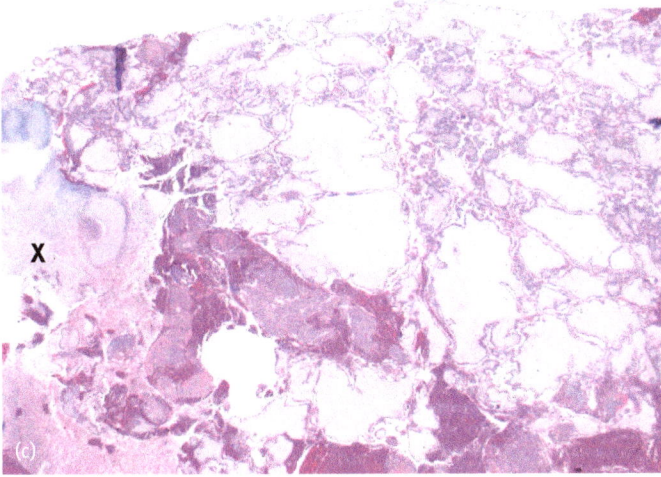

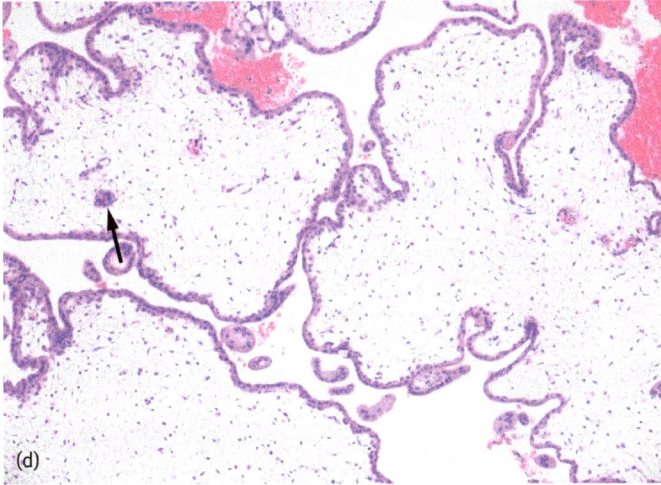

Fig. 12.4: (continued) (c) Low power view representing embryonic tissue (X) and a mixture of hydropic, enlarged villi with normal sized ones within 9th weeks of gestation, (d) hydropic hypovascu-
larized villi with irregular, "fjord like" outline with intravillous trophoblastic inclusions.

Differential Diagnoses

Care should be taken to not misinterpret folded fetal membranes as cistern formation within chorionic villi [20].

The main differential diagnoses include CHM and mesenchymal dysplasia of the placenta, as well as hydropic non-molar abortions [25] (please see pages 250 and 281). The main differential diagnoses and the morphological approach to it are summarized in Table 12.3 and Fig. 12.5. Very rarely PHM may be associated with exaggerated placental site.

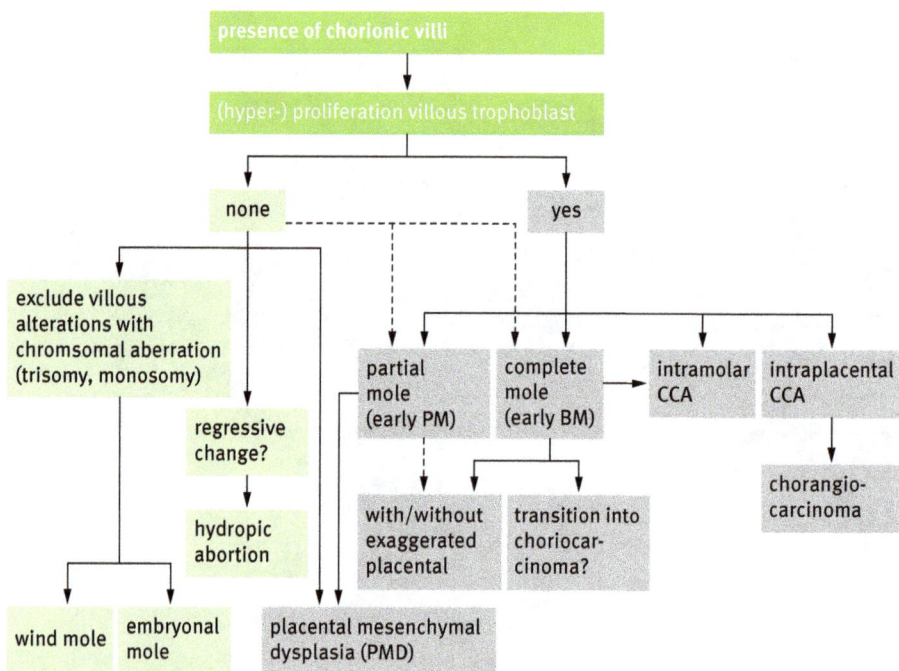

Fig. 12.5: Algorithm for the differential diagnosis of villous gestational trophoblastic disease (please see text, [26].

Table 12.3: Clinico-pathologic features of partial and complete hydatidiform mole and placental mesenchymal dysplasia [1,20,22,26,27].

	partial mole	early complete mole	complete mole	mesenchymal dysplasia
macroscopic findings	inconspicuous, enlarged placenta	inconspicuous	increased tissue amount, cystic villi may be present	increased tissue amount, enlarged placenta
embryo-fetal tissue	present malformation may occur	missing	missing	present malformation may occur
microscopic findings				
– villous stromal edema	yes, focal	inconspicuous, myxoid	diffuse	yes, stromal hyperplasia
– hydropic villi with central cysts	stem villi	may be focally present	present, may diffuse	stem villi
– intravillous vessels	yes (but not canalicular)	primitive vessels (CD 34 + ve)	canalicular vessels may occur	yes, may be dilated
– trophoblastic hyperplasia	weak to moderate and focal	strong circumferential or apolar	strong circumferential or apolar	none or very focal
– trophoblastic atypia	none or very focal	yes, may be prominent and diffuse	yes, may be prominent and diffuse	none
– p57^{KIP2}/PHLDA2	positiv[1]	negative[2]	negativ[2]	positive
genetic background	diandric triploid mostly dispermic (rarely tetraploid)	androgenetic diploid mostly monospermic	androgenetic diploid mostly monospermic	mostly diploid, biparental (trisomy may be present)
clinical signs				
– uterine size	normal	normal	mostly enlarged	normal
– ovarian theca-luteincysts	none	none	yes	none
– HCG-levels	slightly elevated	marked elevation	marked elevation	not elevated
– risk for persisting GTD	0,02–5 %	about 25 %	about 25 %	none

[1] > 10 %, see text
[2] may be positive in mosaic / chimeric conception, see text

Prognosis

There is low risk for the development of persistent GTD and choriocarcinoma, between < 0.02 to 1.7 % [28–30]. But some authors report a risk up to 4 % [19]. Women with a PHM as their first gestational event and with a diagnosis earlier in gestation are more likely to develop post molar GTN [31].

12.3.2 Complete hydatidiform mole (CHM)

CHM are in the majority of cases androgenetic in origin with a diploid karyotype containing paternal chromosomal and maternal mitochondrial DNA (Fig. 12.6) [16].

Clinically: Patients with CHM present with a large for date uterus, dysfunctional uterine bleeding and elevated β-HCG-values. On ultrasound a complex intra-uterine mass containing multiple small cystic spaces may be seen. Rarer symptoms include hyperemesis, hyperthyroidism, pre-eclampsia, pulmonary embolism and ovarian theca-lutein cysts [19,32,33]. In developed countries with routine prenatal care, the majority of patients represent with vaginal bleeding, missed abortion and/or abnormal sonographic findings [33–36].

Macroscopically: In the majority of cases, the D & C evacuations show a voluminous appearance and in a serious number of cases gross villi with cystic changed may be seen (Fig. 12.8a). In contrast, cases of early-CHM (see below) in evacuated tissue lack any suspicious findings on visual inspection.

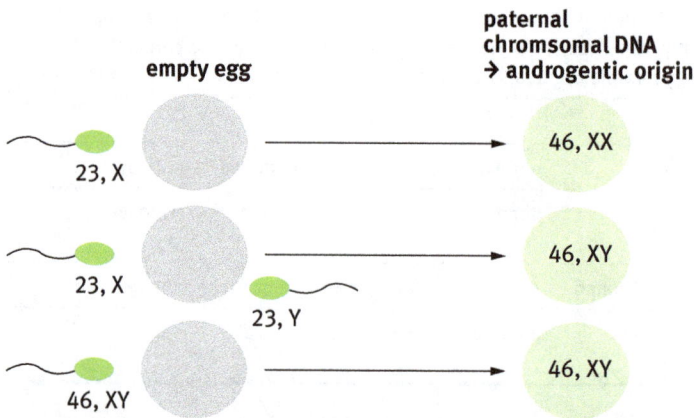

Fig. 12.6: Genetic background of complete hydatidiform mole with androgenetic origin [16–18].

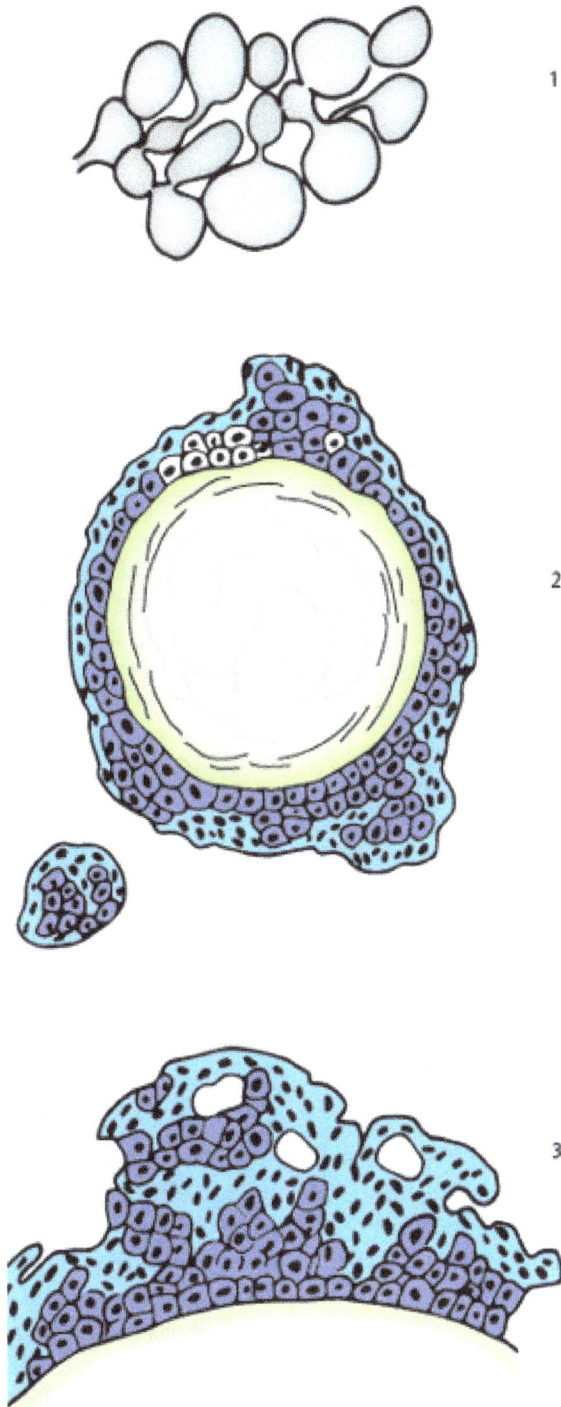

Fig. 12.7: Complete hydatidiform mole (CHM). Schematic presentation of the histological criteria for (classic) complete hydatidiform mole: (1) grape-like macroscopic appearance; (2) microscoically enlarged villi with central cystic alteration and circumferential trophoblastic (hyper-) proliferation; (3) villous trophoblastic hyperplasia, mainly done by the proliferation of the zytotrophoblast, intermingled with some intermediate trophoblastic cells and syncytiotrophoblast.

Morphologically: Well developed CHMs are characterised by [21,37,38] Fig. 12.8:
–   presence of enlarged villi with marked hydropic change and frequent central cyst formation,
–   cysts are surrounded by a rim of loose connective tissue representing variable degree of regressive change,
–   in some cases angioblastic proliferations may be seen representing abortive vessels without forming a vascular lumen,
–   a variable degree of (sometimes pronounced) trophoblastic proliferation may be seen, the predominant cell types represent cyto- and syncytiotrophoblast, intermingled with a variable number of intermediate trophoblastic cells, cytological atypia and mitotic figures are common,
–   embryonic/fetal tissue and non-molar villi are not present in the vast majority of cases.

Because of prolonged intrauterine retention, regressive change may occur within the molar villi, (Fig. 12.8g). These cases embedding of additional tissue may be helpful.

Usually, CHMs are diagnosed around the 11th week of gestation, but due to advances in routine ultrasound and increased use of routine pre-natal care, CHMs are now diagnosed earlier in pregnancy, at approximately the 7th week [11,32,35,36]. In the earlier cases the aforementioned histologic findings are not well established and the diagnosis of *early-CHM* may be challenging [137,138].

Microscopically: The early -CHM is characterized by [2,21,35,39,137,138] Fig. 12.9):
–   smaller sized villi, presenting a phylloid-like appearance,
–   central cistern formation is absent or inconspicuous,
–   villous stroma is typically hypercellular and myxoid and cellular debris of villous stromal cells may be seen on higher magnification,
–   a significant number of cases have stromal blood vessels, sometimes with luminal formation, but nucleated embryonal erythrocytes are rare,
–   marked trophoblastic proliferation is not always present and if absent cause a diagnostic challenge between early-CHM and hydropic abortions.

Immunohistochemistry

CHM is of androgenetic origin and paternally derived. Maternally expressed genes, such as p57, are not present. Immunohistochemical staining for p57, nuclear staining of stromal villous cells and the cytotrophoblast (CT) should be completely negative in CHM (Fig. 12.8e) [40,41]. Diagnostically, up to 10 % of villous stromal cells and/or cytotrophoblastic cells may be positive for p57 to meet the requirements for a diagnosis of CHM [42]. Positively stained nuclei of the extravillous trophoblast and decidual cells may be used as internal positive controls (Fig. 12.8e).

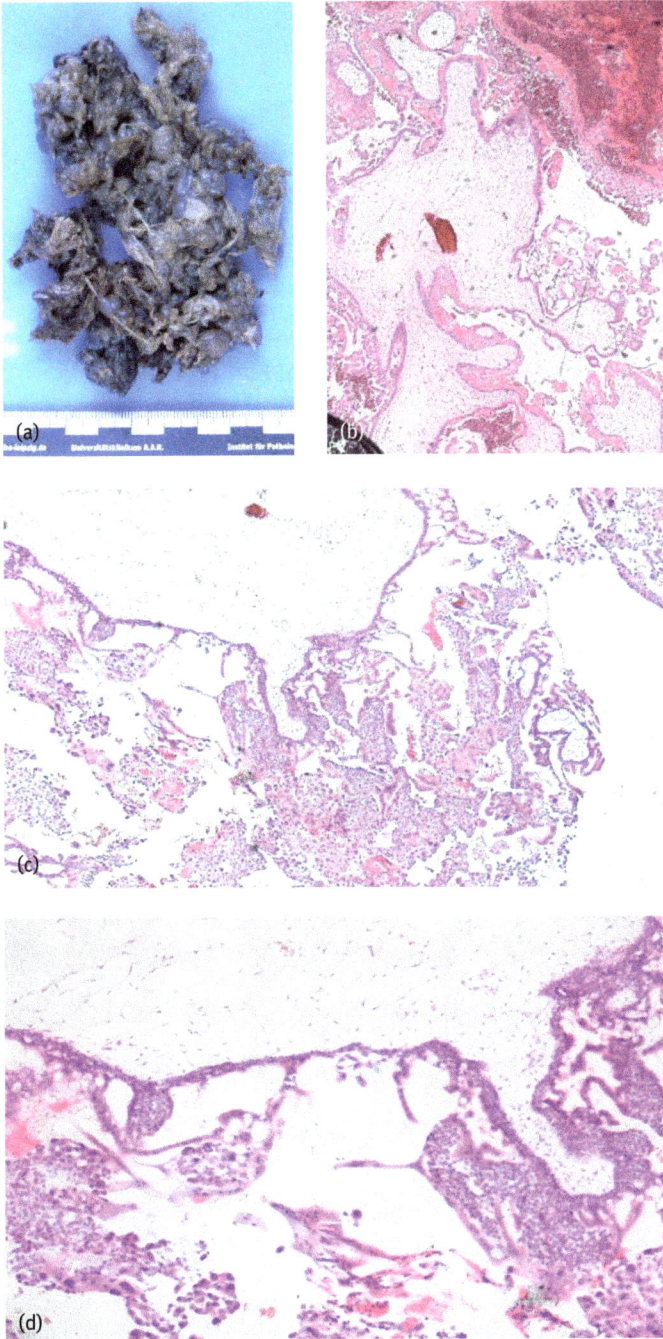

Fig. 12.8: Complete hydatidiform mole (CHM). (a) macroscopic picture of a curettage with CHM representing enlarged villi with cystic ("grape like") appearance, (b) and (c) enlarged, hydropic changed villi with irregular contour accompanied by trophoblastic hyperproliferation; (d) hydropic villous stroma, covered by increased trophoblastic proliferation, mainly by the cyto- and syncytiotrophoblast.

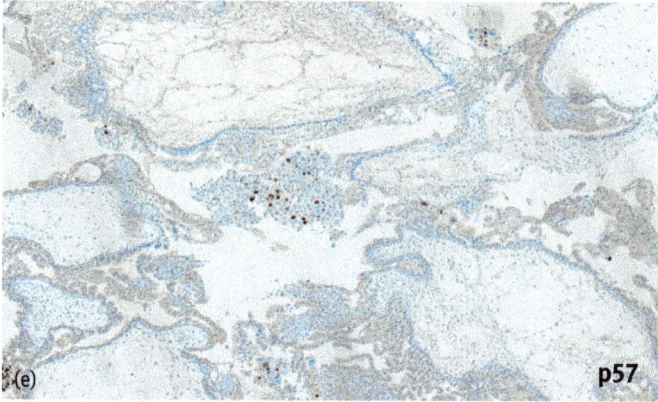

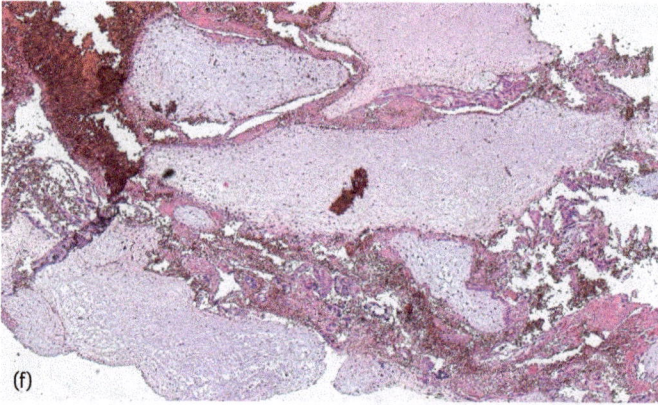

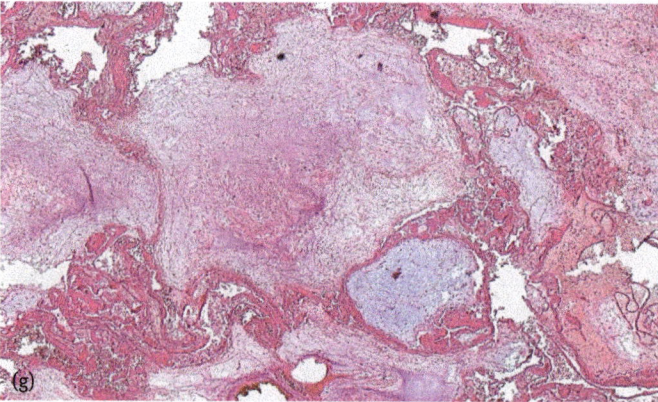

Fig. 12.8: (continued) (e) negative p57 immunostaining of the villous cytotrophoblast and stromal cells, extravillous cytotrophoblastic cells are nuclear positive and serve as positive internal control; (f) molar villi with weak to moderate regressive change, note the pale villous stroma and the eosinophilic change of the villous trophoblastic cells; (g) CHM with heavy regressive change, representing as "ghost villi", note the increased diameter and irregular contour of the villi, villous trophoblast appears as eosinophilic rim, outlining the villous surface.

Rare cases *of androgenetic/biparental mosaic/chimeric CHM* may be challenging in p57-immunochemistry interpretation. These mostly represent a mixture of villi with and without trophoblastic hyperplasia. Villi lacking trophoblastic hyperplasia show a p57-positive cytotrophoblast with negative stromal cells, whereas villi with trophoblastic hyperplasia are uniformly p57-negative in both cell types (Fig. 12.10) [27].

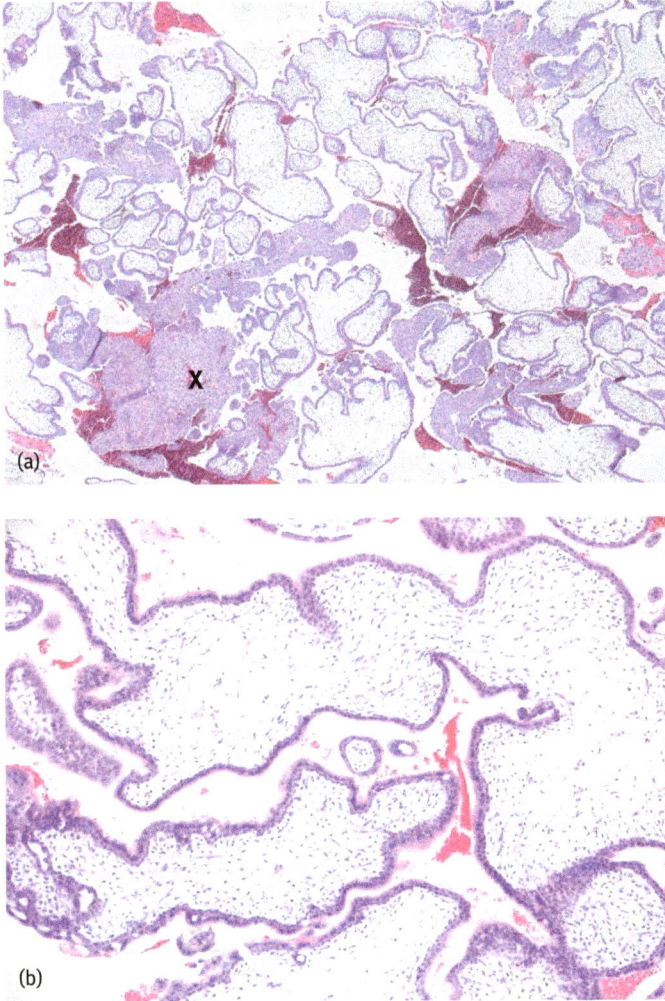

Fig. 12.9: Early complete mole. (a) low power view with slightly enlarged villi with some hydropic change, within intervillous space trophoblastic proliferation is present (X); (b) enlarged villi with hydropic highly cellular stroma and double layered trophoblast on its surface.

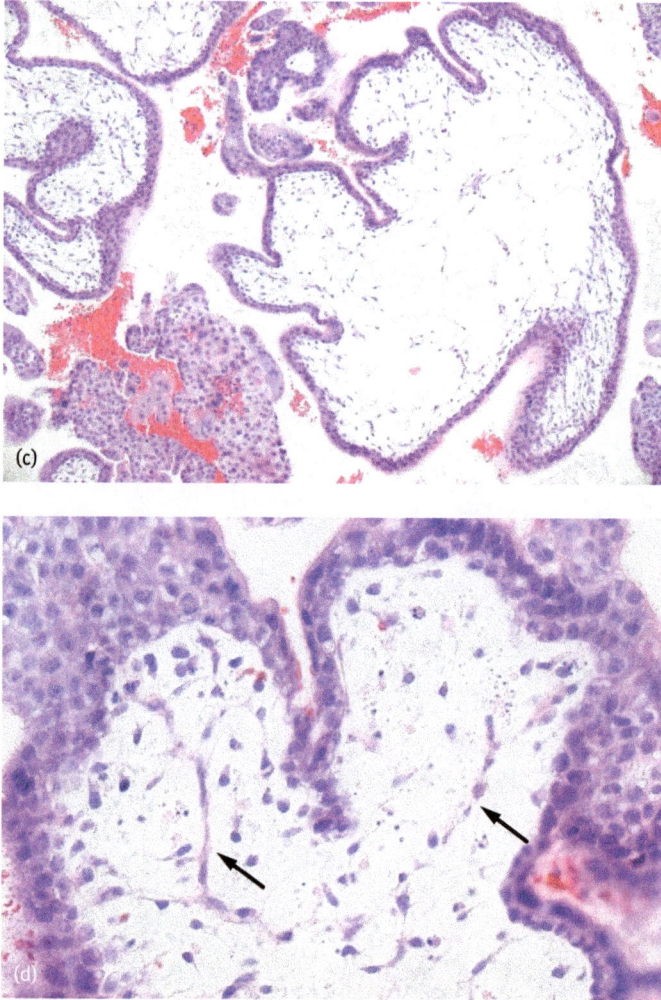

Fig. 12.9: (continued) (c) Hydropic villi with slightly central pseudocystic degeneration; (d) large power with some primitive vessels without luminal development (arrow) and nuclear debris within the hydropic stroma.

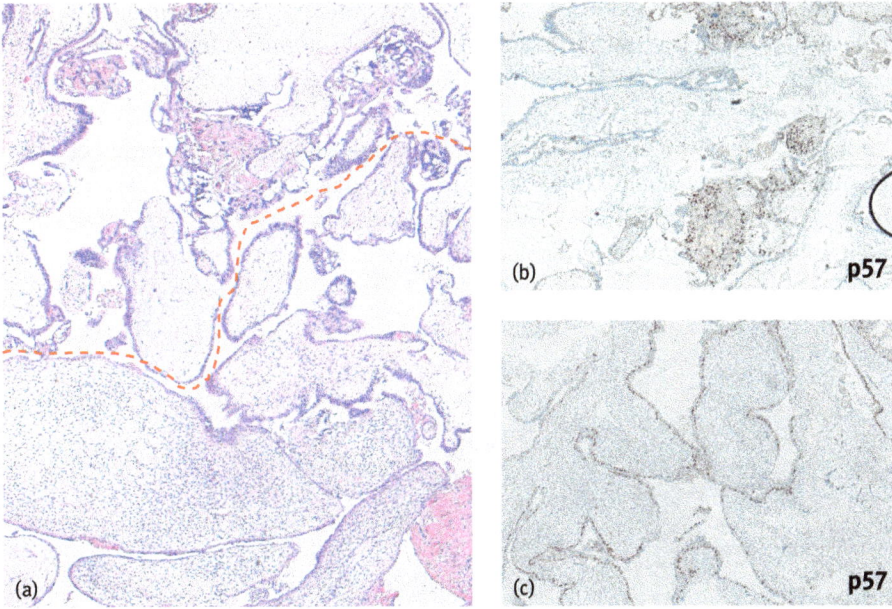

Fig. 12.10: androgenetic/biparental mosaic/chimeric CHM. (a) mixture of chorionic villi with weak trophoblastic hyperplasia and hypocellular hydropic villous stroma (upper half) and hypercellular villi, lacking trophoblastic proliferation; (b) hydropic villi represent complete negative p57-immunostaining within the villous cytotrophoblast and stromal cells; (c) the more cellular chorionic villi, lacking trophoblastic hyperplasia, represent p57-positivity within villous cytotrophoblastic cells but, the villous stromal cells are negative

Differential Diagnoses of Molar Pregnancies

Rarely, CHM may occur in an *ectopic tubal pregnancy* [43]. Some (early) tubal pregnancies can show a prominent trophoblastic proliferation on microscopy [44] and care should be given to not misinterpret this as a GTD (Fig. 12.11). p57 immunohistochemistry may be helpful in these problematic cases.

In isolated cases, trophoblastic proliferation of the fetal membranes may mimic tangential cutting of molar villi with trophoblastic hyperplasia (Fig. 12.12). Embedding of additional tissue and immunohistochemical stains for p57 can be helpful in this setting.

The main differential diagnoses are the *PHM, hydropic abortions* (with and without chromosomal abnormalities) and *mesenchymal dysplasia* of the placenta (see Table 12.3 and Fig. 12.5 [2,25,45]. P57 nuclear staining of the villous cytotrophoblast and stromal cells is retained in PHM, hydropic abortions and placental mesenchymal dysplasia [46].

Exaggerated placental site (see below) is a common finding in early CHM, but may also be associated with "conventional" CHM. The presence of invading intermediate trophoblastic cells in the decidua, and the inner part of the myometrium with replacement of the walls of spiral arteries represents a normal finding, especially in early pregnancy. This finding is neither diagnostic for an exaggerated placental site nor for an invasive mole.

In rare cases, when molar villi are intermingled with normal appearing villi, the possibility of a *twin/multiple pregnancy*, in which one of the placentas is molar and the other is normal should be considered [47]. In those cases clinical information p57-immunostaining and even molecular analyses [41,48,49] may be of diagnostic value.

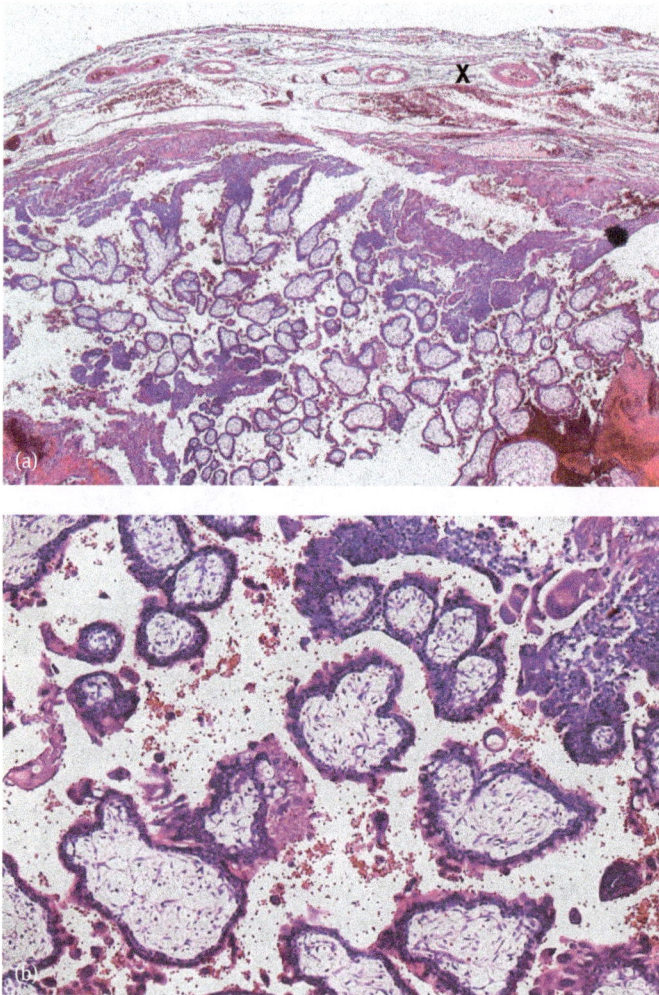

Fig. 12.11: Tubal pregnancy mimicking (early) complete hydatidiform mole. (a) low power view with tubal wall (X) and intraluminal small chorionic villi with mesenchymal, edematous stroma and strong, apolar trophoblastic proliferation; (b) higher magnification from (a).

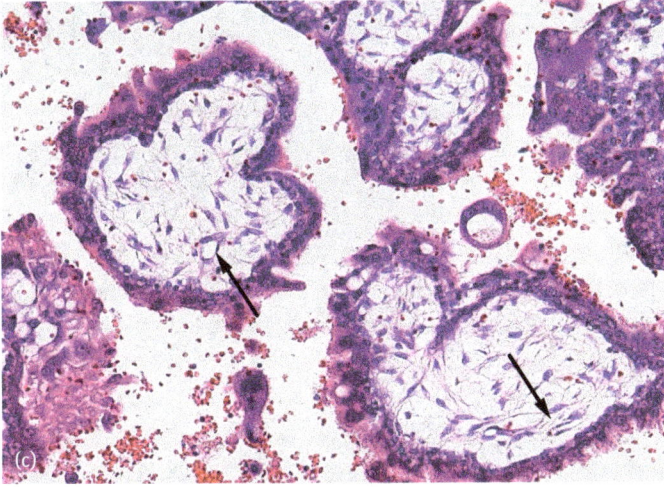

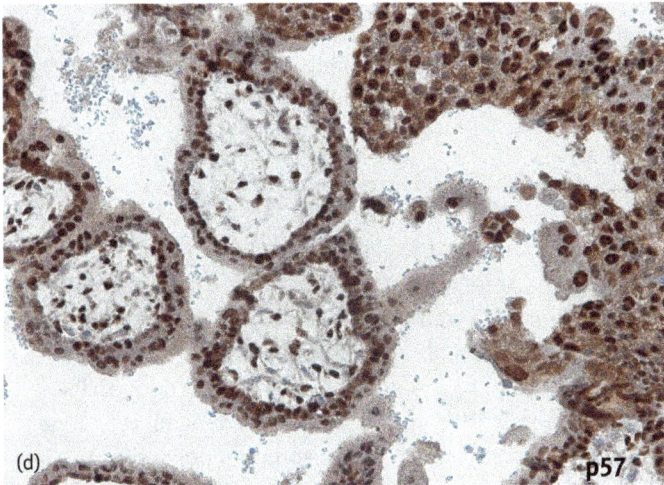

Fig. 12.11: (continued) (c) Chorionic villi with circumferential proliferation of slightly hyperplastic trophoblastic epithelium and small vessels within the villous stroma (arrow); (d) retained strong nuclear positivity for p57 within the villous and extravillous zytotrophoblastic cells and villous stromal cells.

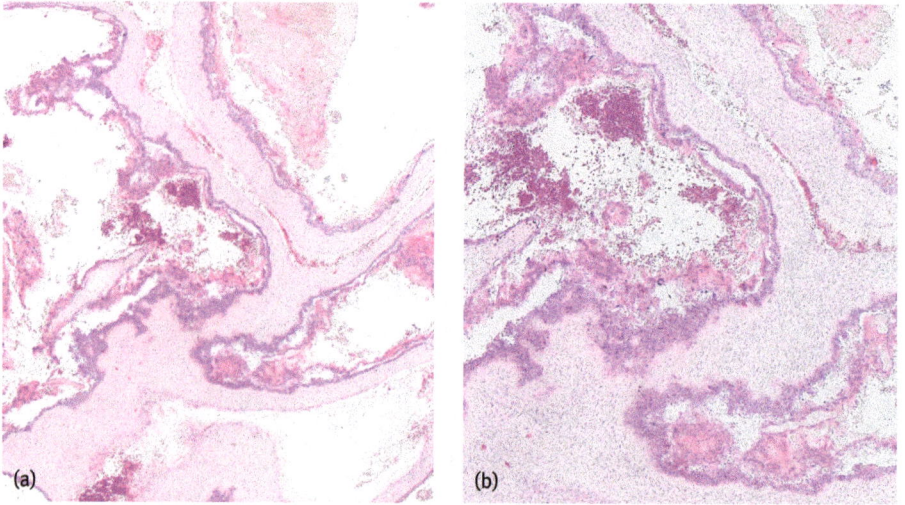

Fig. 12.12: Fetal membranes mimicking complete hydatidiform mole; (a) and (b) fragments of slightly fibrous fetal membranes with (reactive) trophoblastic hyperplasia, mimicking complete hydatidiform mole. Note, there are no hydropic alterations of the stroma and no cistern formation (for details please see text).

Ancillary Techniques

Flow cytometry has been used to determine the ploidy of products of conception [50]. The technique may require fresh tissue for optimal results may be time consuming and is only available at some institutions. Flow cytometry allows the distinction between triploidy (in PHM) and diploidy. The discrimination between CHM, hydropic abortion (with and without trisomy) and placental mesenchymal dysplasia is not possible.

Molecular techniques can be helpful in this setting. Short tandem repeat genotyping, as used in forensics, can determine the parental source of polymorphic alleles and can aid the above mentioned differential diagnoses by discerning androgenic diploidy, diandric (paternal) triploidy and biparental diploidy [49,51,52].

An algorithmic approach using p57 immunohistochemistry and genetic profiling may precisely aid the diagnosis in complex cases [1,48,53].

Such ancillary techniques can play a vital role in the clinical management of patients, especially in early CHM where there are neither morphological nor immunohistochemical features that can reliably predict the subsequent requirement of chemotherapy treatment [54].

12.3.3 Invasive hydatidiform mole (IHM)

Clinically: In IHM there is a strong association with a history of CHM [41].

Recent studies suggest that the risk of IHM after CHM is higher in cases of a heterozygotic/dispermic complete mole [55,65].

Macroscopically: There are no indicative features. In hysterectomy specimens non-specific hemorrhagical nodules within the myometrium may be seen.

Morphologically: IHM is characterized by Fig. 12.13 [21,56]: presence of molar villi within the myometrium, its vascular spaces, or at distant sites e. g. vagina or lung.

Therefore, only hysterectomy specimens or representative biopsies from distant sites are sufficient to allow at diagnosis of IHM. The presence of trophoblastic cells at the placental implantation site, and invading the decidua, and invading the inner part of the myometrium with replacement of the walls of spiral arteries, all represent normal findings. In addition the presence of an "exaggerated placental site" associated with a CHM should not be mistakenly diagnosed as IHM. The presence of exaggerated placental site in association with a CHM is not indicative for the diagnosis of IHM.

The diagnosis of IHM on curettage may be possible, if the tissue contains fragments of myometrium with invasive molar villi. Morphologically, the villi of IHM share the features of CHM villi, however, their size may be smaller and the trophoblastic proliferation may not be so pronounced. Especially after previous chemotherapy villi in CHM can't undergo regressive change and sometimes only ghost molar villi are present histologically.

Differential Diagnosis of IHM
Very rarely the differential diagnosis includes placenta increta/percreta and these can be challenging [57]. However in placenta in- and percreta a decidualization of the endometrium is greatly reduced or missing entirely. Very rarely, an intramural pregnancy [58] may be in the differential. In each of the aforementioned differential diagnoses the placental villi demonstrate no molar changes and nuclear p57 staining is retained. Proliferated trophoblastcic cells of IHM may mimic gestational choriocarcinoma, so careful interpretation, deeper sectioning and adequate embedding of the endo-myometrial junction in hysterectomy specimens after CHM or in suspicion for IHM in mandatory.

12.3.4 Gestational Choriocarcinoma (CC)

Gestational choriocarcinoma represents a highly invasive and aggressive trophoblastic tumor. The current WHO-classification defines CC as a trophoblastic tumor consisting of a trimorphic proliferation of the cytotrophoblast, syncytiotrophoblast, and intermingled with intermediate trophoblastic cells [1] with an absence of chorionic villi. Only in rare cases of CC occurring with villi are reported:

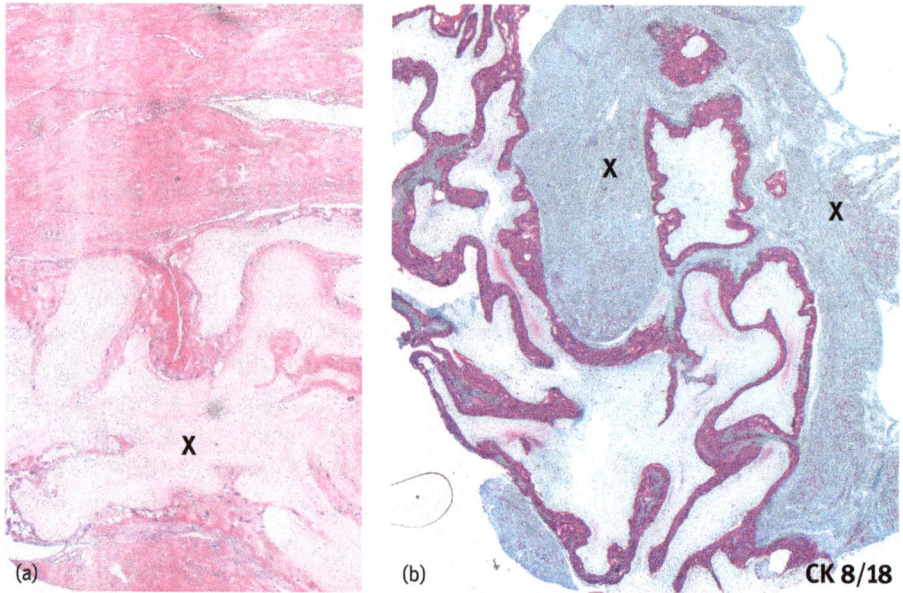

Fig. 12.13: Invasive hydatidiform mole; (a) molar villi with regressive change (X) lying between the smooth muscle fibres of the myometrium; (b) molar villous trophoblast highlighted by positive immunostaining against CK 8/18, the surrounding myometrium (X) with negative staining.

– intraplacental CC [59–61],
– intramolar CC and
– CC in association with tubal pregnancy [43,62].

There is an ongoing debate regarding the diagnosis of intramolar choriocarcinoma. It is well established that CHMs represent a wide spectrum of trophoblastic proliferation and show variation, from one case to another [63] which may be changed by previous chemotherapy and intrauterine retention. Therefore the diagnosis of an intramolar CC should be made with caution. Some authors suggest a diagnostic requirement of an infiltrative and cytologically malignant trophoblastic proliferation that is morphologically indistinguishable from CC which occurs in the presence of villi with molar characteristics [65].

CC is a rare disease with an incidence of 3.1/100.000 births in Europe and North America [9], but in can be as high as 0.4–2/1.000 pregnancies in south-eastern Asian countries [66,67].

In general CC may be associated with any type of pregnancy. Very rarely it occurs within tubal extrauterine pregnancy [43,68,69]. Prior to the introduction of sequential maternal HCG-follow up and effective chemotherapy, about 50 % of CC occurred following a previous complete molar pregnancy, and 25 % after a previous non-molar abortion and 25 % after previous term pregnancy [70]. Currently 50 % of CC will be

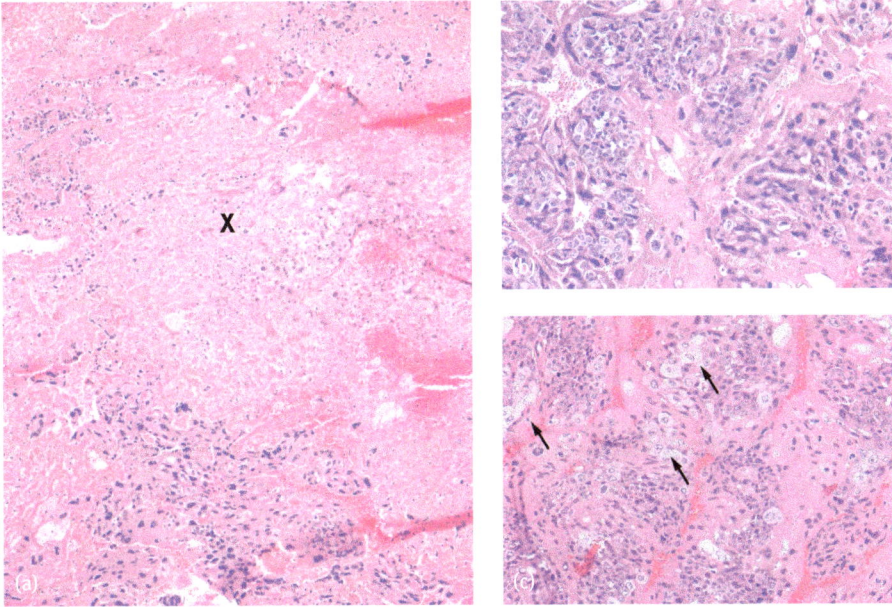

Fig. 12.14: Gestational Choriocarcinoma; (a) low power view representing a trophoblastic proliferation with dirty and hemorrhagic necroses (X); (b) biphasic proliferation of atypical cyto- and syncytiotrophoblastic cells; (c) atypical cyto- and syncytiotrophoblast intermingled by some intermediate trophoblastic cells with clear cytoplasm (arrows).

preceded by term pregnancy and 25 % after previous complete molar pregnancy [71]. The average length of time to CC is 13 months after complete molar pregnancy and 1–3 months following a term pregnancy [72,73]. The risk of postmolar CC is 2–3 % for complete [29,74] and < 0.02 to 1.7 % for partial moles [28–30].

Macroscopically: Both, uterine or metastatic CC typically forms hemorrhagic masses with a variable amount of necrosis and ill-defined borders [75]. In specimens suspicious for CC paraffin blocks should be obtained from the transition zone between the hemorrhagic/necrotic area and the surrounding tissue. Extensive sampling is strongly recommended. If CC is associated with a (third-trimester) placenta, it is frequently interpreted as placental infarction, however the location is unusual central for such infarct [60]). A significant number of CC associated with a placenta, the placenta was macroscopically normal [61].

Morphologically: CC display [1,8,21] Fig. 12.14:
– cohesive sheets of a trimorphic trophoblastic proliferation of intermediate and cytrotrophoblastic cells with a rim of syncytiotrophoblast,
– in the majority of cases marked cytological atypia with brisk mitotic activity is present,

– the Ki-67 labeling-index is high (~90 %) and may be of some value in the differential diagnosis for PSTT and ETT (see Table 12 .4 and 5),
– in cases with previous chemotherapy treatment the number of apoptotic cells may be abundant and may mimic and be misinterpreted as single cell keratinisation,
– vascular invasion is a striking feature of CC. In contrast to other malignant epithelial tumors, CC lacks tumor-associated angiogenesis. CC realise their blood supply via extensive invasion and destruction of pre-existing vessels with secondary formation of hemorrhagic blood lakes which are very characteristic,
– the tumor cells express a broad-spectrum cytokeratines and the syncytiotrophoblast is positive for β-HCG.

Differential Diagnoses
The main differential diagnoses include other trophoblastic lesions (see Table 12.4 and Table 12.5 as well as Fig. 12.15).

After an incomplete evacuation of a complete or partial hydatidiform mole [63] rarely after previous non-molar miscarriage, persisting trophoblastic cells may challenging. In the majority of cases those trophoblastic cell clusters represent parts of "normal", non-GTD associated trophoblastic tissue from the implantation site. After previous mole these cells represent the morphologic equivalent of persisting trophoblastic disease and the diagnosis of CC should be made with caution. In the setting with previous CHM or IM, the presence of lymph-vascular invasion by trophoblastic cells is not considered unequivocally diagnostic of CC [65]. Additional tissue should be embedded and examined in uncertain cases and further clinical information requested, for example, clinical signs of persisting/metastasising GTD and HCG-values.

Other differential diagnoses include poorly differentiated carcinomas of the female genital tract with trophoblastic differentiation [88] and undifferentiated carcinomas which may represent the carcinomatous component of a malignant mixed Müllerian tumor (MMMT, [89,90]. In the majority of cases MMMT is associated with older age and negativity for GATA-3 and variable expression of CK 8/18 (please see Fig. 12.15 and Table 12.4).

Regressive changes, sometimes seen in association with chemotherapy, may cause extensive apoptotic bodies which may be misinterpreted as single cell keratinization in poorly differentiated squamous cell carcinomas (SCC, [91]). Immunohistochemically, the SCC is positive for p63, p40 and CK 5/6, sometimes for CK 18 and may express p16 if they show a HPV-association. In contrast CC positive for CK 8/18, GATA-3 [135] and β-HCG (although β-HCG positivity may be reduced after chemotherapy). Cytotrophoblastic cells in CC stain positively for SALL-4 [79] GATA-3 has been reported to be positive in PSTT [80]. A heavily pre-treated CC may mimic or recur with the morphologic features of ETT [92,93].

epithelial proliferation suspicious for trophoblastic lesion?

yes (p16–, CK 18+++, HLA-G+++)

no

exclude non-trophoblastic lesion
Desmin, Vimentin, CK 18, HMW-CK*, HPL, CD 146, Inhibin α, β-HCG, HMB-45, Ki-67 etc.

no tumorlike lesion

tumor development

EPS
chorionic villi?
giant cells?
mitoses: rare
Ki-67-LI: < 1%
p63–, hPL+++

PSN
hyaline matrix
cellularity
mitoses: rare
IT-Marker +**
Ki-67-LI: 5–10 %
cyclin E–,
p63+++, hPL ±

IPSR*
chorionic villi?
moderate
cellularity
rare mitoses
superficial
invasion

choriocarcinoma
· bi- (tri-) phasic
  pattern
· β-HCG +
· Ki-67-LI: ~ 75 %
  p63+/+++

PSTT
diffuse infiltration
dissecting growth
pattern
high cellularity
mitoses: 0–6/10 HPF
char. vascular
invasion AE 1/3+,
CK 18+
Inhibin α+, HPL+,
CD146+
Ki-67-LI: > 10-30%,
p63–

ETT
pushing border
moderate cellularity
mitoses: 1–10/10HPF
necroses/hyaline
matrix, calcification
may occur preserved
vessels wall
HPL ±, CD 146 focally+
Inhibin α+, CK 18+
Ki-67-LI: 10–25 %
cyclin E++, p63+++

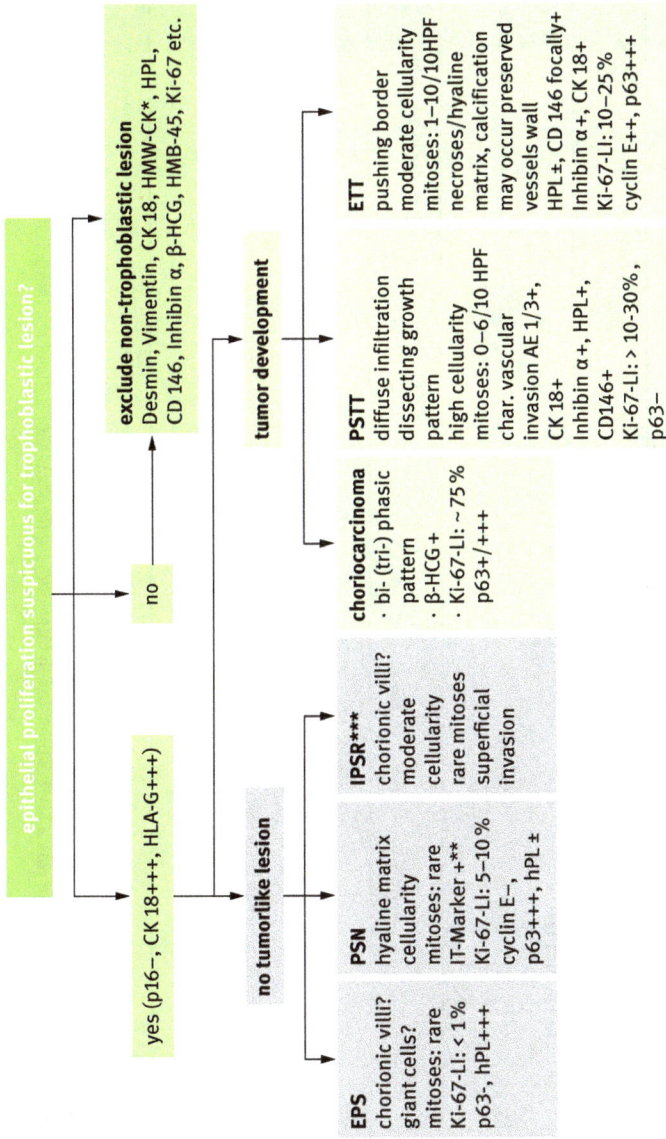

Fig. 12.15: Algorithm for the differential diagnosis of non-villous gestational trophoblastic disease (please see text, Horn & Vogel 2004, Shih 2007, Horn 2013). *HMW-CK = high molecular weight cytokeratines, **IT-Marker = immunohistochemical markers for intermediate trophoblastic cells, ***IPSR = increased placenta site reaction (see page 329 and Fig. 12.23) [18,76,77].

Table 12.4: Immunohistochemical stains for non-villous trophoblastic lesions and its main differential diagnoses [1,51,53,76,78,79–84].

	β-HCG	p63/p40	HPL	PLAP	Inhib-in α	CD 146	EMA	CK 18	HMW-CK¹	HMB-45	GATA-3	SALL-4	cyclin E	HLA-G	Ki-67
1. gestational trophoblastic lesions**															
choriocarcinoma	+++	−	−/+	?	+	−	+	+	+	−	+	+	−	+	~90 %
placental site nodule	−	+	+	?	+	+/−	+/−	+	+	−	+	?	−	+	< 5 %
EPS	focally+	−	+++	focally+	+	++	+	+	+	−	+	−	−	+	< 5 %
PSTT	focally+	−	+++	focally+	+	+++	+	+	+	−	+	−	−	+	10–30 %
ETT	−	+	−/+	−/+	+	focally+	+	+	*	−	+	−	+	+	10–25 %
2. non-trophoblastic lesions															
squamous cell cancer²	−	+	−	−	−	−	+	−/+	+++	−	−/(+)	−	rarely+	focally+	> 50 %
(epitheloid) leiomyo-sarcoma³	−	−	−	−	−	−	(+)	−	−	−	−	−	−	−	variabel (> 50 %)
malignant melanoma	−	−	−	−	−	+	−	−/+	−	+	−	?	focally+	−	high
MMMT/poorly differentiated endometrial carcinomas	−⁴	−/+	−	−	−	−	+	+	+	−	−	−	−/+	−	high

¹HMW-CK: high molecular weight cytokeratines; ²the vast majority of SCC are positive for CK 5/6 and p16, whereas trophoblastic tumors are almost negative; ³leiomyomas and leiomyosarcomas are positive for myogenic markers whereas trophoblastic tumors are negative; ⁴may be + ve in somatic syncytiotrophoblastic cells within the tumor; * it has been reported that HSD3B1 may represent a specific trophoblastic marker [85]; ** it has been shown, that PD-L1 is expressed in a variety of non-villous GTD [86]. In normal trophoblast there was a high expression in intermediate trophoblastic cells of the implantation site [87].

Table 12.5: Useful clinico-pathologic features for the differential diagnosis of non-villous GTD (for details please see text).

	Chorio-carcinoma	PSN	EPS	PSTT	ETT
age	pre-mp[1] (29–31 yrs)	wide range	pre-mp	20–60 yrs	15–48 yrs
previous pregnancy	term, CHM, tubal	each kind	each kind, early CHM	mostly term	mostly term
pre-therapeutical HCG	> 10.000 IU/l	not elevated	< 1.000 IU/l	< 1.000 IU/l	< 1.000 IU/l
clinical symptoms	most cases	none/rarely	none	mostly	none/yes
diagnosis because of	symptoms	incidental	incidental	symptoms	symptoms
tumor present	mostly	none	none	mostly	mostly
tumor location	mostly uterine corpus	isthmic/corpus	corpus	corpus	uterus, extra-uterine
hemorrhagic lesion	YES	none	none	none/focally	none/focally
growth pattern	infiltrative, destructive	none	dissective	dissective	pushing
geographic necroses	none/hemorrhagic ones	none	none	none/rarely	YES
vascular pattern	haemangio-invasion	none[2]	mimicking	"pale rings" normal placental site	well preserved surrounded by trophobl. cells
cellular composition	triphasic (CT & ST & IT)[3]	monomorphic	bimorphic	bimorphic	monomorphic
giant cells	syncytial	none	intermediate trophoblastic type	intermediate trophoblastic type	none/rarely
mitotic activity	high	none	none	variable (mostly ≥ 5/10 HPF)	0–9/10 HPF
Ki-67 index	high > 90 %	mostly < 5 %	< 5 %	10–30 %	10–25 %

[1]pre-mp = pre-menopausal; [2]may be present in atypical PSN; [3]CT = cytotrophoblast, SZ = syncytiotrophoblast, IT = intermediate trophoblast

Prognosis

Gestational CC is a highly aggressive disease but is also highly responsive to effective chemotherapy. Prognosis depends on tumor stage and the FIGO risk score [14,15,94]. In FIGO low-risk disease, post-molar CC represent with increased risk of failure to first-line single-agent methotrexate chemotherapy [95].

12.3.5 Placental Site Trophoblastic Tumor (PSTT)

PSTT represents a rare neoplastic lesion of the implantation site (Ch. 11) [1,76]. The detailed histogenesis is unclear [96] but, the presence of X-chromosome related information may be necessary prerequisite as these tumors lack a Y-chromosome [97–99]. In contrast to CC, which is preferentially associated with CHM or IHM, about two thirds of PSTT develop after normal pregnancy or non-molar abortion with a median latency of 12 to 18 months [78] but this latency extend up to three years [100].

The leading symptoms are vaginal bleeding and enlarged uterus [99,101,102]. The serum β -HCG values may be elevated up to 1.000–2.000 IU/ml [13,99,101,102].

Macroscopically: The findings are very variable with well circumscribed to ill-defined lesions of different size with a reported average of 5 cm [78,99]. The cut surface may be soft, tan to yellow. About half of the cases represent focal hemorrhagic change which is less extensive than in CC. If extensive hemorrhage, necroses and deep infiltrative growth are evident, it may indicate malignant behaviour (see below).

Morphologically: The cellular composition of PSTT is similar to normal placental site reaction and EPS ([21,78,99] Fig. 12.16, Table 12.5):
- densely packed intermediate trophoblastic cells with a variable number of intermediate type trophoblastic giant cells,
- cytoplasm may be amphophilic, eosinophilic, or, sometimes clear,
- the mitotic index often is between 2–4 per 10 HPF [78,103], but may be higher,
- at the infiltrative edge, intermediate trophoblastic cells infiltrate the myometrium individually or in small groups in a dissecting pattern that preserves muscle fibers which may be highly compressed. However cases with a destructive type of infiltration may occur,
- a distinctive vascular invasion is present with the walls of the spiral arteries replaced by mononucleated intermediate trophoblast (IT) cells and fibrinoid eosinophilic material forming "pale eosinophilic rings" maintaining a central lumen. That pale rings may be better visible at low or intermediate power. In several cases these pale rings are incomplete and in other cases the vessels wall is completely replaced by intermediate trophoblast cells. Groups of IT may be present in the lumen of the vessels. The pattern of invasion may be highlighted with CK 18 and the muscle fibers by SMA or vimentin.

Immunohistochemically: The tumor cells are strong and diffuse positive for CK 18, EMA, inhibin, HPL, HLA-G and CD 146 rarely positive for β-HCG and p63 is almost always negative [77]. SALL-4 is negative [79]. GATA-3 has reported to be positive in PSTT [80,135]. The Ki-67 labelling-index is about 10–30 % [76,78].

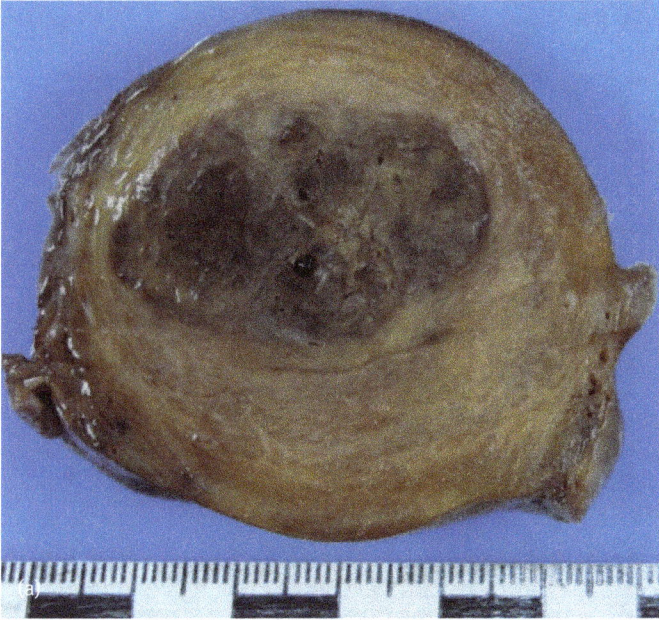

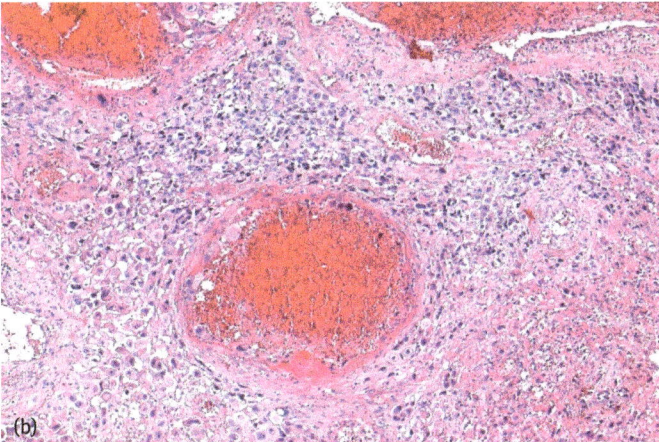

Fig. 12.16: Placental site trophoblastic tumor (PSTT); (a) horizontal cut of a PSTT within the uterine cavity. Note that there is some necrosis but no extensive hemorrhage; (b) distinctive vascular invasion with replacing vessels wall by fibrinoid eosinophilic material and intermediate trophoblastic cells.

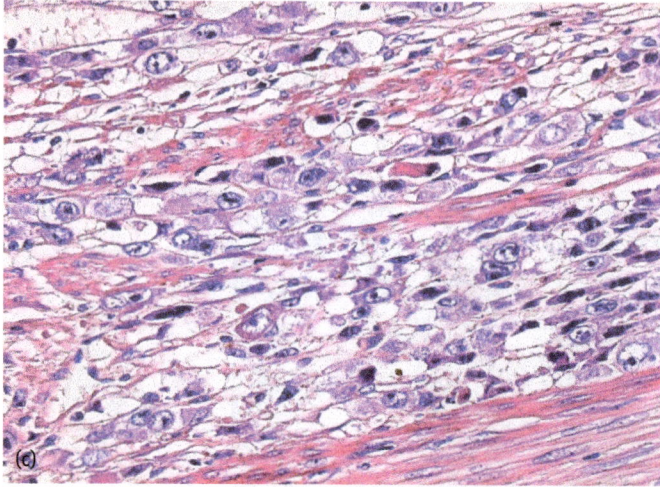

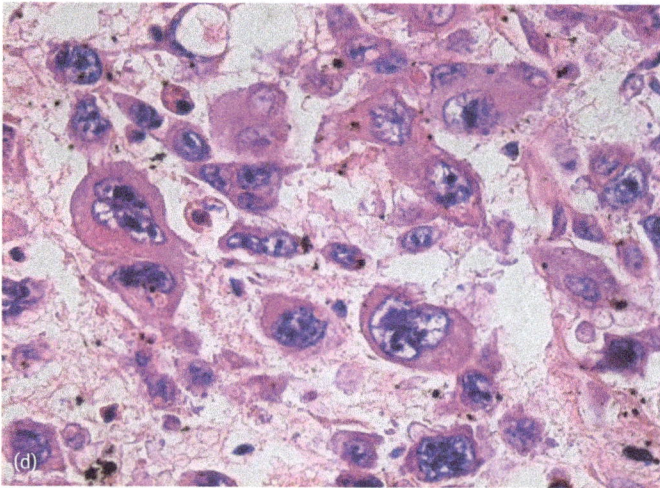

Fig. 12.16: (continued) (c) Intermediate trophoblastic cells infiltrating the myometrium singly and in small groups with a dissecting but not destructive pattern, preserving the muscle fibers; (d) polymorphic intermediate trophoblastic cells, intermingled by intermediate trophoblastic giant cells.

Differential Diagnoses

The main differential diagnoses of PSTT include other trophoblastic tumors (see Table 12.4 and Fig. 12.15). In some cases the distinction between PSTT and exaggerated placental site (EPS) may be challenging. In the majority of cases with EPS non-molar or molar villi are present (sampling issue) and there is no tumor formation. Features favouring PSTT are: presence of tumor by visual inspection, high cellularity with a small number of giant cells of the intermediate trophoblastic type, destructive growth, no chorionic villi (adequate tissue sampling is essential), presence of mitoses, high Ki-67 labelling-index (> 5–10 %).

Poorly differentiated tumors [104], such as epitheloid leiomyoma and leiomyosarcoma should also be considered differentially.

Prognosis

It is generally difficult to predict the clinical behaviour with certainty on morphology [98,99,106]. Factors reported to be associated with malignant behaviour are [1,78,106]:
- advanced tumor stage with extension beyond the uterus,
- older age (> 35 years),
- infiltration of the myometrium > 50 %,
- tumor necrosis (extensive)
- presence of cells with clear rather than amphophilic or eosinophilic cytoplasm,
- marked nuclear and cellular atypia, increased mitotic activity (> 5/10 HPF), Ki-67 mitotic -index > 50 %.

12.3.6 Epitheloid Trophoblastic Tumor (ETT)

ETT is the rarest type of gestational trophoblastic tumors and consists of a neoplastic proliferation of intermediate trophoblastic cells of the chorionic type [1,93,136].

There are several pathogenetic pathways (Fig. 12.17). but the majority of cases may develop *de novo* from retained intermediate trophoblastic cells [96,107]. Molecular analyses suggest that in the majority of cases maternal X-chromosomal linked genetic information is necessary for the development of ETT, however it can also develop in male pregnancies [105,108]. Some ETTs may arise from an atypical PSN [83,93]. A third pathway has been postulated for cases in which CC was (heavily) pre-treated by poly-chemotherapy with the eradication of chemosensitive trophoblastic cells and the

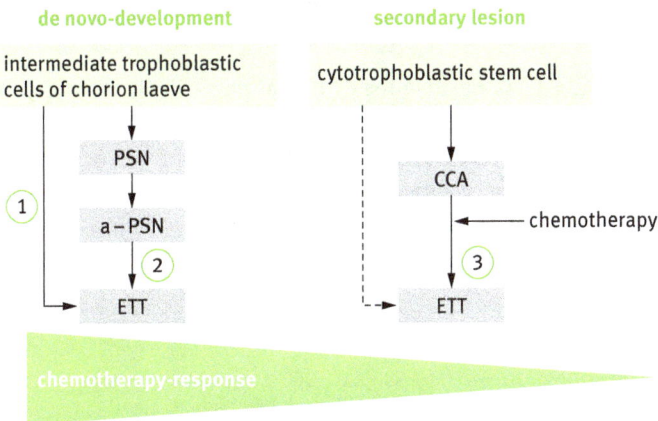

Fig. 12.17: Different pathogenetic pathways within the development of epitheloid trophoblastic tumor [83,92,93,96,107, 109–111].

persistence of resistant cell clones with ETT-like morphology [92,109–111]. The latter pathway may be supported by the fact that CC is a proliferatively active tumor with a Ki-67 mitotic-index of ~90 % (but not 100 %) and ETTs a low proliferative lesion. Additionally, ETTs within the lung has been reported following persisting complete and invasive moles treated by chemotherapy [64,112].

The majority of ETTs occur in pre-menopausal women with a mean age of 36 years [107]. About two thirds of the cases are preceded by term pregnancy, about 15 % by a non-molar abortion and 15 % by molar pregnancy [107,109,113], after a median time interval of 6.2 years [64]. The leading symptoms are dysfunctional bleedings with moderately elevated serum β-HCG values, approximately 2.500 IU/ml [64,101,113]. Some patients present with a uterine tumor and 35–40 % have metastatic disease at time of diagnosis [113–115].

Macroscopically: The majority of cases present with a large tumor of variable size which may be located in the corpus (Fig. 12.18a), isthmus or cervix uteri, sometimes the tumor may be located outside the genitalia e. g. the lung or within a cesarian scar [1,112,116]. The cut surface is variable but frequently shows tan to brown coloration and is solid, sometimes with pseudocystic degeneration, hemorrhage, geographic necroses, sometimes fistula formation and calcification and occurs.

Morphologically: The ETT is characterized by (Fig. 12.18; [1,21,22,64,77,81,107,112]:
– nodular/multinodular growth,
– tumor edge represent a pushing border but, sometimes
– an infiltrative growth may occur,
– deposition of hyaline-like material between tumor cell nodules, representing geographic necroses, sometimes associated with calcification, is characteristic,
– ETT is composed of a relatively uniform population of mononucleated cells with eosinophilic or clear cytoplasm, often with distinct cell membranes and rounded nuclei, that contain distinct nucleoli. Nuclear atypia is generally moderate with a mitotic count of 0–9 mitoses per 10 HPF,
– within the tumor well developed vessels with preserved walls and without vascular invasion are characteristic.

Immunohistochemically: The ETT is positive for cytokeratines, CK 18, HLA-G, p63, H3D3B1, cyclin E and inhibin [1,81,82]. In contrast implantation site IT (and PSTT), are negative or, only show focal expression for HPL, β-HCG and CD 146, and are negative for p16. SALL-4 is also reported to be negative [79]. Although experience is limited, as in testicular ETT [117], GATA-3 has reported to be positive in ETT [80]. Ki-67 mitotic-index ranges between 10–25 % [76,83].

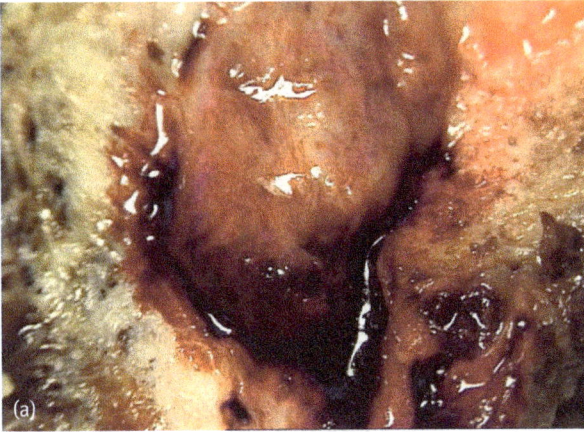

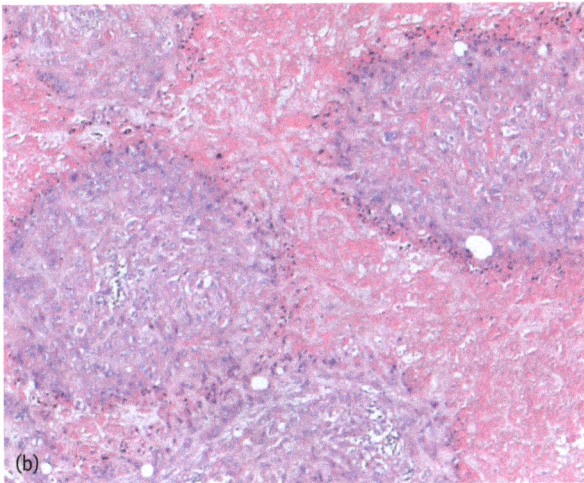

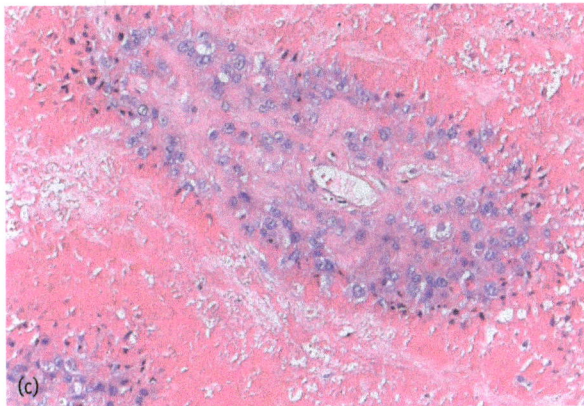

Fig. 12.18: Epitheloid trophoblastic tumor (ETT); (a) ETT protruding in the uterine cavity with polypoid appearance; (b) intermediate trophoblastic cells separated by hyalinised necrotic material in a geographic pattern, there is no hemorrhage between the tumor cells; (c) uniform intermediate trophoblastic cells with prominent nucleoli, well defined nucleolar membranes and pale, eosinophilic cytoplasm, intratumoral vessels are surrounded by these cells with preserving vessel wall without vascular invasion.

Differential Diagnoses

The main differential diagnoses include other trophoblastic tumors (see Tables 12.4 and 12.5 and Fig. 12.15). In some cases the distinction between ETT and atypical PSN may be challenging. When the ETT occurs or involve the uterine cervix, the tumor cells may colonise the endocervical gland and mimic a high-grade squamous intraepithelial lesion [118] or non-keratinising primary squamous cell carcinoma of the cervix. The latter is negative for GATA-3, inhibin, HLA-G and cyclin E and positive for p16 and HPV in the majority of cases.

Prognosis

The prognosis is similar to PSTT with mortality reported to be approximately 10 % of the patients will die of the disease [96,105]. 35–40 % of the patients will present with metastatic disease at time of diagnosis [113–115]. A long time interval between preceding gestations may be unfavourable prognostic factor [114]. The prediction of behaviour on morphology is always not possible in the majority of cases [1] but a mitotic count of > 6 mitoses per 10 HPF may indicate poor prognosis [36].

12.3.7 Intermediate trophoblastic tumor (ITT) and unclassified GTD

The intermediate trophoblast represents a special subtype of trophoblastic cells with an intermediate morphology and biological functions between the more immature cytotrophoblast and the syncytiotrophoblast [119,120].

In GTD there is an overlapping immunohistochemical profile in EPS and PSTT as well as in PSN and ETT [76,82]. Furthermore, staining of HLA-G has been demonstrated in CC, PSTT and ETT [82,121]. In addition, stem cell features haves been reported in different types of GTD [121].

The transition from one entity to another has been documented; atypical PSN into ETT and CC into ETT after treatment with combined chemotherapy [83,93,122].

More recently, trophoblastic lesions with mixed morphologic features of CC, PSTT and ETT, and even IM, in a single lesion were seen [110,115,123,124]. For lesions with morphologic features of the intermediate trophoblast, the term intermediate trophoblastic tumor (ITT) may be appropriate [4,21,82].

In some trophoblastic lesions the amount of trophoblastic tissue that is available for morphologic analysis is inappropriate or the morphology is inconclusive for a definitive diagnosis. In these cases, the term unclassified GTD may be used and the patient should be monitored by serial β-HCG analyses and undergo examination for the presence of metastatic disease.

12.3.8 Placental Site Nodule (PSN)

The PSN represent a benign non-neoplastic lesion caused by the retention of inter-mediate trophoblastic cells after any type of pregnancy [1]. The retained IT-cells are thought to be of the chorionic type of IT [76,111]. In the majority of cases, the PSN is an incidental finding in uterine curettages, endo-cervical biopsies or hysterectomy specimens in a variety of clinical settings. About two thirds of the lesions have been reported to occur at the lower uterine segment [125,126] sometimes associated with irregular/dysfunctional uterine bleeding [75]. Rarely PSN can occur within the Fallo-pian tube [127,128].

Macroscopically: The PSN is not visible with a reported size ranging between 0.4 and 1.0 cm on histology [125,126].

Morphologically: PSN is typically characterised by [1,21,125,126]; Fig. 12.19:
–   a singular or multiple, nodular or plaque-like and well circumscribed lesion with a pushing border,
–   the presence of a hyalinised eosinophilic matrix which may contain hemosiderin,
–   a variable number of haphazardly distributed intermediate type trophoblastic cells arranged in small clusters, cords or as single cells with regressive changes and atypia, sometimes bi- or multinucleated cells may occur in a low number. The number of trophoblastic cells may be very scanty and can be highlighted by cytokeratin staining.
–   mitoses only rarely occur.

Immunohistochemically, the intermediate trophoblastic cells of the PSN are positive for cytokeratin 18, pan-cytokeratines, EMA, inhibin-α, GATA-3 and HLA-G [82–84]. They express p63 but unlike ETT, lack cyclin E expression [81]. The Ki-67 mitotic index is usually low (< 5 %; [76])
      Lesions which do not meet the histomorphologic criteria of "typical" PSN, but falls short of ETT have been referred to as *atypical PSN* (a-PSN; [77,81,83]). That term is found in the current WHO-classification [1] but is not well defined. Compiling liter-ature data [81,83,116,120,129,130], they are characterized by (Fig. 12.20):
–   intermediate trophoblastic cells with moderate to marked atypia (enlarged nuclei with hyperchromatic often smudgy chromatine).
–   increased proliferative activity (mitoses and elevated Ki-67 mitotic index),
–   high cellularity,
–   ill-defined borders,
–   increased size (usually > 0.4 cm).

Morphologic features of "usual" and atypical PSN are summarized in Table 12.6.

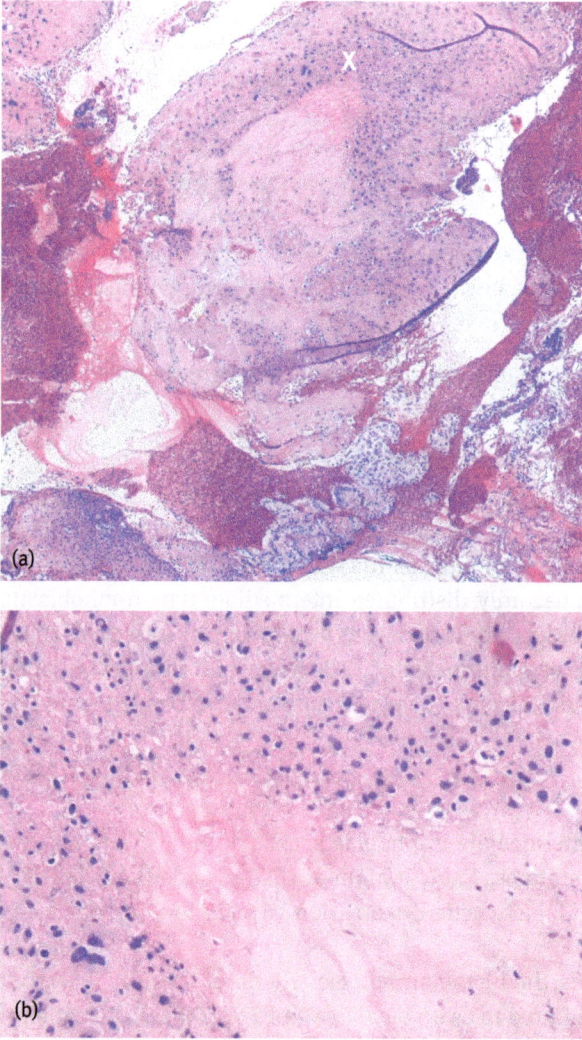

Fig. 12.19: Placental site nodule (PSN); (a) fragmented tissue containing a nodular lesion with smooth borders (X); (b) cellular trophoblastic lesion in a background of hyalinized matrix containing mononuclear trophoblastic cells with some nuclear hyperchromasia and pleomorphisms.

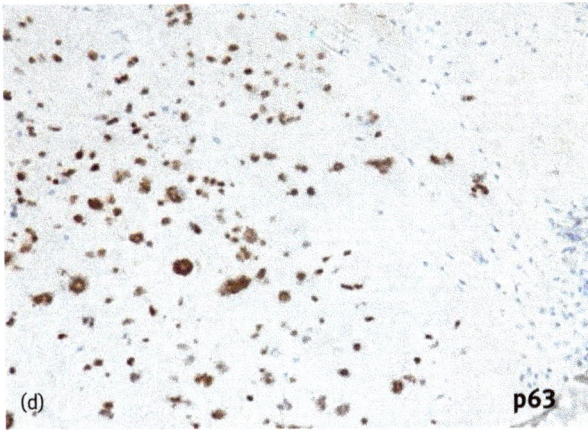

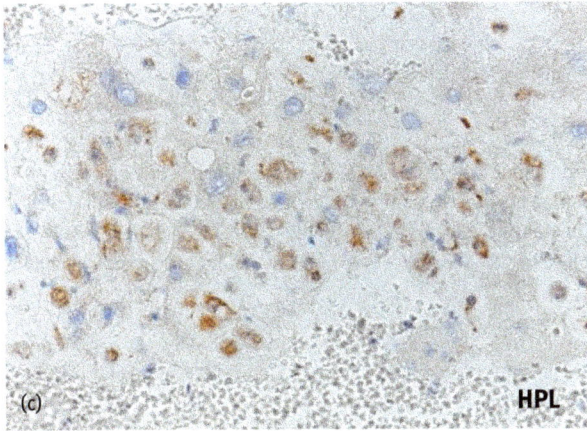

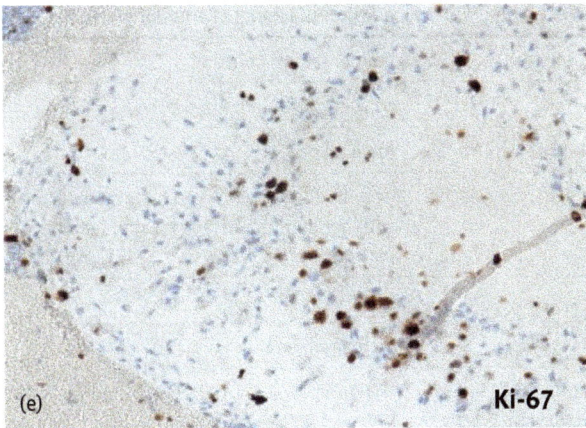

Fig. 12.19: (continued) (c) and (d) intermediate trophoblastic cells with immunohistochemical positive reaction for HPL and p63; (e) intermediate trophoblastic cells with low proliferative activity, highlighted by Ki-67 staining.

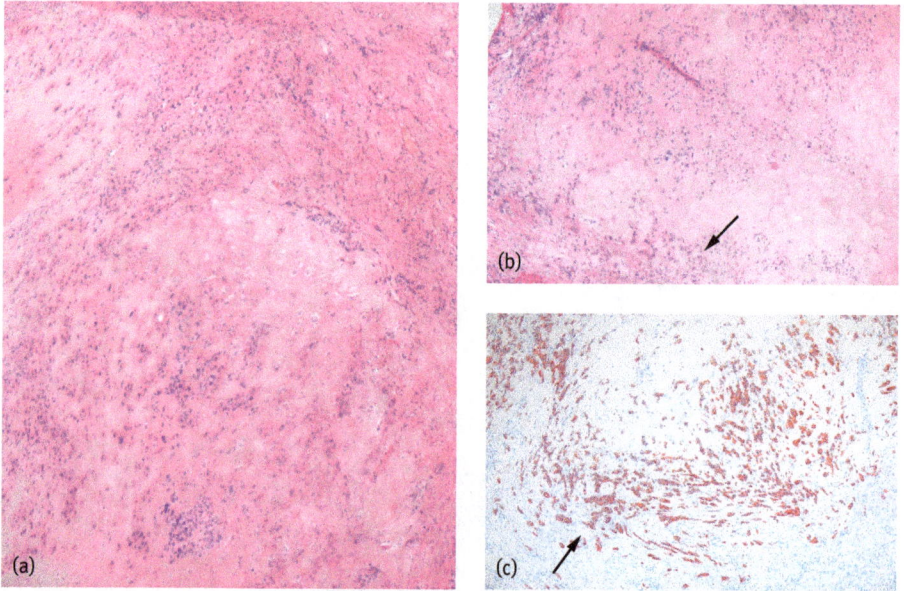

Fig. 12.20: Atypical placenta site nodule (a-PSN); (a) and (b) low and medium power view representing a nodular shaped lesion with pushing border, containing a high number of trophoblastic cells, embedded in a hyalinized matrix, sometimes the lesion is not well demarcated (arrow); (c) (intermediate) trophoblastic cells highlighted by CK 8/18 indicating a highly cellular lesion with irregular borders (arrow).

Table 12.6: Morphologic features of placental site nodule (PSN) and atypical placental site nodule (a-PSN).

	placental site nodule (PSN)	atypical placental site nodule (a-PSN)
appearance	incidental, microscopic	incidental, microscopic
outline	pushing border	pushing AND ill defined borders
cellularity	variable, may be hypocellular	increased
cellular atypia	may be present, "regressive type"	yes, moderate to marked (enlarged nuclei with hyperchromatic, often smudged chromatine)
mitoses	none	present
lesions size	small	increased (mostly > 0.4 cm)
immunohistochemistry	+ve for: pan-CK, CK 18, GATA-3, p63; cyclin E -ve	+ ve for: pan-CK, CK 18, GATA-3 p63, cyclin E?*
Ki-67	mostly < 5–8 %	increased (> 5 %, but lower as 10 % in ETT??)

*cyclin E has been reported as positive in ETT, but negative in "usual" PSN [81]

Differential Diagnoses

A PSN may be misinterpreted as an eosinophilic variant of a high grade squamous intraepithelial lesion however, the PSN is negative for p16 and HPV. Rarely PSN and cervical squamous cell cancer can coexist [131]. PSNs must be differentiated from *retained decidua* with regressive changes (Fig. 12.21). Intermediate trophoblastic cells of the PSN may be highlighted using CK 8/18 or GATA-3 staining but are negative for vimentin. Hemosiderin pigment is more often seen in retained decidua, it can also occur in PSN.

Unlike ETT, PSN lacks cyclin e-expression [81]. It has been suggested that ETT may develop from a-PSN [81,83,129], so in small biopsies or challenging cases the differential diagnosis between these two lesions is not possible [81].

Prognosis

The typical PSN represent a benign lesion and follow up control is not indicated. But a-PSN may represent a step in transition to ETT [81,83,129] or may associated with other types of GTD and serial b-HCG measurements may be warranted [129].

12.3.9 Exaggerated Placental Site (EPS)

EPS represents a lesion with an exuberant but non-neoplastic proliferation of the intermediate trophoblast at the implantation site. The current WHO-classification states that an EPS represents part of the normal spectrum of implantation site changes [1].

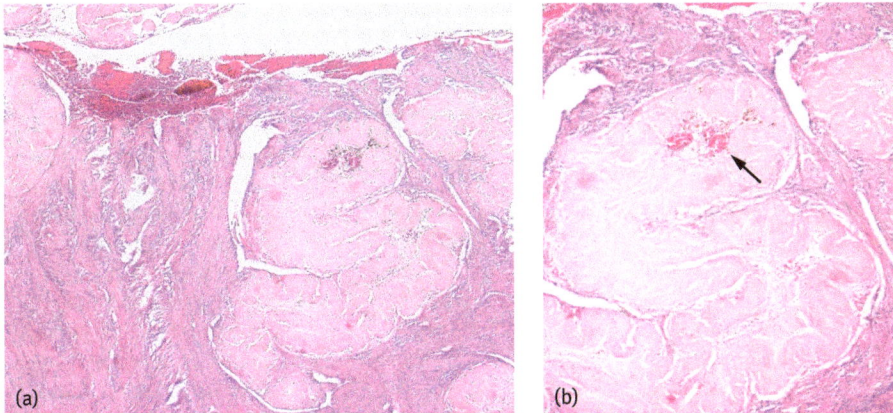

Fig. 12.21: Retained decidual tissue mimicking placental site nodule; (a) low power view representing well demarcated multinodular lesion within the uterine myometrium with hyaline appearance; (b) hyalinized matrix with some fresh and older (arrow) hemorrhagic change. Note, there are no cells within the hyalinized stroma (see text).

EPS can be found in association with normal pregnancy, abortion and complete hydatidiform moles and is mostly seen in the first trimester. Very rare cases have been seen in association with PHM [24]. Biologically, there may be a difference between EPS in non-molar gestations and those with molar disease. There are no specific symptoms and EPS is usually an incidental finding [126].

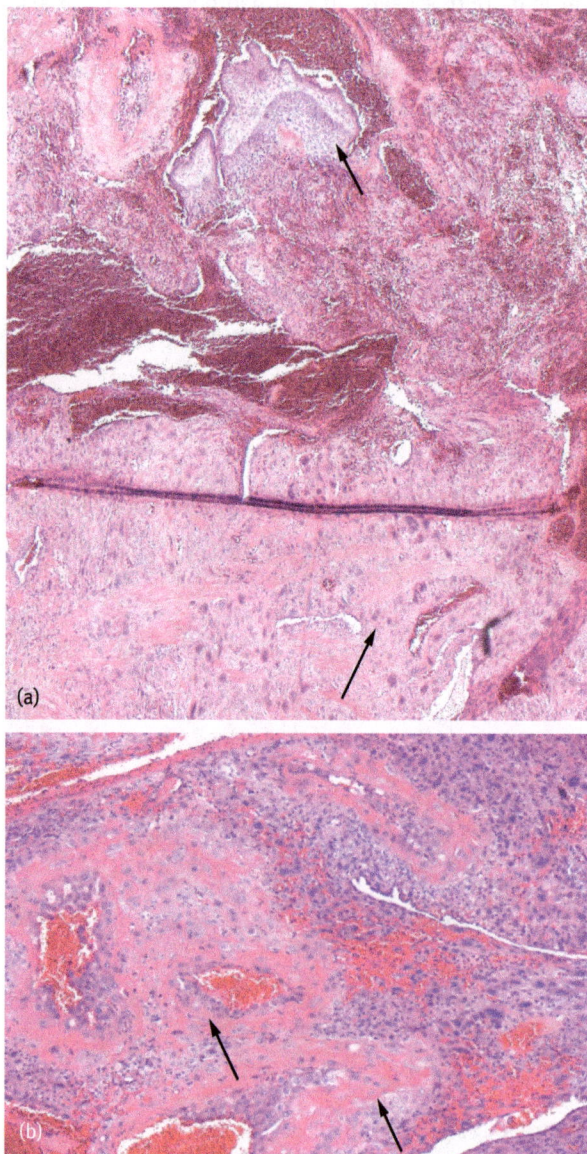

Fig. 12.22: Exaggerated placental site (EPS); (a) low power view representing first trimester chorionic villi (arrow) and placental implantation site; (b) placental implantation site with highly cellular intermediate trophoblastic proliferation and spiral arteries (arrows), vessels wall is replaced by fribrinoid material and intermediate trophoblastic cells.

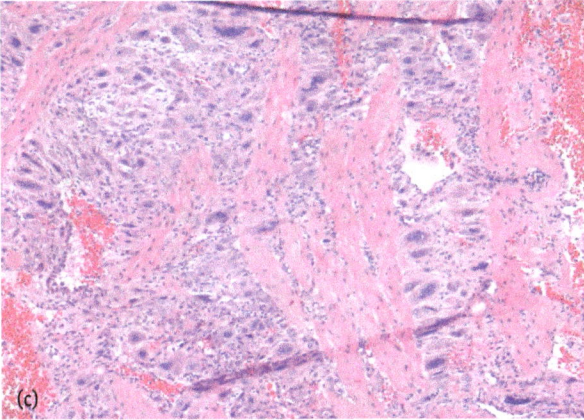

Fig. 12.22: (continued) (c) Highly cellular lesion with high number of intermediate trophoblastic cells dissecting the smooth muscle fibres of the myometrium.

Morphologically EPS is characterised by Fig. 12.22 [1,21,77,126]:

- an extensive trophoblastic infiltration of the decidua and the underlying myometrium by intermediate trophoblastic cells without destructive growth, mimicking the patterns of normal placental site,
- endometrial glands are surrounded by the infiltrative growing cells, and the cells infiltrate between smooth muscle fibers of the myometrium by intermediate cells that demonstrate no destructive growth and sometimes heavily compressed but not destroyed. This present a "dissecting pattern of infiltrative growth" rather than a destructive one,
- the vessels walls of the spiral arteries are replaced by fibrinoid material, and intermediate trophoblastic cells,
- chorionic villi may be found in the majority of cases,
- in contrast to a normal placental site, the number of intermediate trophoblast giant cells is increased.

Immunohistochemically the amount of trophoblastic proliferation can be highlighted by CK 18, GATA-3 or pan-cytokeratines. As in normal placental site, the Ki-67 labeling index is < 5 % [77,93,107].

Differential Diagnosis

Fig. 12.23: The main differential diagnosis is the distinction from *increased placental site reaction* (IPSR) That lesion is characterized by highly cellular proliferation of mononucleated intermediate trophoblastic cells without an increase of the number of intermediate trophoblastic giant cells. Especially in cases with deep curetting, the trophoblastic proliferation may be present within superficial myometrium (Fig. 12.23a, b and d). This feature is not indicative for EPS or PSTT, respectively. The intermediate trophoblastic cells within increased placental site reaction may represent increased proliferative activity, which may be higher in the trophoblastic cells within the decidua when compared to the trophoblastic cells within the myometrium (Fig. 12.23c and g). Morphologic features of EPS and increased placental site reaction (IPSR) are summarized in Table 12.7.

In fractional curettings the distinction from PSTT may be challenging or impossible [132]. The presence of chorionic villi favours the diagnosis of EPS over PSTT. Additional embedding of tissue may be helpful. Lack of tumor formation and low Ki-67 (< 5 %) may separate EPS form PSTT [77,93,107]. The trophoblastic proliferation of a placenta increta, especially at wrong implantation localisation, e. g. cesarian section, may mimic EPS [133].

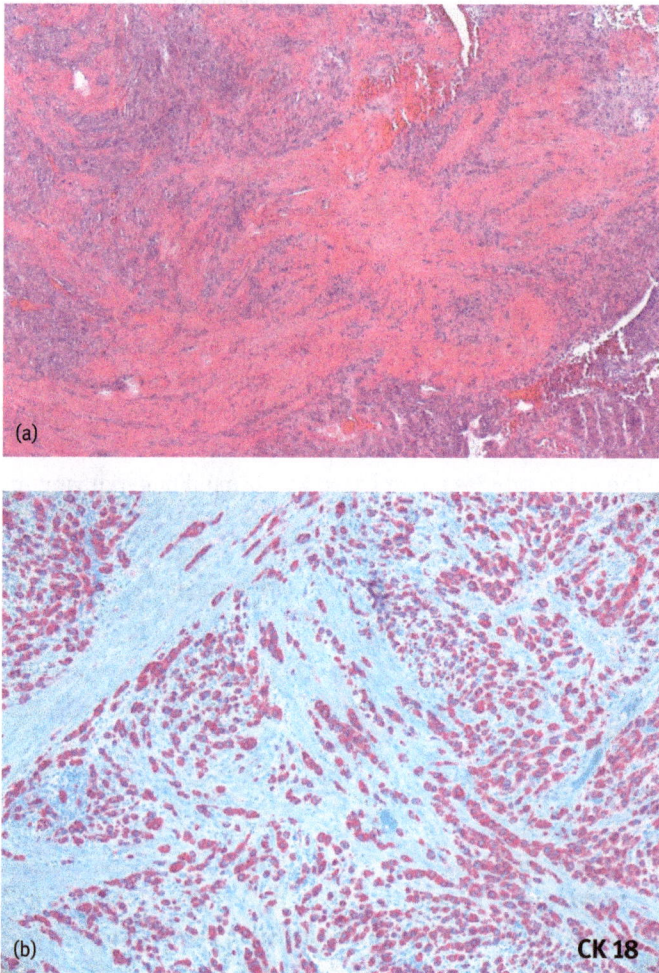

Fig. 12.23: Increased placental site reaction mimicking exaggerated placental site (EPS); (a) highly cellular proliferation of intermediate trophoblastic cells dissecting smooth muscle fibres of the myometrium; (b) highlighting the mononucleated intermediate trophoblastic cells by CK 18-immunostaining.

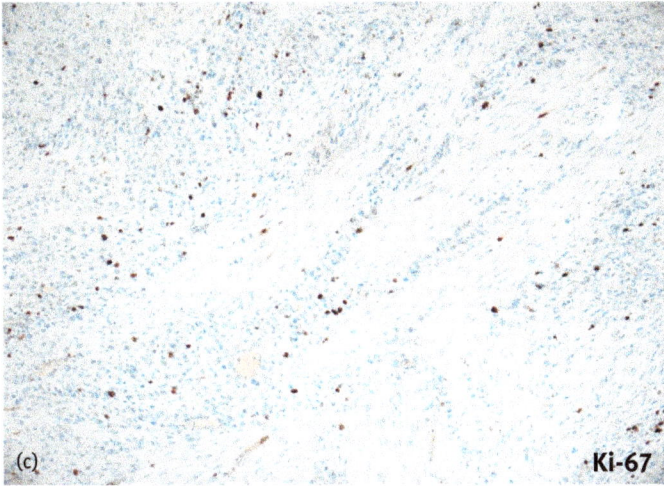

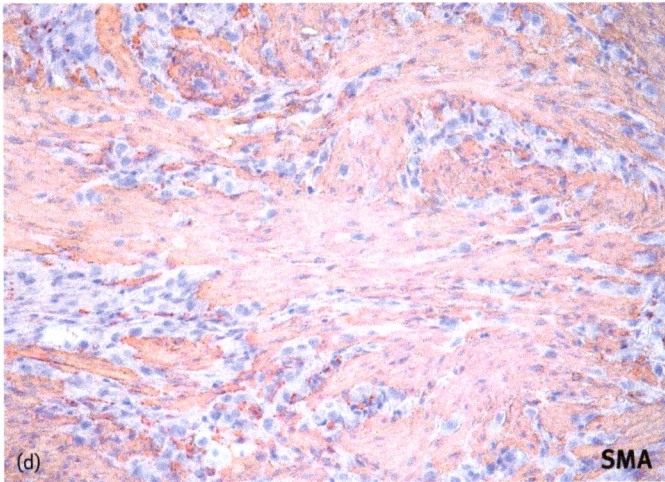

Fig. 12.23: (continued) (c) Low, but increased proliferative activity of the trophoblastic cells growing within the myometrium, indicated by Ki-67-immunstaining (compare to Fig. 12.23g); (d) dissected myometrial cells, highlighted by immunostaining for smooth muscle actin (SMA), trophoblastic cells are negative.

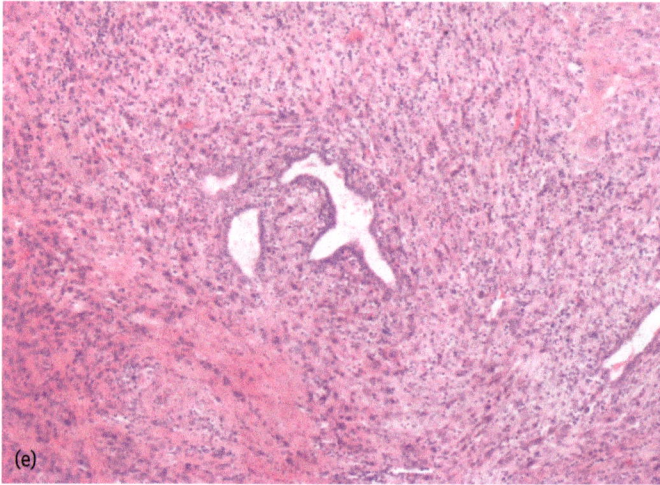

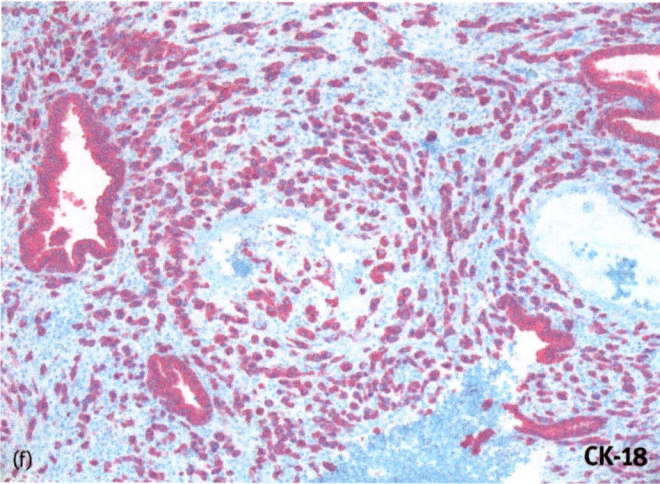

Fig. 12.23: (continued) (e) Highly cellular proliferation of intermediate trophoblastic cells within the decidua, surrounding endometrial glands without destructive growth; (f) highlighting the trophoblastic cells by CK 18-immunostaining.

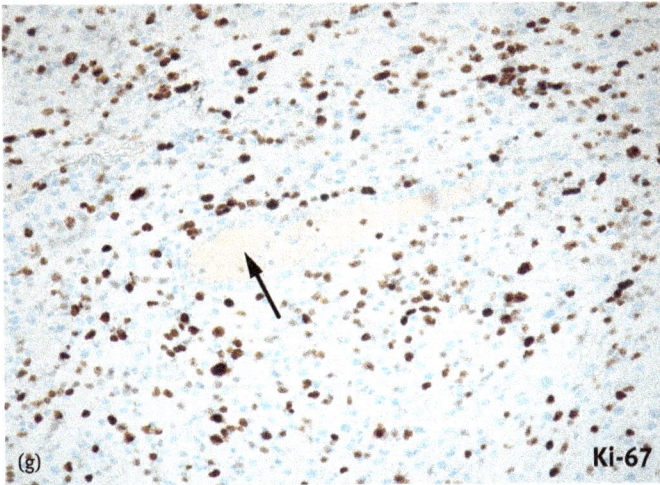

Fig. 12.23: (continued) (g) highly increased proliferative activity of the trophoblastic cells growing within the decidua, indicated by Ki-67-immunstaining (note the higher proliferative activity of the intermediate trophoblastic cells within the decidua, when compared to the intermediate trophoblastic cells within the myometrium [see Fig. 12.23c]).

Table 12.7: Morphologic features of exaggerated placental site (EPS) and increased placental site reaction (IPSR).

	exaggerated placental site (EPS)	increased placental site reaction (IPSR)
appearance	microscopic	microscopic
association with	mostly (early) CM and any kind of (early) pregnancy	any kind of pregnancy (mostly 1st trimester)
chorionic villi	may be present	mostly present
growth pattern	non-destructive, dissecting	non-destructive, dissecting
cellular trabeculation	may be present	none
celluarity	increased, intermediate trophoblastic	increased, intermediate trophoblastic
celluar composition	mononuclear and intermediate tropho blastic giant cells with increased number of giant cells	mononuclear and intermediate tropho blastic giant cells no increase of giant cells
intermediate trophoblastic giant cells	numerous	present, but rare, not prominent
spiral arteries	vessels wall replaced by fibrinoid material and intermediate trophoblastic cells mimicking normal placental implantation site	vessels wall replaced by fibrinoid material and intermediate trophoblastic cells as seen in normal placental implantation site
endometrial glands	surrounded by intermediate trophoblastic cells	surrounded by intermediate trophoblastic cells

Table 12.7: (continued) Morphologic features of exaggerated placental site (EPS) and increased placental site reaction (IPSR).

	exaggerated placental site (EPS)	increased placental site reaction (IPSR)
myometrial cells	dissected and compressed by inter-mediate troblastic cells	dissected and compressed by inter-mediate troblastic cells
immunohistochemistry	+ve for: pan-CK, CK 18, GATA-3	+ve for: pan-CK, CK 18, GATA-3
Ki-67	mostly < 5 %	high, esp. in cytotrophoblast as in normal placental implantation site (~80 %)

Prognosis

EPS represents a benign lesion in almost all cases. But if the EPS is associated with an early CHM there is an increased risk for the development of persistent GTD. In this context the risk is more likely correlated to the trophoblastic proliferation of the CHM rather than the occurrence of the EPS itself [77]. At this time there is no evidence that EPS represents a precursor lesion of PSTT [132,134].

References

[1] Hui P, Baergen R, Cheung ANY, et al. Gestational Trophoblastic Disease. In: Kurman RJ, Carcangiu ML, Herrington CS, Young RH (Eds.) WHO Classification of Tumours of Female Reproductive Organs. IARC Lyon 2014, pp. 158–67
[2] Sebire NJ, May PC, Kaur B, Seckl MJ, Fisher RA. Abnormal villous morphology mimicking a hydatidiform mole associated with paternal trisomy of chromosomes 3,7,8 and unipaternal disomy of chromosome 11. Diagn Pathol. 2016;11:20.
[3] Atrash HK, Hogue CJ, Grimes DA. Epidemiology of hydatidiform mole during early gestation. Am J Obstet Gynecol. 1986;154(4):906–909.
[4] Brown J, Naumann RW, Seckl MJ, Schink J. 15 years of progress in gestational trophoblastic disease: Scoring, standardization, and salvage. Gynecol Oncol. 2017;144(1):200–207.
[5] Smith HO, Hilgers RD, Bedrick EJ, et al. Ethnic differences at risk for gestational trophoblastic disease in New Mexico: A 25-year population-based study. Am J Obstet Gynecol. 2003;188(2):357–366.
[6] Tham BW, Everard JE, Tidy JA, Drew D, Hancock BW. Gestational trophoblastic disease in the Asian population of Northern England and North Wales. BJOG. 2003;110:555–559.
[7] Martin BH, Kim JH. Changes in gestational trophoblastic tumors over four decades. A Korean experience. J Reprod Med. 1998;43:60–68.
[8] Smith HO, Kohorn E, Cole LA. Choriocarcinoma and gestational trophoblastic disease. Obstet Gynecol Clin North Am. 2005;32(4):661–684.
[9] Lybol C, Thomas CM, Bulten J, et al. Increase in the incidence of gestational trophoblastic disease in The Netherlands. Gynecol Oncol. 20111;121(2):334–338.
[10] Eysbouts YK, Bulten J, Ottevanger PB, et al. Trends in incidence for gestational trophoblastic disease over the last 20 years in a population-based study. Gynecol Oncol. 2016;140(1):70–75.
[11] Lurain JR, Singh DK, Schink JC. Management of metastatic high-risk gestational trophoblastic neoplasia: FIGO stages II-IV: risk factor score > or = 7. J Reprod Med. 2010;55:199–207.

[12] Kuyumcuoglu U, Guzel AI, Erdemoglu M, Celik Y. Risk factors for persistent gestational trophoblastic neoplasia. J Exp Ther Oncol. 2011;9:81–84.
[13] Horn LC, Ulrich U. Gestationsbedingte Trophoblasterkrankungen. In: Ulrich U (Ed.) Gynäkologische Onkologie. de Gruyter Berlin, Boston 2013, pp192-232.
[14] Seckl MJ, Sebire NJ, Berkowitz RS. Gestational trophoblastic disease. Lancet. 2010;376(9742):717–729.
[15] Agarwal R, Alifrangis C, Everard J,et al. Management and survival of patients with FIGO highrisk gestational trophoblastic neoplasia: the U. K. experience, 1995–2010. J Reprod Med. 2014;59(1–2):7–12.
[16] Hoffner L, Surti U. The genetics of gestational trophoblastic disease: a rare complication of pregnancy. Cancer Genet. 2012;205:63–77.
[17] Murphy KM, Descipio C, Wagenfuehr J, et al. Tetraploid partial hydatidiform mole: a case report and review of the literature. Int J Gynecol Pathol. 2012;31(1):73–79.
[18] Horn LC. Gestationsbedingte Trophoblasttumoren. In: Dietel M, Klöppel G (Eds.) Remmele – Pathologie. Mamma, Weibliches Genitale, Schwangerschaft und Kindererkrankungen. Springer, Berlin, Heidelberg, 2013, pp. 633–658.
[19] Sun SY, Melamed A, Joseph NT, et al. Clinical Presentation of Complete Hydatidiform Mole and Partial Hydatidiform Mole at a Regional Trophoblastic Disease Center in the United States Over the Past 2 Decades. Int J Gynecol Cancer. 2016;26(2):367–370.
[20] Buza N, Hui P. Partial hydatidiform mole: histologic parameters in correlation with DNA genotyping. Int J Gynecol Pathol. 2013;32(3):307–315.
[21] Horn LC, Einenkel J, Höhn AK. Classification and Morphology of Gestational Trophoblastic Disease. Curr Obstet Gynecol Rep. 2014;3:44–54.
[22] Cheung AN. Pathology of gestational trophoblastic diseases. Best Pract Res Clin Obstet Gynaecol. 2003;17:849–868.
[23] Wells M. The pathology of gestational trophoblastic disease: recent advances.Pathology. 2007;39:88–96.
[24] Horn LC, Vogel M, Schmidt D, Ulrich UA. Trophoblasttumorregister der Arbeitsgemeinschaft Gynäkologische Onkologie (AGO). Geburtshilfe Frauenheilk. 2009;69:834–835.
[25] Wilson Y, Bharat C, Crook ML, et al. Histological comparison of partial hydatidiform mole and trisomy gestation specimens. Pathology. 2016;48(6):550–554.
[26] Vogel M, Horn LC. Gestational trophoblastic disease, Villous gestational trophoblastic disease. Pathologe. 2004;25(4):269–279.
[27] Lewis GH, DeScipio C, Murphy KM, et al. Characterization of androgenetic / biparental mosaic / chimeric conceptions, including those with a molar component: morphology, p57 immnohistochemistry, molecular genotyping, and risk of persistent gestational trophoblastic disease. Int J Gynecol Pathol. 2013;32(2):199–214.
[28] Medeiros F, Callahan MJ, Elvin JA, et al. Intraplacental choriocarcinoma arising in a second trimester placenta with partial hydatidiform mole. Int J Gynecol Pathol. 2008;27:247–251.
[29] Seckl MJ, Fisher RA, Salerno G, et al. Choriocarcinoma and partial hydatidiform moles. Lancet 2000;356:1443–1144.
[30] Wielsma S, Kerkmeijer L, Bekkers R, et al. Persistent trophoblast disease following partial molar pregnancy. Aust N Z J Obstet Gynaeco. 2006;46:119–123.
[31] Worley MJ Jr, Joseph NT, Berkowitz RS, Goldstein DP. Women with a partial mole during their first pregnancy and diagnosed earlier in gestation are at increased risk of developing gestational trophoblastic neoplasia. Int J Gynecol Cancer. 2014;24(5):941–945.
[32] Berkowitz RS, Goldstein DP. Clinical practice. Molar pregnancy. N Engl J Med. 2009;360:1639–1645.
[33] Berkowitz RS, Goldstein DP. Current management of gestational trophoblastic diseases. Gynecol Oncol. 2009;112:654–662.

[34] Fowler DJ, Lindsay I, Seckl MJ, Sebire NJ. Histomorphometric features of hydatidiform moles in early pregnancy: relationship to detectability by ultrasound examination. Ultrasound Obstet Gynecol. 2007;29(1):76–80.

[35] Hou JL, Wan XR, Xiang Y, Qi QW, Yang XY. Changes of clinical features in hydatidiform mole: analysis of 113 cases. J Reprod Med. 2008;53:629–633.

[36] Lurain JR. Gestational trophoblastic disease II: classification and management of gestational trophoblastic neoplasia. Am J Obstet Gynecol. 2011;204:11–18.

[37] Fox H. Differential diagnosis of hydatidiform mole. Gen Diagn Pathol. 1997;143:117–125.

[38] Paradinas FJ. The histological diagnosis of hydatidiform moles. Curr Diagn Pathol. 1994;1:24–31.

[39] Sebire NJ. Histopathological diagnosis of hydatidiform mole: contemporary features and clinical implications. Fetal Pediatr Pathol. 2010;29(1):1–16.

[40] Fukunaga M. Immunohistochemical characterization of cyclin E and p27KIP1 expression in early hydatidiform moles. Int J Gynecol Pathol. 2004;23:259–264.

[41] Hui P, Martel M, Parkash V. Gestational trophoblastic diseases: recent advances in histopathologic diagnosis and related genetic aspects. Adv Anat Pathol. 2005;12:116–125.

[42] Castrillon DH, Sun D, Weremowicz S, et al. Discrimination of complete hydatidiform mole from its mimics by immunohistochemistry of the paternally imprinted gene product p57KIP2. Am J Surg Pathol. 2001;25:1225–1230.

[43] Horn LC, Bilek K, Pretzsch G, Baier D. Choriocarcinoma in extrauterine tubal pregnancy. Geburtshilfe Frauenheilkd. 1994;54(6):375–377.

[44] Burton JL, Lidbury WA, Gillespie AM, et al. Over-diagnosis of hydatidoform mole in early tubal ectopic pregnancy. Histopathology. 2001;38:409–417.

[45] Parveen Z, Tongson-Ignacio JE, Fraser CR, Killeen JL, Thompson KS. Placental mesenchymal dysplasia. Arch Pathol Lab Med. 2007;131:131–137.

[46] Ulker V, Aslan H, Gedikbasi A, et al. Placental mesenchymal dysplasia: a rare clinicopathologic entity confused with molar pregnancy. J Obstet Gynaecol. 2013;33(3):246–249.

[47] Lin LH, Maestá I, Braga A, et al. Multiple pregnancies with complete mole and coexisting normal fetus in North and South America: A retrospective multicenter cohort and literature review. Gynecol Oncol. 2017;145(1):88–95.

[48] Hui P, Buza N, Murphy KM, Ronnett BM. Hydatidiform Moles: Genetic Basis and Precision Diagnosis. Annu Rev Pathol. 2017;12:449–485.

[49] Ronnett BM, DeScipio C, Murphy KM. Hydatidiform moles: ancillary techniques to refine diagnosis. Int J Gynecol Pathol. 2011;30:101–116.

[50] Lage JM, Mark SD, Roberts DJ, et al. A flow cytometric study of 137 fresh hydropic placentas: correlation between types of hydatidiform moles and nuclear DNA ploidy. Obstet Gynecol. 1992;79:403–410.

[51] Banet N, Descipio C, Murphy KM, et al. Characteristics of hydatidiform moles: analysis of a prospective series with p57 immunohistochemistry and molecular genotyping. Mod Pathol. 2014;27(2):238-254.

[52] Hui P. Molecular diagnosis of gestational trophoblastic disease. Expert Rev Mol Diagn. 2010;10:1023–1034.

[53] Buza N, Hui P. Immunohistochemistry and other ancillary techniques in the diagnosis of gestational trophoblastic diseases. Semin Diagn Pathol. 2014;31(3):223–232.

[54] Petts G, Fisher RA, Short D, et al. Histopathological and immunohistochemical features of early hydatidiform mole in relation to subsequent development of persistent gestational trophoblastic disease. J Reprod Med. 2014;59(5–6):213–220.

[55] Baasanjav B, Usui H, Kihara M, et al. The risk of post-molar gestational trophoblastic neoplasia is higher in heterozygous than in homozygous complete hydatidiform moles. Hum Reprod. 2010;25(5):1183–1191.

[56] Buza N, Hui P. Gestational trophoblastic disease: histopathological diagnosis in the molecular era. Diagnostic Histopathology. 2010;16:526–537.

[57] Parra-Herran C, Djordjevic B. Histopathology of Placenta Creta: Chorionic Villi Intrusion into Myometrial Vascular Spaces and Extravillous Trophoblast Proliferation are Frequent and Specific Findings With Implications for Diagnosis and Pathogenesis. Int J Gynecol Pathol. 2016;35(6):497–508.

[58] Kirk E, McDonald K, Rees J, Govind A. Intramural ectopic pregnancy: a case and review of the literature. Eur J Obstet Gynecol Reprod Biol. 2013;168(2):129–133.

[59] Caldas RF, Oliveira P, Rodrigues C, et al. Intraplacental Choriocarcinoma: Rare or Underdiagnosed? Report of 2 Cases Diagnosed after an Incomplete Miscarriage and a Preterm Spontaneous Vaginal Delivery. Case Rep Med. 2017;2017:7892980.

[60] Ganapathi KA, Paczos T, George MD, et al. Incidental finding of placental choriocarcinoma after an uncomplicated term pregnancy: a case report with review of the literature. Int J Gynecol Pathol. 2010;29:476–478.

[61] Jiao L, Ghorani E, Sebire NJ, Seckl MJ. Intraplacental choriocarcinoma: Systematic review and management guidance. Gynecol Oncol. 2016;141(3):624–631.

[62] Wan J, Li XM, Gu J. Primary choriocarcinoma of the fallopian tube: a case report and literature review. Eur J Gynaecol Oncol. 2014;35(5):604–607.

[63] Horn LC, Kowalzik J, Bilek K, Richter CE, Einenkel J. Prognostic value of trophoblastic proliferation in complete hydatidiform moles in predicting persistent disease. Pathol Res Pract. 2006;202(3):151–156.

[64] Allison KH, Love JE, Garcia RL. Epithelioid trophoblastic tumor: review of a rare neoplasm of the chorionic-type intermediate trophoblast. Arch Pathol Lab Med. 2006;130:1875–1877.

[65] Bynum J, Murphy KM, DeScipio C, et al. Invasive Complete Hydatidiform Moles: Analysis of a Case Series With Genotyping. Int J Gynecol Pathol. 2016;35(2):134–141.

[66] Altieri A, Franceschi S, Ferlay J, Smith J, La Vecchia C. Epidemiology and aetiology of gestational trophoblastic diseases. Lancet Oncol. 2003;4(11):670–678.

[67] Poen HT, Djojopranoto M. The Possible Etiologic Factors of Hydatidiform Mole and Choriocarcinoma: Preliminary Report. Am J Obstet Gynecol. 1965;92:510–513.

[68] Jwa SC, Kamiyama S, Takayama H, et al. Extrauterine Choriocarcinoma in the Fallopian Tube Following Infertility Treatment: Implications for the Management of Early-Detected Ectopic Pregnancies. J Minim Invasive Gynecol. 2017;24(5):855–858.

[69] Rotas M, Khulpateea N, Binder D. Gestational choriocarcinoma arising from a cornual ectopic pregnancy: a case report and review of the literature. Arch Gynecol Obstet. 2007;276(6):645–647.

[70] Bagshawe KD, Golding PR, Orr AH. Choriocarcinoma after hydatidiform mole. Studies related to effectiveness of follow-up practice after hydatidiform mole. Br Med J. 1969;27;3(5673):733–737.

[71] Soper JT. Gestational trophoblastic disease. Obstet Gynecol. 2006;108(1):176–187.

[72] Banerjee D, Barsode SD, Basu P. Management of Gestational Trophoblastic Diseases-An Update. Rev Recent Clin Trials. 2015;10(4):255–262.

[73] Goldstein DP, Berkowitz RS. Current management of gestational trophoblastic neoplasia. Hematol Oncol Clin North Am. 2012;26(1):111–131.

[74] Matsui H, Iizuka Y, Sekiya S. Incidence of invasive mole and choriocarcinoma following partial hydatidiform mole. Int J Gynaecol Obstet. 1996;53(1):63–64.

[75] Baergen R. Gestational choriocarcinoma. Gen Diagn Pathol. 1997;143:127–141.

[76] Shih IeM. Trophogram, an immunohistochemistry-based algorithmic approach, in the differential diagnosis of trophoblastic tumors and tumorlike lesions. Ann Diagn Pathol. 2007;11:228–234.

[77] Shih IM, Kurman RJ. The pathology of the intermediate trophoblastic tumors and tumorlike lesions. Int J Gynecol Pathol. 2001;20:31–47.

[78] Baergen RN, Rutgers JL, Young RH, Osann K, Scully RE. Placental site trophoblastic tumor: A study of 55 cases and review of the literature emphasizing factors of prognostic significance. Gynecol Oncol. 2006;100:511–520.

[79] Stichelbout M, Devisme L, Franquet-Ansart H, et al. SALL4 expression in gestational trophoblastic tumors: a useful tool to distinguish choriocarcinoma from placental site trophoblastic tumor and epithelioid trophoblastic tumor. Hum Pathol. 2016;54:121–126.

[80] Mirkovic J, Elias K, Drapkin R, et al. GATA3 expression in gestational trophoblastic tissues and tumours. Histopathology. 2015;67(5):636–644.

[81] Mao TL, Seidman JD, Kurman RJ, Shih IeM. Cyclin E and p16 immunoreactivity in epithelioid trophoblastic tumor-an aid in differential diagnosis. Am J Surg Pathol. 2006;30:1105–1110.

[82] Kalhor N, Ramirez PT, Deavers MT, Malpica A, Silva EG. Immunohistochemical studies of trophoblastic tumors. Am J Surg Pathol. 2009;33:633–638.

[83] Tsai HW, Lin CP, Chou CY, et al. Placental site nodule transformed into a malignant epithelioid trophoblastic tumour with pelvic lymph node and lung metastasis. Histopathology. 2008;53:601–604.

[84] Singer G, Kurman RJ, McMaster MT, Shih IeM. HLA-G immunoreactivity is specific for intermediate trophoblast in gestational trophoblastic disease and can serve as a useful marker in differential diagnosis. Am J Surg Pathol. 2002;26:914–920.

[85] Chou YY, Jeng YM, Mao TL. HSD3B1 is a specific trophoblast-associated marker not expressed in a wide spectrum of tumors. Int J Gynecol Cancer. 2013;23(2):343–347.

[86] Bolze PA, Patrier S, Massardier J, et al. PD-L1 Expression in Premalignant and Malignant Trophoblasts From Gestational Trophoblastic Diseases Is Ubiquitous and Independent of Clinical Outcomes. Int J Gynecol Cancer. 2017;27(3):554–561.

[87] Veras E, Kurman RJ, Wang TL, Shih IM. PD-L1 Expression in Human Placentas and Gestational Trophoblastic Diseases. Int J Gynecol Pathol. 2017;36(2):146–153.

[88] Horn LC, Hänel C, Bartholdt E, Dietel J. Mixed serous carcinoma of the endometrium with trophoblastic differentiation: analysis of the p53 tumor suppressor gene suggests stem cell origin. Ann Diagn Pathol. 2008;12(1):1–3.

[89] Horn LC, Dallacker M, Bilek K. Carcinosarcomas (malignant mixed Mullerian tumors) of the uterus. Morphology, pathogenetic aspects and prognostic factors. Pathologe. 2009;30(4):292–301.

[90] Lopez-Garcia MA, Palacios J. Pathologic and molecular features of uterine carcinosarcomas. Semin Diagn Pathol. 2010;27(4):274–286.

[91] Horn LC, Bilek K, Nenning H. Postpartal gestational choriocarcinoma fatally misdiagnosed as squamous cell cancer of the uterine cervix. Gen Diagn Pathol. 1997;143:191–196.

[92] Lu B, Zhang X, Liang Y. Clinicopathologic Analysis of Postchemotherapy Gestational Trophoblastic Neoplasia: An Entity Overlapping With Epithelioid Trophoblastic Tumor. Int J Gynecol Pathol. 2016;35(6):516–524.

[93] Shih IeM. Gestational trophoblastic neoplasia--pathogenesis and potential therapeutic targets. Lancet Oncol. 2007;8:642–645.

[94] Neubauer NL, Strohl AE, Schink JC, Lurain JR. Fatal gestational trophoblastic neoplasia: An analysis of treatment failures at the Brewer Trophoblastic Disease Center from 1979–2012 compared to 1962–1978. Gynecol Oncol. 2015;138(2):339–342.

[95] Strohl AE, Lurain JR. Postmolar choriocarcinoma: An independent risk factor for chemotherapy resistance in low-risk gestational trophoblastic neoplasia. Gynecol Oncol. 2016;141(2):276–280.

[96] Horowitz NS, Goldstein DP, Berkowitz RS. Placental site trophoblastic tumors and epithelioid trophoblastic tumors: Biology, natural history, and treatment modalities. Gynecol Oncol. 2017;144(1):208–214.

[97] Hui P, Wang HL, Chu P, Yang B, et al. Absence of Y chromosome in human placental site trophoblastic tumor. Mod Pathol. 2007;20:1055–1060.
[98] Zhao J, Lv WG, Feng FZ, et al. Placental site trophoblastic tumor: A review of 108 cases and their
implications for prognosis and treatment. Gynecol Oncol. 2016;142(1):102–108.
[99] Zhao J, Xiang Y, Wan XR, Cui QC, Yang XY. Clinical and pathologic characteristics and prognosis
of placental site trophoblastic tumor. J Reprod Med. 2006;51:939–944.
[100] Lan C, Li Y, He J, Liu J. Placental site trophoblastic tumor: lymphatic spread and possible target
markers. Gynecol Oncol. 2010;116:430–437.
[101] Moutte A, Doret M, Hajri T, et al. Placental site and epithelioid trophoblastic tumours: diagnostic pitfalls. Gynecol Oncol. 2013;128(3):568–572.
[102] Schmid P, Nagai Y, Agarwal R, et al. Prognostic markers and long-term outcome of placental-
site trophoblastic tumours: a retrospective observational study. Lancet 2009;374:48–55.
[103] Santoro G, Laganà AS, Micali A, et al. Historical, morphological and clinical overview
of placental site trophoblastic tumors: from bench to bedside. Arch Gynecol Obstet.
2017;295(1):173–187.
[104] Horn LC, Göretzlehner G, Dirnhofer S. Placental site trophoblastic tumor (PSTT) initially misdiagnosed as cervical carcinoma. Pathol Res Pract. 1997;193:225–230.
[105] Zhao S, Sebire NJ, Kaur B, Seckl MJ, Fisher RA. Molecular genotyping of placental site and epithelioid trophoblastic tumours; female predominance. Gynecol Oncol. 2016;142(3):5 b01-7.
[106] Piura B. Placental site trophoblastic tumor--a challenging rare entity. Eur J Gynaecol Oncol.
2006;27:545–551.
[107] Shih IM, Kurman RJ. Epithelioid trophoblastic tumor: a neoplasm distinct from choriocarcinoma and placental site trophoblastic tumor simulating carcinoma. Am J Surg Pathol.
1998;22(11):1393–1403.
[108] Yap KL, Hafez MJ, Mao TL, et al. Lack of a y-chromosomal complement in the majority of gestational trophoblastic neoplasms. J Oncol. 2010;364508.
[109] Hamazaki S, Nakamoto S, Okino T, et al. Epithelioid trophoblastic tumor: morphological and
immunohistochemical study of three lung lesions. Human Pathol. 1999;30:1321–1327.
[110] Luk WY, Friedlander M. A fibroid or cancer? A rare case of mixed choriocarcinoma and epithelioid trophoblastic tumour. Case Rep Obstet Gynecol. 2013;2013:492754.
[111] Shih IM, Kurman RJ. p63 expression is useful in the distinction of epithelioid trophoblastic
and placental site trophoblastic tumors by profiling trophoblastic subpopulations. Am J Surg
Pathol. 2004;28:1177–1183.
[112] Macdonald MC, Palmer JE, Hancock BW, Tidy JA. Diagnostic challenges in extrauterine epithelioid trophoblastic tumours: a report of two cases. Gynecol Oncol. 2008;108:452–454.
[113] Palmer JE, Macdonald M, Wells M, Hancock BW, Tidy JA. Epithelioid trophoblastic tumor: a review of the literature. J Reprod Med. 2008;53:465–475.
[114] Davis MR, Howitt BE, Quade BJ, et al. Epithelioid trophoblastic tumor: A single institution case
series at the New England Trophoblastic Disease Center. Gynecol Oncol. 2015;137(3):456–461.
[115] Zhang X, Zhou C, Yu M, Chen X. Coexisting epithelioid trophoblastic tumor and placental site
trophoblastic tumor of the uterus following a term pregnancy: report of a case and review of
literature. Int J Clin Exp Pathol. 20151;8(6):7254–7259.
[116] Liang Y, Zhou F, Chen X, Zhang X, Lü B. Atypical epithelioid trophoblastic lesion with cyst and
fistula formation after a cesarean section: a rare form of gestational trophoblastic disease. Int J
Gynecol Pathol. 2012;31(5):458–462.
[117] Idrees MT, Kao CS, Epstein JI, Ulbright TM. Nonchoriocarcinomatous Trophoblastic Tumors of the Testis: The Widening Spectrum of Trophoblastic Neoplasia. Am J Surg Pathol.
2015;39(11):1468–1478.
[118] Fadare O, Parkash V, Carcangiu ML, Hui P. Epithelioid trophoblastic tumor: clinicopathological
features with an emphasis on uterine cervical involvement. Mod Pathol. 2006;19(1):75–82.

[119] Cierna Z, Varga I, Danihel L Jr, et al. Intermediate trophoblast--A distinctive, unique and often unrecognized population of trophoblastic cells. Ann Anat. 2016;204:45–50.

[120] Kurman RJ, Shih IeM. Discovery of a cell: reflections on the checkered history of intermediate trophoblast and update on its nature and pathologic manifestations. Int J Gynecol Pathol. 2014;33(4):339–347.

[121] Feng HC, Tsao SW, Ngan HY, et al. Overexpression of prostate stem cell antigen is associated with gestational trophoblastic neoplasia. Histopathology. 2008;52:167–174.

[122] Chen BJ, Cheng CJ, Chen WY. Transformation of a post-cesarean section placental site nodule into a coexisting epithelioid trophoblastic tumor and placental site trophoblastic tumor: a case report. Diagn Pathol. 2013;8:85.

[123] Shen DH, Khoo US, Ngan HY, et al. Coexisting epithelioid trophoblastic tumor and choriocarcinoma of the uterus following a chemoresistant hydatidiform mole. Arch Pathol Lab Med. 2003;127(7):e291-293.

[124] Yoo SH, Kim KR, Robboy SJ. Invasive hydatidiform mole of the lung with an implantation site intermediate trophoblast: Report of a case supporting the pathways of trophoblast differentiation. Pathol Int. 2016;66(7):413–414.

[125] Huettner PC, Gersell DJ. Placental site nodule: A clinicopathologic study of 38 cases. Int J Gynecol Pathol. 1994;13:191–198.

[126] Young RH, Kurman RJ, Scully RE. Proliferations and tumors of intermediate trophoblast of the placental site. Semin Diagn Pathol. 1988;5(2):223–237.

[127] Campello TR, Fittipaldi H, O'Valle F, Carvia RE, Nogales FF. Extrauterine (tubal) placental site nodule. Histopathology. 1998;32(6):562–565.

[128] Choi JJ, Emmadi R. Incidental placental site nodule in a fallopian tube. Int J Surg Pathol. 2014;22(1):90–92.

[129] Kaur B, Short D, Fisher RA, et al. Atypical placental site nodule (APSN) and association with malignant gestational trophoblastic disease; a clinicopathologic study of 21 cases. Int J Gynecol Pathol. 2015;34(2):152–158.

[130] McCarthy WA, Paquette C, Colavita M, Lawrence WD. Atypical Placental Site Nodule Arising in a Postcesarean Section Scar: Case Report and Review of the Literature. Int J Gynecol Pathol. 2019;38(1):71–75.

[131] Luna DV, Dulcey I, Nogales FF. Coexistence of placental site nodule and cervical squamous carcinoma in a 72-year-old woman. Int J Gynecol Pathol. 2013;32(3):335–337.

[132] Yeasmin S, Nakayama K, Katagiri A, et al. Exaggerated placental site mimicking placental site trophoblastic tumor: case report and literature review. Eur J Gynaecol Oncol. 2010;31:586–589.

[133] Cramer SF, Heller DS. Placenta Increta Presenting as Exaggerated Placental Site Reaction. Pediatr Dev Pathol. 2017;20(2):152–157.

[134] Dotto J, Hui P. Lack of genetic association between exaggerated placental site reaction and placental site trophoblastic tumor. Int J Gynecol Pathol. 2008;27:562–567.

[135] Banet N, Gown AM, Shih IeM, et al. GATA-3 expression in trophoblastic tissues: an immunohistochemical study of 445 cases, including diagnostic utility. Am J Surg Pathol. 2015;39(1):101–108.

[136] Horn LC, Bilek K. Histologic classification and staging of gestational trophoblastic disease. Gen Diagn Pathol. 1997;143:87–101.

[137] Keep D, Zaragoza MV, Hassold T, Redline RW. Very early complete hydatidiform mole. Hum Pathol. 1996;27(7):708–713.

[138] Sebire NJ, Makrydimas G, Agnantis NJ, et al. Updated diagnostic criteria for partial and complete hydatidiform moles in early pregnancy. Anticancer Res. 2003;23(2C):1723–1728.

13 Multiple pregnancy

In a multiple pregnancy two or more embryos develop simultaneously from one or more zygotes.

The frequency of spontaneous multiple pregnancies in Europe is estimated according to Hellin's law [1]:
- twins (a): 1:85,
- triplets (a^2): 1:7225,
- quadruplets (a^3): 1:614,125,
- quintuplets (a^4): 1:52,200,625.

The proportion of multiple pregnancies from natural conception is more than 12%; however, only 2% survive until term [2]. Due to modern treatments for sterility and assisted reproduction, the incidence of multiple pregnancies is increasing. One sonographically confirmed twin vanishes spontaneously (vanishing twin) in ca. 66% of multiple pregnancies.

13.1 Twin pregnancy – chorionicity and zygosity

In a twin pregnancy the two placentas may be completely separated or fused (Fig. 13.1). In a German study of 561 twin pregnancies, between gestational weeks 15 and 42, separate placentas were reported in 29% and fused placentas in 71% [3]. From international literature, separate placentas are reported in 34% to 37% of twin pregnancies [4–6] and a fused dichorionic-diamniotic (DiDi) twin placenta in 33% to 39% of pregnancies. Monochorionic twin placentas are assumed to occur in 14% to 30% of twin pregnancies [4]; from material (Pediatric Pathology and Placentology, Charité Berlin) [3] monochorionic twin placentas were seen in ca. 37% of twin pregnancies. Monochorionic-monoamniotic (MoMo) placentas are estimated to be 1–3% of all twin placentas.

https://doi.org/10.1515/9783110452600-013

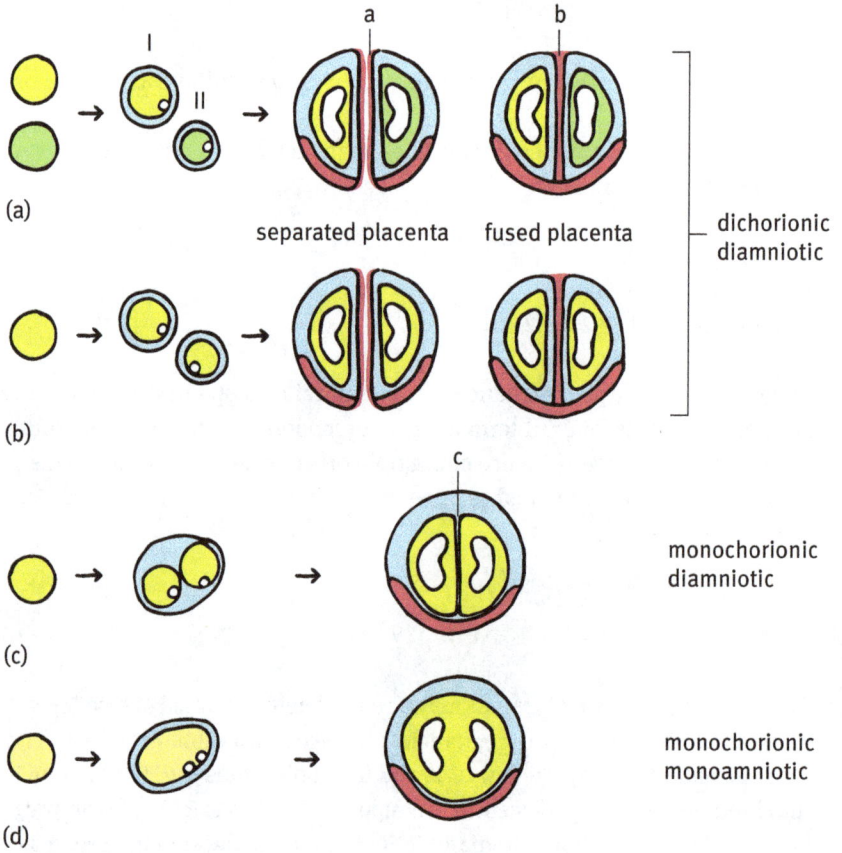

Fig. 13.1: Placentation in twin placentas. (a) Two ovaries (I and II) with an ovulation in each that develops separately into two separate dichorionic-diamniotic (DiDi) twin placentas (secondary fusion of the placentas may occur); (b) two ovulations in one ovary: Separate or fused dichorionic-diamniotic (DiDi) twin placenta; (c) ovulation of a twin follicle: Fused monochorionic-diamniotic (MoDi) placenta; (d) ovulation of an oocyte with two nuclei: Fused monochorionic-monoamniotic (MoMo) placenta.

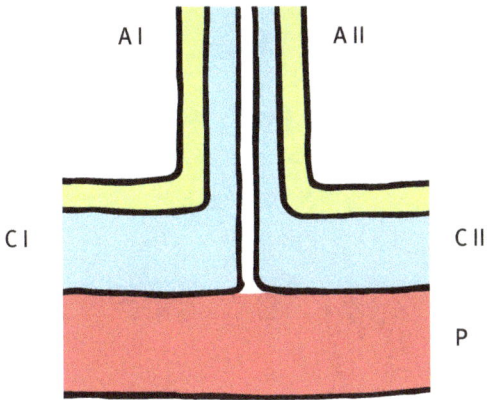

(a) dichorionic diamniotic

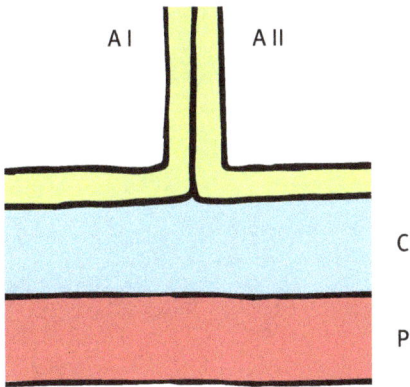

(b) monochorionic diamniotic

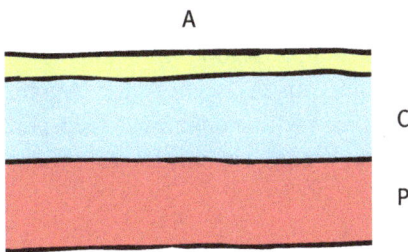

(c) monochorionic monoamniotic

Fig. 13.2: Illustration of the morphological appearance of the dividing membrane. (a) In a dichorionic-diamniotic (DiDi) placenta, the dividing membrane consists of an amniotic (A) and a chorionic (C) membrane from each twin (I and II); (b) the dividing membrane of monochorionic-diamniotic (MoDi) twin placenta consists of only one chorionic membrane and two amniotic membranes; (c) in monochorionic-monoamniotic (MoMo) twin placenta a dividing membrane is missing. (P) Placenta.

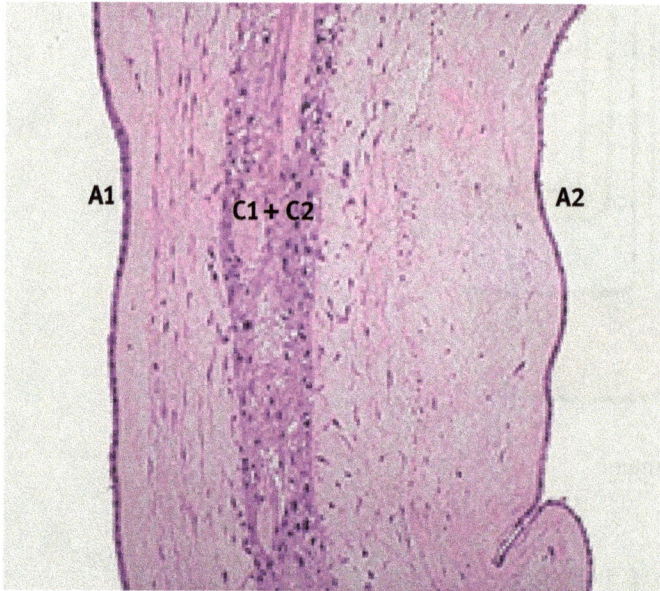

Fig. 13.3: Morphology of a dichorionic-diamniotic (DiDi) dividing membrane in a secondary fused twin placenta. Amniotic membrane (A1), chorionic membrane (C1), chorionic membrane (C2), amniotic membrane (A2).

13.1.1 Placentation shape and zygosity

In ca. 80 % of twin pregnancies it is possible to determine zygosity after delivery by use of the following criteria [7]:
–   gender of children,
–   placental morphology (Table 13.1),
–   non-morphological diagnoses, such as blood group,
–   immunohistochemistry and tissue type characterization; through DNA typing on frozen or formalin fixed tissue samples from the placenta or umbilical cord of both twins.

Separated twin placentas are seen in 24 % of monozygotic twins and a secondary fused dichorionic-diamniotic (DiDi) twin placenta in 28 % of monozygotic twins. Monochorionic placentas are almost always seen with monozygotic twins; examples of monochorionic placentas and dizygosity are reported in only few exceptional cases of secondary chorionic resorption [8].

Dizygotic twins

Dizygotic twins develop from two oocytes fertilized by two spermatocytes. Conjugation of the oocytes may be the result of several conditions [9]:
– one ovulation in each ovary,
– two ovulations in one ovary,

Each of the zygotes develops separately, with one placenta, amniotic sac and umbilical cord, and are independently implanted in the uterus. If the blastocysts implant close to each other the placenta may fuse into one dichorionic-diamniotic (DiDi) twin placenta (Table 13.1).

Monozygotic twins

These develop from a single oocyte fertilized by a single spermatocyte. Mitotic division of the zygote determines placenta formation (Table 13.1) and the following patterns are seen:
– Separation within the first three days (Morula Stage), before differentiation of tropho- and embryoblast: The two developing concepti have separate umbilical cords but share a single placenta and amniotic sac. Implantation may proceed as in dizygotic twins.
– Separation between day 3 and 8 post conception (p. c.), the blastocyst stage prior to amniotic differentiation. Division is limited to the embryoblast and amnion and a monochorionic-diamniotic (MoDi) placenta develops.
– Separation between day 8 and 13 p. c. Separation of the fertilized egg after chorionic and amniotic development. Only the embryoblast can divide and the two embryos share a single amniotic sac. A monochorionic-monoamniotic (MoMo) twin placenta develops.
– Separation after day 13 p. c. Late separation of the embryoblast causes incomplete separation of the twins (conjoined twins; pagus and duplicitas). Examination shows a fused placenta with one amniotic sac and one, or rarely two umbilical cords, but with only one point of insertion of the cord on the chorionic plate.
– In rare cases separation starts before amniotic development is finished and results in an incompletely separated amniotic sac joined by rudimentary amniotic strands. Secondary development of an amniotic sac due to spontaneous, or traumatic, rupture and resorption of the primary separating wall has a similar appearance and should be considered.

Table 13.1: Placenta shape, zygosity and timing of zygotic division.

placenta	dividing membrane	vessel anastomosis	sex	zygosity	zygotic division
separate	dichorionic-diamniotic (*DiDi*)	none	different / same	dizygotic	fertilization
separate	dichorionic-diamniotic (*DiDi*)	none	same	monozygotic	morula (first 3 days p. c.)
secondary fused	dichorionic-diamniotic (*DiDi*)	seldom	different / same	dizygotic	fertilization
secondary fused	dichorionic-diamniotic (*DiDi*)	rare	same	monozygotic	morula (first 3 days p. c.)
primary fused	monochorionic-diamniotic (*MoDi*)	often	same	monozygotic	blastocyst before amniotic development (3–8 days p. c.)
primary fused	monochorionic-monoamniotic (*MoMo*)	common	same	monozygotic	blastocyst after amniotic development (8–13 days p. c.)
primary fused	monochorionic-monoamniotic (*MoMo*)	fused umbilical cord	same	monozygotic	13 days p. c. (or few days later)

Findings in twin placentas

Weight of dichorionic and monochorionic twin placentas, according gestational age, is usually less than single placentas.

Basal/maternal plate of monochorionic placentas is smaller than that of dichorionic placentas. The placental index, based on placental weight and area, from week 28 onward, is 2 in monochorionic placentas and less than 2 in dichorionic placentas.

Shape anomalies in twin placentas are reported to be seen in 18 %, and this is a similar frequency to placentas from other risk pregnancies. Marginal and velamentous umbilical cord insertions are more often reported in twin placentas (14.8 % and 7.8 % respectively). A marginal insertion is seen in 22.2 % of monochorionic and 10.9 % of dichorionic placentas, whereas a velamentous umbilical cord insertion was seen in 10 % of monochorionic and 0.9 % dichorionic placentas.

Solitary umbilical cord artery (SUA) was found in 1.8 % of dichorionic and 2.9 % of monochorionic placentas. Additionally, 3 % of all twin placentas were seen with aneurysms of the chorionic plate (unpublished material from the Department for Pediatric Pathology and Placentology, Charite, Berlin).

Circulatory disturbance in twin placentas was found as often as in singleton placentas, but it correlates more often with maternal circulatory disturbance and preeclampsia.

Villous maturation disorders grades 2 and 3, (Ch. 7) were found in ca. 60 % of all twin placentas. Pre-term accelerated villous maturation was seen in 35 % of cases.

Normal villous maturation for gestational age was seen in 57 % of twin placentas and maturation disorders were seen in 43 %.

Differences between dichorionic and monochorionic placentas:
- accelerated villous maturation was seen in 45 % of dichorionic placentas and 26 % of monochorionic placentas,
- villous maturation arrest was seen in 5.1 % of dichorionic placentas and 12.7 % of monochorionic placentas,
- retarded villous maturation was seen in 11.4 % of dichorionic placentas and 19 % of monochorionic placentas
- chorangiosis type I was seen in 2.2 % of dichorionic placentas and 7.3 % of monochorionic placentas.

Chorangiomas were found macroscopically in 0.6 % of dichorionic placentas and 1.4 % of monochorionic placentas.

Inflammation of amniotic and parenchymatous type was seen as often as in singleton placentas.

Signs of intrauterine hypoxia were seen in 15 % of all twin placentas; presenting as macroscopic meconium discoloration of the chorionic plate and amniotic membranes (30 %) and histologically as meconium phagocytosis (50 %) and a subchorionic infiltration of maternal granulocytes (35 %).

Consequences for the fetus
- *Pre-term deliveries are increased:* 40–65 % of twins are born prematurely.
- *Fetal growth restriction:* Birth weight of twins is less than in singleton pregnancies. In gestational week 38, the 50th percentile value of twin birth weight is identical to the 10th percentile of singleton pregnancies [10].
- *Hypertension in pregnancy (preeclampsia):* Preeclampsia in twin pregnancy is seen ca. 30 % more often than in singleton pregnancy [11]. It is assumed that utero-placental ischemia, caused by the discordance of increased fetal volume and increased uterine wall thickness, may play a role.
- *Abortion rates and perinatal mortality* are increased in twin pregnancy. There is a 3 to 13 fold higher risk of fetal death of a twin when compared to singleton pregnancies. Of 10,204 twin pregnancies, both twins died in 3 % and one twin in 4.2 % [12]. Risk of intrauterine fetal death for twin 2 is 1.6 times greater than for twin 1 [13]. The death of both twins was seen in in 50 % of pregnancies, the death of only one twin in 18 % and death of the second twin in 32 % [3].

13.2 Dichorionic twin placentas

This type of chorionicity is characterized by a thick dividing membrane which separates the placentas and individual amniotic sacs.

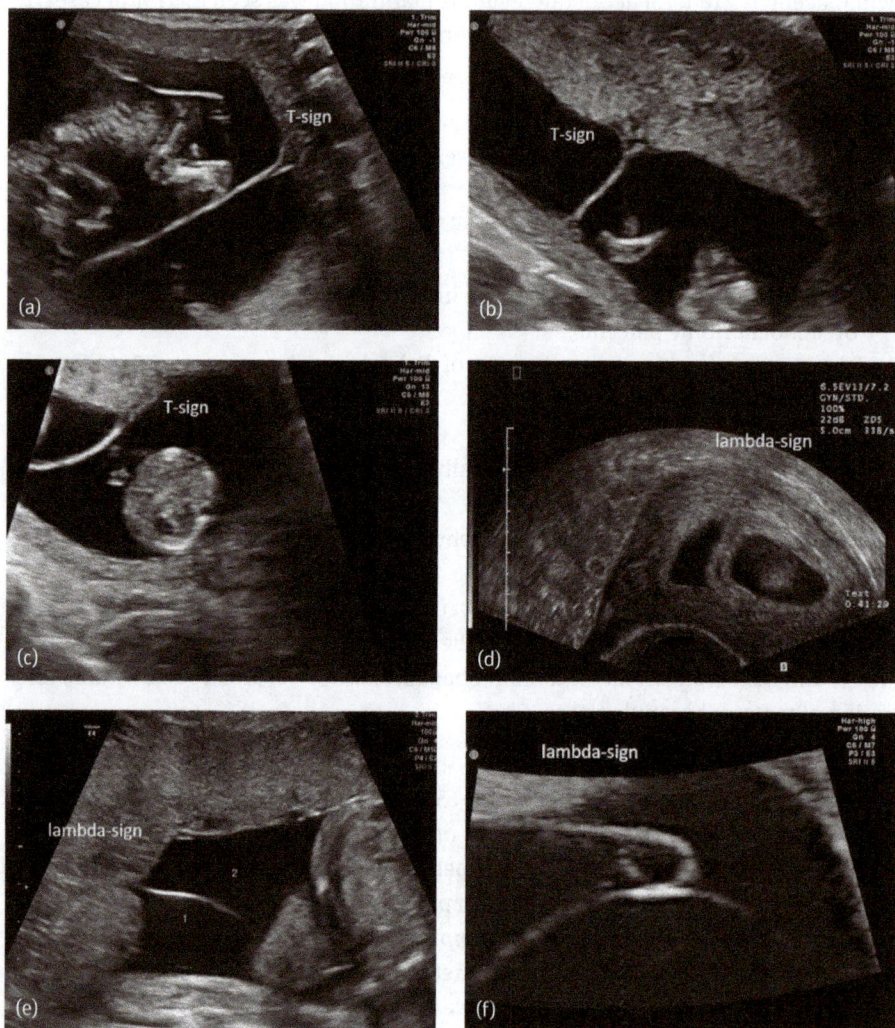

Fig. 13.4: Ultrasound examinations of twin placentas in the first trimester after 7 weeks of gestation, can determine amnionicity and chorionicity. A–C: The "T" sign refers to a monochorionic placenta with a double amniotic membrane in which the inter twin membrane extends from the placenta at a 90 degree angle and abruptly stops. E–F: The "twin peak" or "lambda" sign is a triangular projection which identifies dichorionic twin placentas and is best seen at weeks 10–14 of gestation. In monochorionic-monoamniotic (MoMo) twins the inter twin membrane is absent. Two separate placentas indicate dichorionic twins; however, a bi-lobed or succenturiate lobed placenta can be mistaken as two separate placentas and mask a monochorionic placentation (by courtesy of Prof. Dr. Th. Braun, Clinics for Obstetrics, Charité Berlin, Germany).

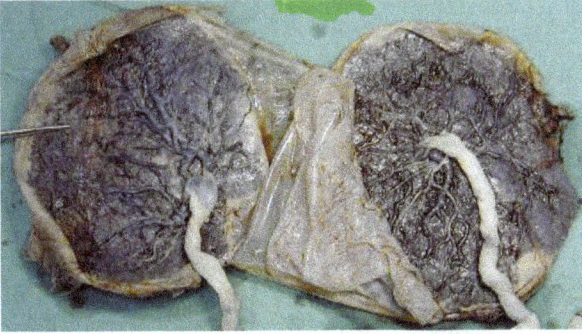

Fig. 13.5: Separate dichorionic-diamniotic (DiDi) twin placentas in gestational week 37, delivery of a healthy boy and girl.

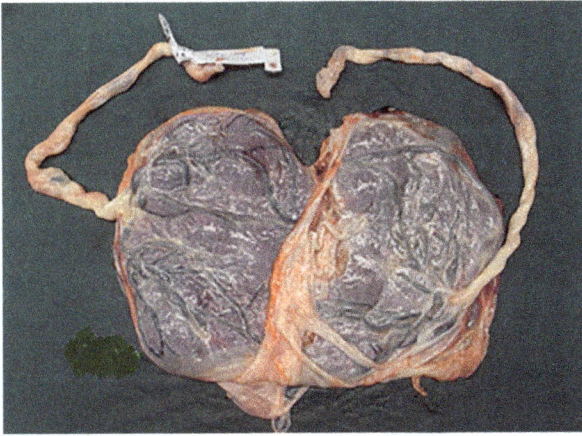

Fig. 13.6: Secondary fused dichorionic-diamniotic (DiDi) twin placenta in gestational week 34, delivery of two healthy boys.

Fused placentas with two amniotic sacs

In this situation the two placentas are fused and look like a single placenta. On the fetal surface two amniotic sacs develop and are separated by a dividing membrane of chorion. Fused placentas with two amniotic sacs can be dichorionic or monochorionic. Examination of the dividing membrane will allow one to distinguish dichorionic from monochorionic:

– Dichorionic placentas show a separating membrane which is macroscopically thick and adherent to the chorionic plate. Histological examination proves fusion with the identification of two chorionic and two amniotic membranes.
– Monochorionic placentas show a thin and very loose dividing membrane which is macroscopically transparent on the placental surface.

13.3 Monochorionic twin placentas

In monochorionic twin placentas the placental disc looks like a single placenta. The amniotic sac may be separated or fused and may show a dividing membrane with one chorionic layer and two amniotic layers monochorionic-diamniotic (MoDi), or have no membrane at all, monochorionic-monoamniotic type (MoMo).

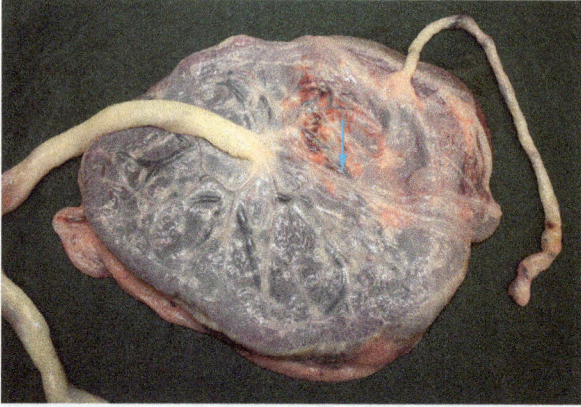

Fig. 13.7: Single placenta with a thin dividing membrane (arrow) in monochorionic-diamniotic (MoDi) twin placenta.

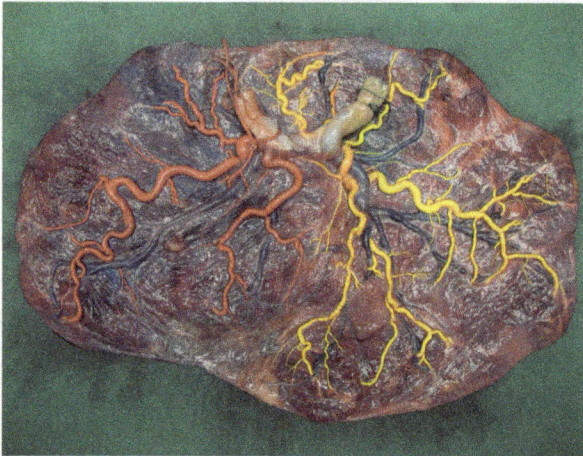

Fig. 13.8: Single placenta without a dividing membrane monochorionic-monoamniotic (MoMo) twin placenta with umbilical cords inserting close to one another. Monochorionic-monoamniotic twin placenta in gestational week 33. Twin 1, APGAR 8-8-10, 2015 g; Twin 2, APGAR 8-8-9, 1875 g. No histological evidence of fetal-fetal vessel anastomoses after dye injection (Twin 1: artery with red dye and vein with blue dye; Twin 2: artery with yellow dye and vein with green dye).

13.3.1 Vessel anastomoses between the twins

Vessel anastomoses indicate that the circulatory systems of the twins are in communication. Superficial anastomoses on the chorionic surface should to be differentiated from deep anastomoses within the villous system.

Anastomoses are characteristic for monochorionic placentas. Monochorionic placentas demonstrated anastomoses in 85 % of cases, of which 72–79 % were superficial (6). Deep intraparenchymal anastomoses develop in fetal cotyledons, and anastomoses are reported in 15 % of twin placentas.

Anastomoses can be highlighted by dye injection and protocols for the examination of twin placentas, when anastomoses are clinically suspected, are relatively standardized between institutions. Fresh placentas are differentially injected with dyes into each umbilical artery and vein. After dye injection and formalin fixation, the placentas are macroscopically mapped for superficial anastomoses and sections are taken for histological analysis.

Development of anastomoses
Vessel anastomoses are assumed to develop following the first contractions of the embryonic heart and the onset of fetal blood circulation.

The direction and pressure of blood flow determines the differentiation into venous and arterial vessels, while blood volume and flow influence vessel persistency/atrophy. It is assumed that the start of fetal heart contractions is of greater influence than the influence of blood volume and flow, as heart contractions influence the primary direction of the blood flow in anastomoses [5]. Fetal vasoactive substances may regulate expansion and size of anastomoses.

Superficial anastomoses
Superficial anastomoses develop as linear connections on the chorionic plate between the segmental and sub-segmental vessels of both circulatory systems. The number of anastomoses is often between two to four, and rarely greater than 10. The distance between the umbilical cord insertion and the anastomoses often measures between 5 and 15 cm. Anastomoses are often of the arterial-arterial type (A-A) and the arterial-venous type (A-V), the latter regularly within the fetal cotyledons. Vessel shunts are usually located in the chorionic plate and show a small distance, only a few mm, between the shunting artery and vein. Superficial venous-venous (V-V) anastomoses are rare.

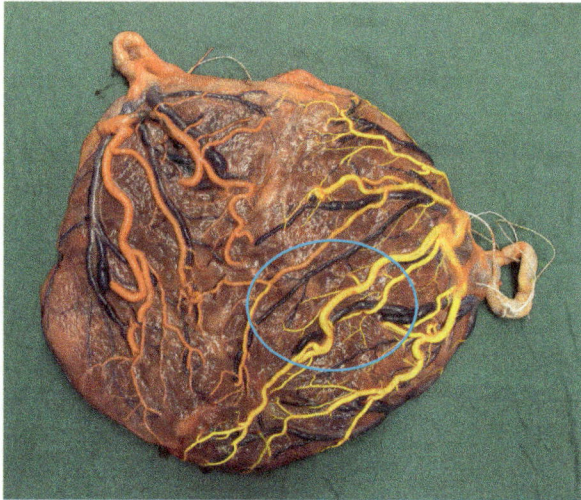

Fig. 13.9: Superficial fetal-fetal anastomosis on the chorionic plate between an artery marked by red dye (twin 1) and an artery with yellow dye (twin 2). A-A anastomosis (circle).

The reported frequency of the different anastomotic types varies:
- Arterioarteriell anastomoses (A-A): 25–57 %
- Arteriovenous anastomoses (A-V): 15–30 %
- Venovenous anastomoses (V-V): 5–20 %

In 40 % of placentas a combination of different anastomotic subtypes is found, most often A-A combined with A-V.

Visualization of anastomoses is almost impossible if IUFD of one twin occurs in early pregnancy, as in cases of fetus papyraceus.

Vessel anastomoses in fused dichorionic twin placentas are extremely rare. In exceptional cases of velamentous umbilical cord insertions at the dividing membrane, vasa aberrantia may cross the membrane and anastomose with the fetal vessels of the other twin. Single cases of deep intravillous anastomoses have been reported [14] but are of no clinical significance [6].

Rare cases of anastomoses are reported between twins of different genders with a partial development of a monochorionic placenta [15] and in blood cell chimerism in dichorionic twins [16,17].

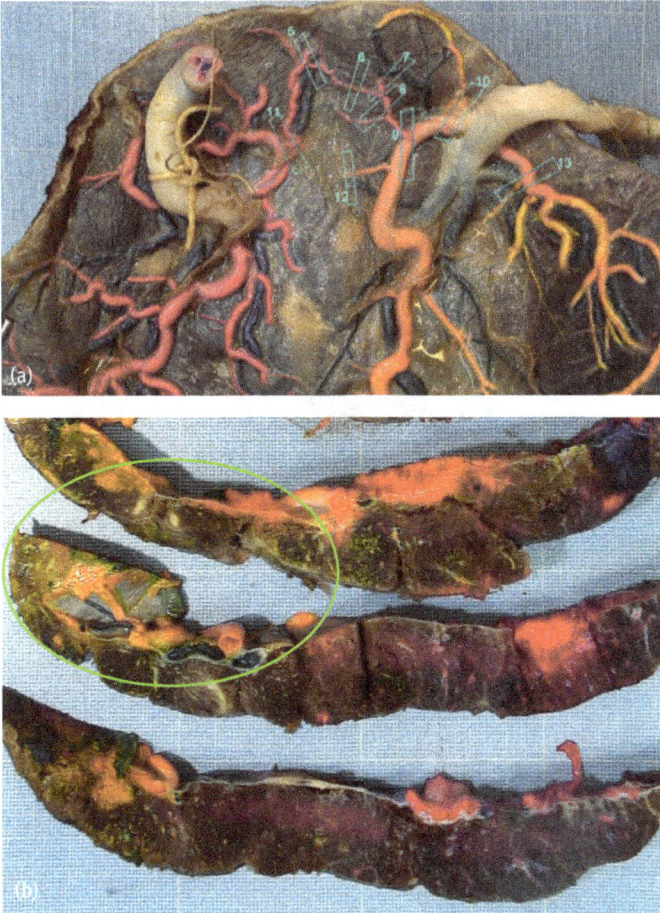

Fig. 13.10: (a) Superficial fetal-fetal vessel anastomoses with orange dye around the umbilical cord of twin 2; the orange dye coloration is due to mixing of the dye colors injected into the vessels of twin 1 and twin 2. Monochorionic-diamniotic (MoDi) twin placenta in gestational week 36 + 6 with induced delivery due to preeclampsia. Delivery of two boys. Anastomotic sampling marked 9 to 13. (b) Macroscopic slices. Suspect regions for fetal-fetal vessel anastomoses (green circle).

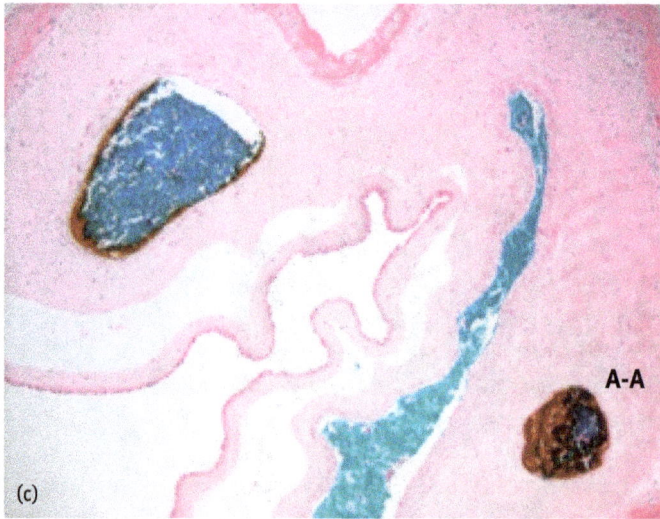

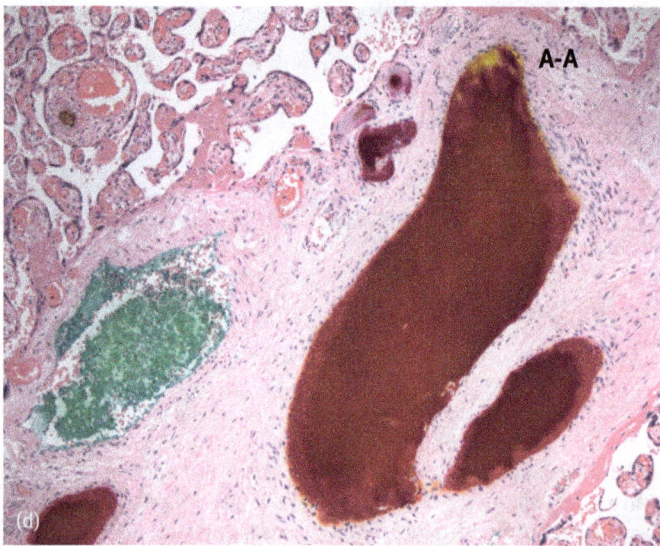

Fig. 13.10: (continued) (c) Dye injection showing an A-A anastomosis and a V-A anastomosis. Red, blue and yellow dye injected in the chorionic vessels: red (artery UC twin 1) and yellow (artery UC twin 2) A-A; blue (vein UC twin 1) and yellow (artery UC twin 2) V-A. (d) Histology of a stem villus (LPF). Red and yellow dye in the stem villous vessels: Red (artery UC twin 1) and yellow (artery UC twin 2), diagnostic for A-A.

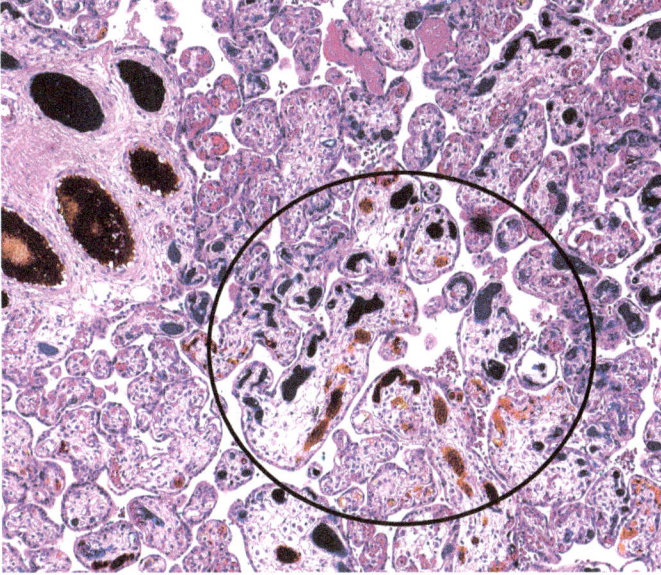

Fig. 13.11: Deep arteriovenous anastomoses (A-V) in stem, intermediate and terminal villi with red and yellow ink in the villous vessels (circle). Monochorionic-diamniotic (MoDi) placenta in gestational week 29. Twins APGAR 3-4-8 and 2-24-9.

Hemodynamic consequences

Vessel anastomoses may cause hemodynamic redistribution of the blood volume of both twins. The direction and extent of the shunt depends on the type, number, size and location of the anastomosis/anastomoses.

Arteriovenous (A-V) anastomoses are often closely related to the vessel branching of both placentas and cause a transfusion from the arterial donor to the venous acceptor side. Multiple arteriovenous anastomoses may cause a bi-directional transfusion to both twins.

Arterial (A-A) and venous (V-V) anastomoses close to the chorionic plate enable the direct reversal of blood flow. Pure arterial (A-A) anastomoses can more frequently stimulate a compensatory reversal of blood flow from the acceptor to the donor in a twin-to-twin transfusion syndrome (TTTS). This reversal of blood flow correlates with a better prognosis in TTTS

Venous anastomoses and the death of one twin may cause ischemic and thromboembolic organ changes in the surviving twin. This is believed to be caused by the transportation of the dead twin's thromboplastin through the venous shunt to the surviving twin.

Fetal consequence of vessel anastomoses depends on:
- heart ejection fraction,
- blood volume and blood pressure,
- local vessel regulation by vasoconstrictive and vasodilatative substances.

13.4 Twin-to-twin transfusion syndrome (TTTS)

Twin-to-twin transfusion syndrome (TTTS) describes an exchange of blood from one fetus to the other via placental vessel anastomoses. Depending on onset of the shunt and the duration of the transfusion, a chronic or acute TTTS may be diagnosed.

TTTS was reported in 11% of 286 twin pregnancies [18]. Ca 6% of all twin pregnancies, between gestational week 15 and 42, showed TTTS. 14% of these cases were monochorionic placentas with TTTS seen in 27% of fetal abortions, 17% stillbirths and 56% live born children [3].

A single case of TTTS was seen in a fused dichorionic-diamniotic twin placenta with velamentous insertion of both umbilical cords in the dividing membrane. Vasa aberrantia from the velamentous vessel insertions crossed the membrane and anastomosed with the fetal vessels of the other twin.

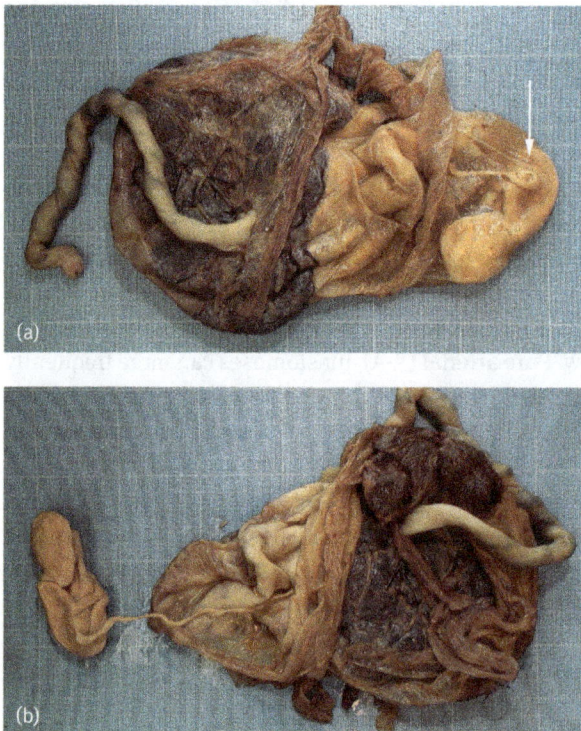

Fig. 13.12: (a) Monochorionic-diamniotic (MoDi) placenta in gestational week 41 with fetus papyraceus in the amniotic sac (arrow). (b) Placenta and opened amniotic sac. Fetus papyraceus with a thin umbilical cord. Death in ca. Gestational Week 16.

Table 13.2: Fetal-fetal transfusion syndromes onset and consequences for the fetus.

onset	chronic TTTS	onset	acute TTTS
early embryonic	acardius	prenatal	acute blood loss in the donor
early fetal	fetus papyraceus		acute volume overload in the acceptor
middle to late fetal	anemia and hypotrophy of the donor		
late fetal	anemia of the donor (no Fetal Growth Restriction [FGR])		

13.4.1 Acute twin-to-twin transfusion syndrome

To be distinguished are:
- acute twin-to-twin transfusion,
- acute transfusion in a chronic transfusion syndrome,
- acute transfusion in discordant twin growth.

Acute twin-to-twin transfusion
Acute TTTS is seen in the prenatal period and characterized by an acute intrauterine transfer of blood volume from one twin (donor) to the other (recipient, acceptor). It is reported to occur in less than 5% of transfusion syndromes. A prerequisite for this to occur is a direct shunt of the superficial arteries or veins in the chorionic plate, and it often occurs in combination with deep villous anastomoses. Blood flow in the anastomoses is balanced until the onset of the acute blood transfusion. The trigger for the transfusion can be:
- acute intrauterine hypoxia or intrauterine shock in a twin,
- during delivery with an acute transfusion from the unborn (non-delivered) twin to the delivered twin.

Findings:
- arterial (A-A) and venous (V-V) anastomoses on the chorionic plate and deep villous anastomoses
- recipient placenta is dark red,
- donor placenta and fetus are pale red (anemic)
- children are almost the same size
- recipient fetus is congested,
- hemoglobin/hematokrit changes in the umbilical cord blood are diagnostic in the surviving twin.

Acute transfusion in chronic transfusion syndromes

Seen in:

– *Reversal of blood flow:* spontaneously due to the death of one twin (therapeutic fetocide and other causes) occurring in the presence of large vessel anastomoses; resulting in the blood flow from the surviving twin passing to the deceased twin.
– *Shunt shift:* blood flow shifts in arteriovenous or veno-arterial anastomoses with affection of both twins. The clinical follow up of an identified shunt is Flow Ultrasound evaluation; for risk calculation, estimated prognosis and appraisal for therapeutic intervention. Post-partum evaluation depends on ultrasound and placental examination.

Acute transfusion occurring in discordant twin growth

This is a special situation in which growth restriction of a twin occurs despite a balanced transfusion or in cases without identifiable anastomoses. If intrauterine death of the smaller twin occurs blood may be acutely transferred to it. This is documented in 8 % of TTTS autopsies [4].

13.4.2 Chronic twin-to-twin transfusion syndrome

The outcome of a chronic TTTS in early pregnancy results in acardius and fetus papyraceus, whereas onset in middle or late pregnancy will cause characteristic changes in the placenta and the fetus (Table 13.3 and 13.4):

Table 13.3: Differences between the acceptor and donor placenta in Chronic TTTS.

	acceptor	donor
vessel anastomosis A-V, A-A, (V-V)		
umbilical cord	thick	thin
cut surface	greyish-red	pale greyish-red
villous maturation	mature / premature choranglosis II	villous maturation arrest, villous maturation retardation
villous lesion		stromal fibrosis
villous trophoblast		nuclear pyknosis, syncytial knots
intervillosum	normal	microfibrin deposition
amniotic fluid	polyhydramnion	oligohydramnion

Table 13.4: Differences in the donor and acceptor Twin in chronic TTTS.

acceptor	donor
normal/overweight	growth restricted
plethora	anemia
cardiomegaly	compensatory > extramedullary blood cell development
hepatomegaly	reticulocytosis
acute involution Adrenal Glands	progressive Involution Adrenal Glands
transudation	hydrops fetalis, acute hemorrhagic shock

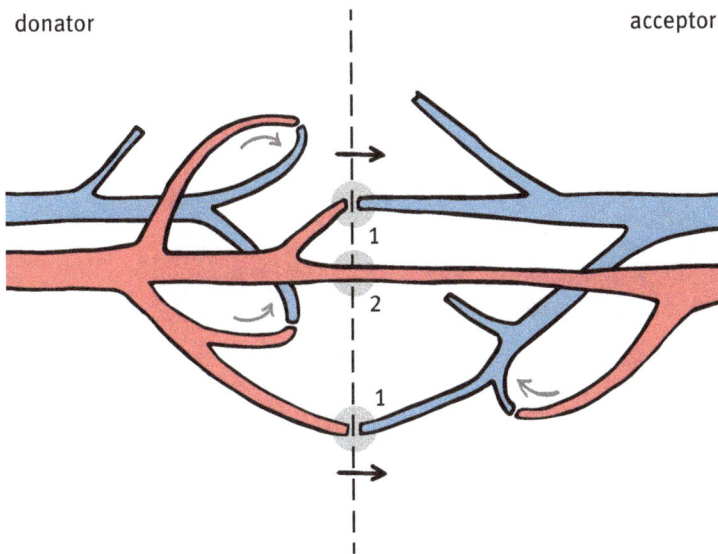

Fig. 13.13: Characteristic vessel anastomoses in chronic TTTS: 1 Arterio-Venous (AV), 2 Arterio-Arterial (AA).

Morphology

Typically, cases of chronic TTTS occur in monochorionic twin placentas with: several A-V anastomoses, weight discordant twins (> 15 % difference), polyhydramnion of one twin and oligohydramnion of the other, and an unambiguous difference of hemoglobin and hematocrit values in the fetuses (> 5 g/l). In more than 50 % of chronic TTTS the A-V anastomotic type predominates. A-A anastomoses may be seen, to a lesser extent, and rarely V-V anastomoses are found on the chorionic plate.

Macroscopically, the donor and recipient portions of the placenta are often clearly demarcated by color differences. The darker placental portion generally corresponds to the recipient, whereas the paler area corresponds to the donor. In long standing transfusion syndromes a difference in the size of both the donor and recipient placental areas may be seen; the smaller portion corresponds to the hypotrophic donor twin and often has a thinner umbilical cord, while the recipient portion of the placenta is often thicker and edematous.

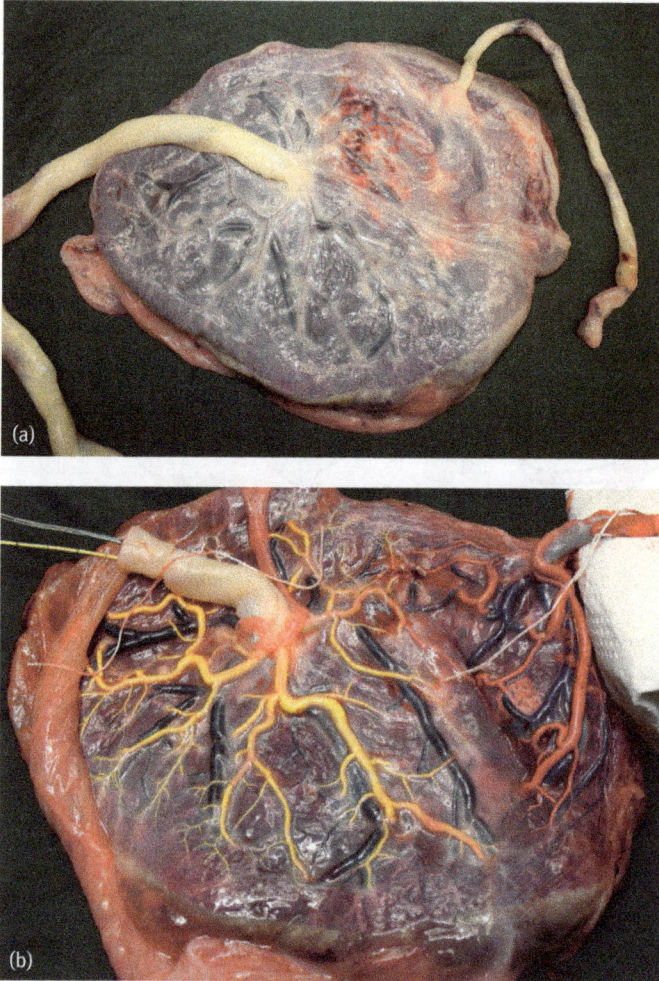

Fig. 13.14: (a) Chronic TTTS in a monochorionic-diamniotic (MoDi) placenta with an edematous umbilical cord of the recipient twin (left) and a thin cord of the donor twin (right). Placenta in gestational week 31. Twin 1 growth restricted and with cardiac malformation. (b) Placenta after dye injection: Edematous umbilical cord acceptor twin with yellow and green dye (left); donor twin umbilical cord with red and blue dye (right).

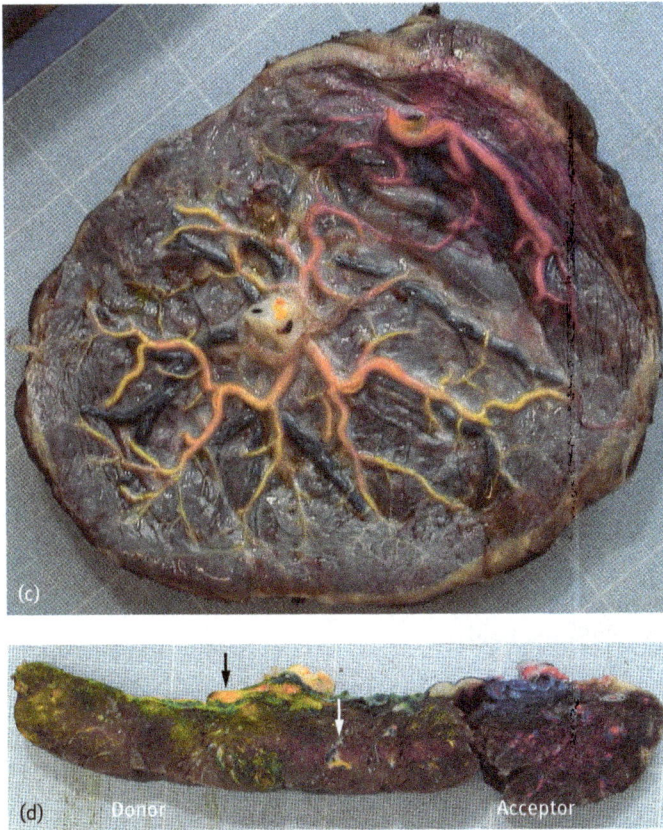

Fig. 13.14: (continued) (c) Placenta after formalin fixation: Edematous umbilical cord with vessels containing orange dye, suggesting superficial anastomoses (arrows). (d) Cut sections of a placenta after formalin fixation, arrow marked anastomoses. Donor portion of the placenta (left) and acceptor portion of placenta (right).

The demarcation between recipient and donor placenta is not always readily apparent as parenchymal islands of the donor twin may lie within the recipient territory and vice versa. These represent deep anastomoses which develop in the cotyledon between both placentas [19].

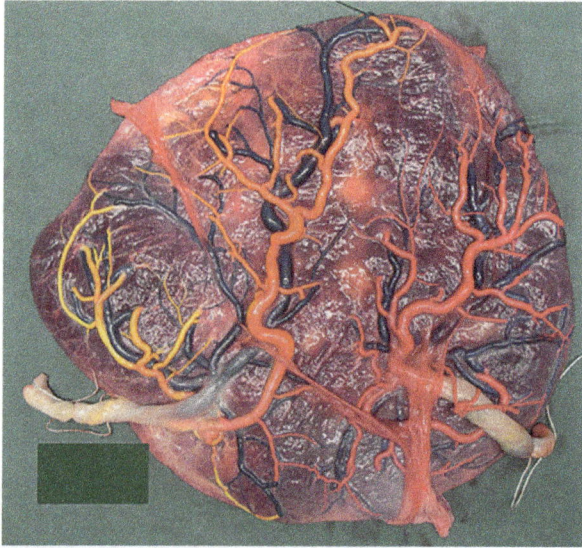

Fig. 13.15: Congested twin placenta with evidence of vessel anastomoses (orange dye mix).

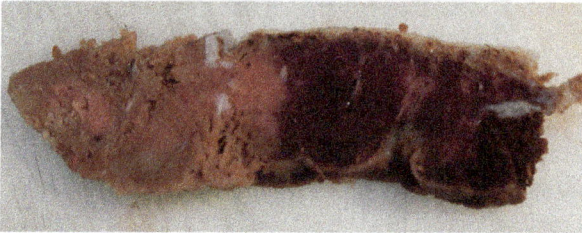

Fig. 13.16: Cut surface of a monochorionic twin placenta with chronic TTTS: Dark-red color of the recipient placenta and pallor of the donor placenta

Histologically The recipient placental area contains mature villous structures, in contrast to the donor placental area which shows immature villi with arrested or re-tarded maturation, or even villous stromal fibrosis. Depending on intravillous anastomoses, both donor and recipient areas may show adjacent mature and immature villi.

Villous maturation disorders with increased vessel proliferation and congestion are typical in the recipient placenta. If the recipient fetus is edematous, the placental portion may show villous stromal edema also. Donor placental villi may show typical secondary changes, such as: collapse sclerosis of the stem villous vessels, stromal fibrosis, regressive nuclear knots on the villous surface and increased inter- and periv-illous microfibrin depositions. The shorter the length of the inter-fetal blood shunt, the less difference between villous maturation disorders is seen and vice versa.

Doppler Ultrasound of the umbilical cord arteries may show normal or decreased blood flow caused by increased vessel resistance in the donor placenta [20]. The direction of the shunt is not always possible to identify [21].

The donor's amniotic sac often shows less amniotic fluid (oligohydramnion) with/without amnion nodosum of the placenta. The acceptor twin is more often sur-

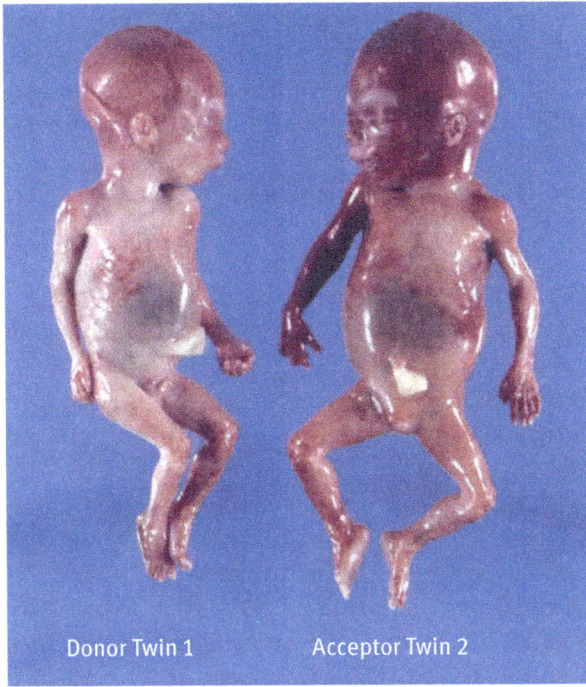

Donor Twin 1   Acceptor Twin 2

Fig. 13.17: TTTS twins. Twin 1: donor, pale and anemic (left); twin 2: acceptor, congested (right).

rounded by increased amniotic fluid (polyhydramnion), possibly due to increased fetal urine production in the acceptor.

13.4.3 Discordance of fetal growth / weight in twin pregnancies without TTTS

In the majority of twins with growth discordance, the placenta is of the dichorionic-diamniotic type [22]. Vessel anastomoses are normally absent but, if present, are of little hemodynamic significance.

In 75 % of these twin pregnancies, the placenta of the smaller twin is small and underweight and often shows distal villous hypoplasia. Additionally, in half of the placentas an extensive inter- and perivillous microfibrin deposition may be seen, and this may be macroscopically visible as gitterinfarcts. The placental territory corresponding to the larger twin often displays only minimal pathological changes which are without clinical significance.

Causes of death of a twin without twin-twin transfusion syndrome (TTTS)

It is not always possible to fully diagnose the cause of death in a twin pregnancy, even following a detailed histological examination; preceded by a through macroscopic assessment of umbilical cord and its insertion and the number, size and type of anastomoses.

In the majority of cases involving the death of both twins the cause is chronic TTTS.

Causative factors in the death of a twin without TTTS are:

- *Acute placental insufficiency* caused by acute pre-term placental rupture of the deceased twin's placenta.
- *Hemorrhagic shock due to bleeding* into a low implanted placenta or a placenta previa, or bleeding from a ruptured aberrant vessel in the placental margin or the free membrane.
- *Morphology of a restricted placental perfusion capacity* or *chronic placental insufficiency* with fetal growth restriction of the twin prior to death.
- *Umbilical cord complications* causing fetal death shortly before, or during delivery: velamentous umbilical cord insertion, umbilical cord prolapse with strangulation and compression of the fetal vessels, and umbilical cord or chorionic plate venous thrombosis. Death in monoamniotic twins may also be caused by umbilical cord entanglement and knots.
- *Ascending amniotic inflammation* occurs especially in the amniotic sac of twin 1 in early intrauterine death, slight maceration may or may not be present.
- *Lethal malformation.* Malformations of both twins, occurring as specific developmental disorders in monochorionic twin pregnancies, are more often seen in early gestational weeks.

13.5 Acardiac twins

A fetus with either a completely absent, or incompletely developed, fetal heart defines acardius. It is frequently seen in combination with other, partly high grade, malformations. This condition is exclusively seen in monozygotic pregnancy [5,23]. An acardius is seen in ca. 1 % of all monochorionic twin pregnancies (less than 1 in 34,000 deliveries).

Classification

Hemiacardius (acardius anceps): partially developed head with facial clefts and lacking a heart

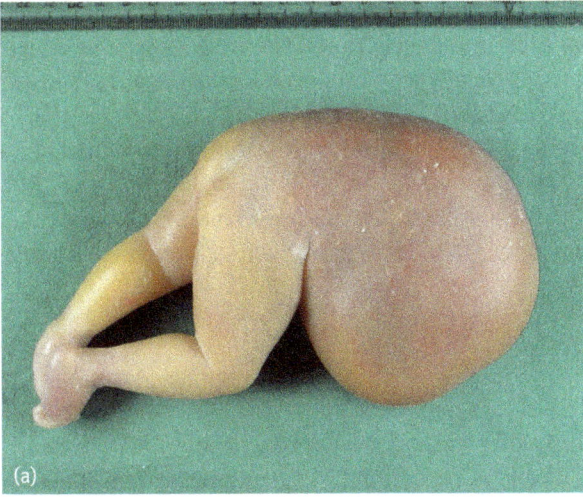

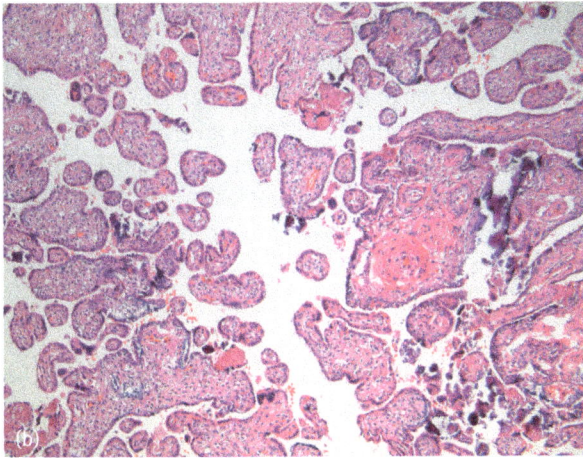

Fig. 13.18: (a) Acardiac twin of a monochorionic twin pregnancy, cesarean section in gestational week 27. Twin 2 normal. (b) Morphology of the placental parenchyma in an acardiac twin with stem villous hypoplasia and retention changes.

Holoacardius:

- *Acardius amorphus:* skin coated tissue mass containing an admixture of tissues without organ differentiation. Distinguishing this from a placental teratoma may not be possible but the presence of an umbilical cord and the degree of skeletal organization favors acardius amorphous.
- *Acardius acephalus:* missing head, missing upper extremities, rudimentary thoracic cavity, missing thoracic organs, abdominal cavity with remnants of intestinal organs and well developed lower extremities.
- *Acardius acormus:* fetal head is attached to the placenta. The trunk is partly or completely absent and extremities are not present.

Morphology

Acardius is, without exception, seen in monochorionic placentas with large superficial vessel anastomoses, characteristically side by side A-A and V-V anastomoses, which are close to the umbilical cord insertion.

The acardius has a filiform and short umbilical cord that often contains only a single artery.

On histological examination, the placental portion corresponding to the acardius shows stem villous vessel hypoplasia, villous maturation arrest, stroma edema and retention changes.

Pathogenesis

There are two suggested hypotheses for acardius:
- Acardiac malformation is caused by a primary maldevelopment of the fetal heart.
- An inter-embryonic shunt develops concurrently with embryonic placental circulation. This causes a complete reversal of blood flow in the malformed embryo and subsequent cardiac maldevelopment. In this early embryonic TTTS, a shunt develops between the acardius and its intrauterine twin partner. The hemodynamically healthy twin pumps blood through the A-A and V-V anastomoses causing the reversal of normal blood flow in the recipient: "twin reversed-arterial-perfusion sequence", TRAP [24]. The retrograde circulation in the umbilical cord of the acardius can be demonstrated by Doppler ultrasound [25].

13.6 Fetus papyraceus and Vanishing twin

Fetus papyraceus: Intrauterine death of a twin in the middle ⅓ of pregnancy with the remnants remaining in utero alongside the viable and developing twin. Growth stagnation, retention phenomena and compression of the deceased twin by the surviving twin are visible.

Fetus papyraceus is diagnosed in 2–3 % of all twin pregnancies.

Vanishing twin: It is diagnosed on ultrasound as an embryonic/fetal loss before gestational week 15 in a multiple pregnancy (Table 13.2). Loss of one fetus without a known cause is reported to occur in 60–70 % of diagnosed twin pregnancies [5]. Rudiments of the residual amniotic sac are sometimes still seen at term. The placenta of the living child may show:
- *Circumscribed fibrin depositions on* the chorionic plate (not subchorionic) or at the placental margin with ghost like rudimentary embryonic elements.
- *Well defined cystic lesions in* the chorionic plate or at the placental margin. The cyst wall may show chorionic membrane remnants, rarely ghost villi and may, or may not, contain fibrin.

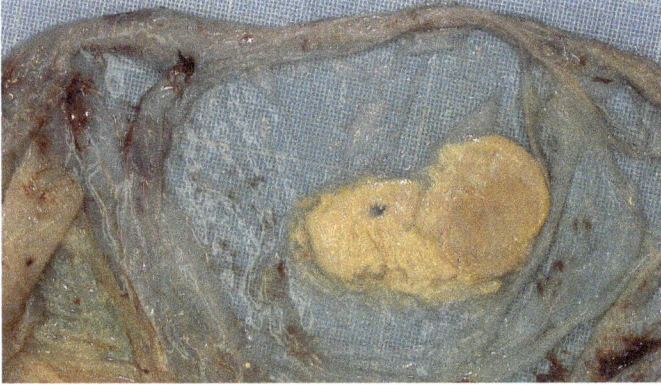

Fig. 13.19: IVF pregnancy with monochorionic-diamniotic twin pregnancy with death of one twin at ca. gestational week 11. The dead fibrous twin lies encapsulated in the membrane (vanishing twin).

- Fibrin deposition, *cystic formation and/or embryo (or only rudiments)* in the free amniotic membrane that is with or without chorionic remnants. Separate to the main placenta.

Pathogenesis
- Early onset of chronic TTTS with the death of one fetus, thrombotic occlusion of the vessel anastomoses close to the chorionic plate or stem villous vessel obliteration by connective tissue.
- Pre-term death of one twin, frequently without a known cause.

Potential causes
- umbilical cord complications: velamentous insertion, umbilical cord torsion, short umbilical cord and umbilical cord entanglement following vessel obstruction in monoamniotic twin placentas
- maternal-placental vascular malperfusion, preterm partial placental abruption of the placenta belonging to the fetus papyraceus
- latrogenic feticide

Morphology
The fetus papyraceus usually lies on the chorionic plate. It is often flattened and compressed in the amniotic sac (fetus compressus) and varies in size, between 1 and 20 cm (CRL/SSL). The size is used to help estimate the gestational age at which embryonic/fetal death occurred.

The umbilical cord is extremely thin, sometimes only filiform. The placenta of the fetus papyraceus is clearly demarcated by its light color and firm sclerotic consistency, when compared to the developing twin placenta. The differential diagnosis of a marginal chronic circulatory disorder should be excluded.

Consequence for the surviving fetus
A fetus papyraceus usually does not interfere with the development of the surviving child. Aplasia cutis and/or intestinal atresia in the surviving child are reported in isolated cases [26].

Fetus papyraceus can be diagnosed in monochorionic and dichorionic placentas; confirming that the condition has no correlation with fetal vessel anastomoses.

13.7 Triplet and greater multiple pregnancy

Triplets can be mono-, di- or trizygotic. Placentation is analogous to mono- or dizygotic twins.

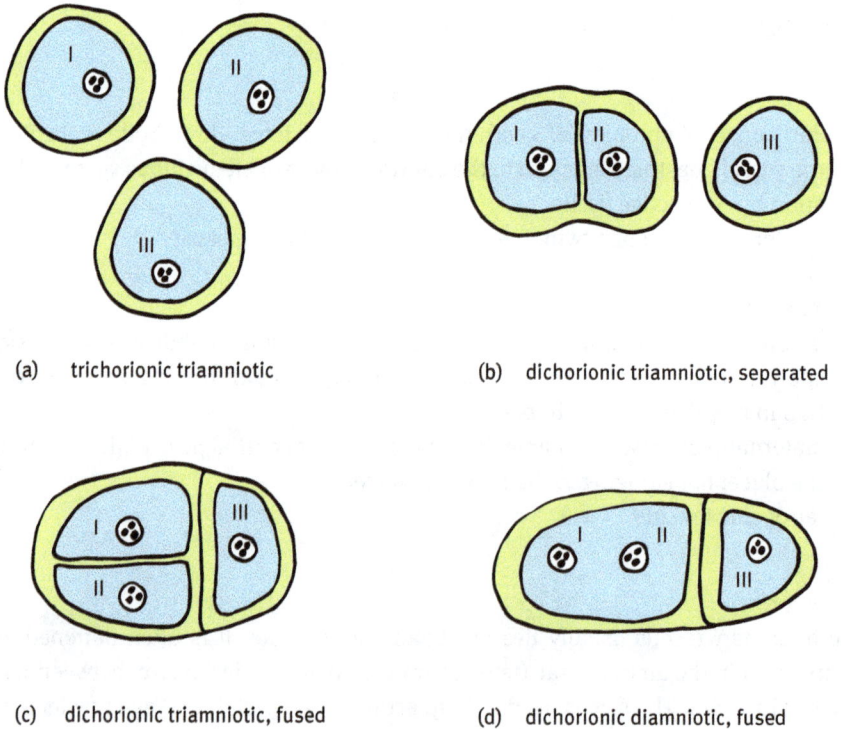

(a) trichorionic triamniotic

(b) dichorionic triamniotic, seperated

(c) dichorionic triamniotic, fused

(d) dichorionic diamniotic, fused

Fig. 13.20: Illustration of the placenta in multiple pregnancy: (a) Trichorionic-triamniotic separated placentas; (b) dichorionic-triamniotic placenta separated placentas; (c) dichorionic-triamniotic fused placenta; (d) dichorionic-diamniotic fused placenta.

To be distinguished are:
- Three separate placentas with chorionic and amniotic membranes (trichorionic-triamniotic).
- Two fused placentas and a separate single placenta; this can occur in trichorionic-triamniotic and dichorionic-triamniotic placentation.
- A single placenta; many forms of placentation are possible: trichorionic-triamniotic triplet placentas, dichorionic-di/triamniotic and monochorionic-mon/di/triamniotic triplet placentas.

From selected material, over a 10 year period in Berlin (Charité Pediatric Pathology and Placentology) a triplet placenta is found in 0.05 % of pregnancies:
- trichorionic triplet placentas: 41 %
- dichorionic triplet placenta: 48 %
- monochorionic triplet placenta: 11 %

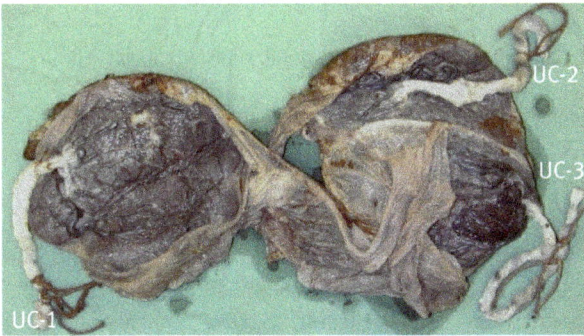

Fig. 13.21: Single placenta (UC 1) and a monochorionic-diamniotic twin placenta (UC 2 and UC 3): Dichorionic-triamniotic, separated triple placenta.

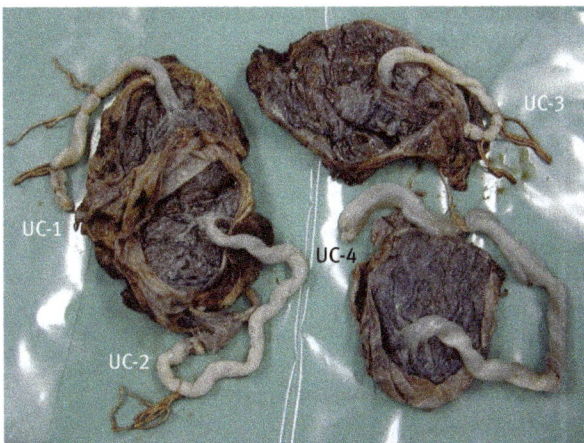

Fig. 13.22: Monochorionic-diamniotic twin placenta (UC 1 and UC 2) and two single placentas (UC 3 and UC 4): trichorionic-quadroamniotic, separated quadruple placenta.

13.7.1 Placental shape and zygosity

– Trichorionic triplet placentas may have trizygotic, dizygotic and monozygotic triplets.
– Dichorionic triplet placentas are assumed to be dizygotic, analogous to twin pregnancies. They lack chorion in the partition wall.
– Each monochorionic triplet placenta is assumed to be monozygotic, due to a common yolk sac.

Vessel anastomoses

Analogous to twin pregnancies observed in dichorionic and monochorionic triplet placentas.

References

[1] Fellman J, Eriksson AW. On the history of Hellin's law. Twin Res Hum Genet. 2009;12(2):183–190.
[2] Boklage CE. Survival probability of human conceptions from fertilization to term. Int J Fertil. 1990;35(2):75, 9–80, 1–94.
[3] Schuhmacher C. Morphologie der Zwillingsplazenta und ihre Bedeutung für das Kind. Berlin; 1991.
[4] Baldwin W. Pathology of multiple pregnancy. Berlin, Heidelberg, New York Tokyo: Springer; 1994.
[5] Benirschke K, Burton GJ, Baergen RN. Pathology of the Human Placenta. 6 ed. Heidelberg, NY, London: Springer; 2012.
[6] Perrin EVDK. Pathology of the placenta. Churchill Livingstone: New York; 1984.
[7] Potter EL. Twin Zygosity and Placental Form in Relation to the Outcome of Pregnancy. American journal of obstetrics and gynecology. 1963;87:566–577.
[8] Strong SJ, Corney G. The placenta in twin pregnancy. Pergamon Oxford. 1967.
[9] Martius G. Lehrbuch der Geburtshilfe. 11. ed. Stuttgart: Thieme; 1985.
[10] Bazso J, Dolhany B, Pohanka O. [Weight increase in twins during the 28th to 42 d week of pregnancy]. Zentralbl Gynakol. 1970;92(20):628–633.
[11] Giffei IM. Zwillingsschwangerschaft In: Dudenhausen JW, editor. Praxis der Perinatalmedizin. Stutgart: Thieme; 1984. p. 226–230; 351–353.
[12] Magnus P, Arntzen A, Samuelsen SO, Haldorsen T, Bakketeig LS. No correlation in post-neonatal deaths for twins. A study of the early mortality of twins based on the Norwegian Medical Birth Registry. Early human development. 1990;22(2):89–97.
[13] Spellacy WN, Handler A, Ferre CD. A case-control study of 1253 twin pregnancies from a 1982–1987 perinatal data base. Obstetrics and gynecology. 1990;75(2):168–171.
[14] Robertson EG, Neer KJ. Placental injection studies in twin gestation. American journal of obstetrics and gynecology. 1983;147(2):170–174.
[15] Nylander PP, Osunkoya BO. Unusual monochorionic placentation with heterosexual twins. Obstetrics and gynecology. 1970;36(4):621–625.
[16] Benirschke K, Kim CK. Multiple pregnancy. 2. The New England journal of medicine. 1973;288(25):1329–1336.

[17] Benirschke K, Kim CK. Multiple pregnancy. 1. The New England journal of medicine. 1973;288(24):1276–1284.

[18] Grischke EM, Boos R, Schmidt W, Bastert G. [Twin pregnancies with fetofetal transfusion syndrome]. Z Geburtshilfe Perinatol. 1990;194(1):17–21.

[19] Schatz F. Die Akardii und ihre Verwandten. Berlin: Hirchwald; 1898.

[20] Vetter K. Considerations on growth discordant twins. J Perinat Med. 1993;21(4):267–272.

[21] Seelbach-Gobel B, Kaesemann H, Roos T. [Doppler ultrasonography differential diagnosis in twin pregnancies]. Z Geburtshilfe Perinatol. 1992;196(1):26–32.

[22] Eberle AM, Levesque D, Vintzileos AM, et al. Placental pathology in discordant twins. American journal of obstetrics and gynecology. 1993;169(4):931–935.

[23] Kloos K, Vogel M. Pathologie der Perinatalperiode. Stuttgart: Thieme; 1974.

[24] Van Allen MI, Smith DW, Shepard TH. Twin reversed arterial perfusion (TRAP) sequence: a study of 14 twin pregnancies with acardius. Semin Perinatol. 1983;7(4):285–293.

[25] Kirkinen P, Herva R, Rasanen J, Airaksinen J, Ikaheimo M. Documentation of paradoxical umbilical blood supply of an acardiac twin in the antepartum state. J Perinat Med. 1989;17(1):63–65.

[26] Wagner DS, Klein RL, Robinson HB, Novak RW. Placental emboli from a fetus papyraceous. J Pediatr Surg. 1990;25(5):538–542.

14 Placental findings accompanying fetal and maternal disease

14.1 Placental changes associated with fetal death

The WHO defines stillbirth (intrauterine fetal death IUFD) as a baby born with no signs of life between gestational week 20 and 28 and with a birth-weight between 350 and 1000 g in high and low income countries [1].

A unified stillbirth classification system does not exist, and this results in variation in the reported causes of fetal death and a wide range in the reported rate of fetal death, between 1.3 and 8.8 per 1000 deliveries [2–4].

Fetal growth restriction is defined as a failure to achieve a genetically predetermined size potential and is considered to be one of the major complications of pregnancy. In contrast, small for gestational age (SGA) fetuses are of weight less than a specified percentile, usually the 10th, when compared to all fetuses at a specific gestation age. Identification of SGA infants is important because these infants are at an increased risk of perinatal morbidity and mortality [5].

Autopsies of 940 stillbirths with a weight > 1000 g (Department of Pediatric Pathology and Placentology, Charité, Berlin, Germany) showed intrauterine growth restriction and intrauterine anoxia or infection in 70 %. In nearly 95 % of cases, morphologic placental examination revealed a cause of fetal death, or pathological findings that were associated with the cause of death.

14.1.1 Pathogenic changes

In general, two groups of placental changes with differing biological significance have to be differentiated:
- changes which cause/are responsible for the stillbirth
- changes which are secondarily related to the stillbirth.

Investigations that correlated placental examination and fetal autopsy findings with detailed clinical/anesthetic information showed that placental examination can pinpoint the cause of death as: manifest placental insufficiency, latent decreased functionality, intrauterine infection or umbilical cord complication in 75 % of stillbirths [6]. This corresponds with statistics from the stillbirth classification system CODAC (Causes of Death and Associated Conditions) which records placental complications as a cause of fetal death in more than 80 % of stillbirths (Table 14.1).

The cause of placental changes, such as villous immaturity or premature placental abruption, and its contribution to intrauterine fetal death may remain unknown. In less than 50 % of stillbirths are clinical risk factors identified.

https://doi.org/10.1515/9783110452600-014

Table 14.1: Causes of fetal deaths (> 1000 g, n = 940) [7].

causes of fetal death	number	%
acute placental insufficiency	289	29.9
chronic placental insufficiency	169	18.0
limited placental function and other causes of anoxia	121	12.8
infection of amniotic type	60	6.4
infection specific type	13	1.4
umbilical cord complication	62	6.6
fetal malformation	74	7.9
hemorrhagic shock	34	3.6
TTTS	27	2.9
hydrops universalis	20	2.1
obstetric complications	7	0.7
anoxia of unknown cause	46	4.9
Unknown cause of death	26	2.6

According to a study of 487 placentas, from intrauterine fetal deaths in gestational week 13 to 41, a chronic placental insufficiency due to villous immaturity, chronic vascular malperfusion and/or endangiitis obliterans was seen in 54 %. Stillbirth was caused by pre-term placental abruption in 24 %, by inflammation of the membranes in 11 % and was of unknown cause in 13.7 % [8].

Stillbirths due to acute placental insufficiency were seen in [9]:
- 9 % of intrapartum deaths,
- 46 % of stillbirths without maceration,
- 58 % of pre-terms,
- 35 % of fetuses with growth restriction.

Morphology correlating with acute placental insufficiency in stillbirth was seen in:
- 15 % of placentas with a clinically diagnosed acute placental insufficiency; large foci of fetal vascular malperfusion without previous structural damage. However, 80 % showed changes due to pre-term abruption.
- 60 % of placentas had an acute fetal vascular malperfusion with associated pre-ceding changes: growth restriction, maturation disorders and/or chronic fetal vascular malperfusion.
- 25 % of placentas had an acute vascular malperfusion associated with a chronic placental insufficiency (global insufficiency).

(Department of Pediatric Pathology and Placentology, Charité, Berlin, Germany)

Stillbirths due to chronic placental insufficiency were seen in ca. 20 % of:
– Associated fetal growth restriction, vascular malperfusion and facultative villous maturation disorders in ca. 60 %.
– Placental growth and villous maturation disorders (grade 3) are found in ca. 30 %.
– Endangiopathia obliterans with villous stromal fibrosis and/or maturation disorders can be associated with placental growth disorders and chronic intervillous vascular malperfusion in ca. 10 %.
– Stillborns were diagnosed as:
  – Macerated in 79 %,
  – Pre-term in 62 %
  – Growth restricted in 98 % (less than 10th weight percentile for gestational age).

Latent decreased placental functionality was seen in more than 10 % of stillbirths. In these cases undergoing stress (birth activity, uterus contraction, uteroplacental circulatory disorders) which may otherwise have been tolerated in a normal, healthy placenta can cause hypoxic episodes or lethal intrauterine anoxia. In this group a decreased placental diffusion capacity was seen due to:
– reduced surface of the metabolic exchange membrane (in ca. 90 %)
– reduction of the intra/intervillous vessel volume (in ca. 10 % of the cases). Fetuses in this group showed:
  – intrapartum fetal death in 17 %,
  – stillbirth with maceration in 65 %,
  – pre-term delivery in 35 %,
  – fetal hypotrophy in 21 %.

Placental inflammation due to maternal infection, before or during delivery, as a cause of fetal death was seen in 8 %. Approximately 85 % died due to amniotic infection syndrome and 15 % due to listeriosis, toxoplasmosis or syphilis infection. Fetuses in this group showed:
– intrapartum death in 8 %,
– stillbirth without maceration in 52 %,
– pre-term delivery in 68 %,
– fetal hypotrophy in 31 %.

Intrauterine and intrapartum *umbilical cord entanglement* as cause of fetal death was seen in 7 % of cases, and this was morphologically characterized as umbilical cord and placental changes due to fetal vascular circulatory interruption. Characteristic indentations may remain on the portions of the fetus entrapped by the cord.

Umbilical cord complications:
– umbilical cord entanglement with fetal strangulation in 45 %,
– umbilical cord prolapse with vascular compression in 20 %,

- true umbilical knots with subsequent circulatory disorders in 14 %,
- occlusive venous thrombi in 21 %.

Fetuses associated with umbilical cord complications showed:
- intrapartum death in 28 %
- stillbirth without maceration in 62 %
- pre-term delivery in 48 %
- fetal hypotrophy in 10 %

Intrauterine anoxia without identifiable causes in the placenta or umbilical cord was seen in 4.9 % (Table 14.1). In these cases the quality of obstetric monitoring, drug therapy and, if applicable, surgical treatment should be evaluated. Intrapartum death due to a traumatic event is rare. Metabolic causes are mostly due to diabetes mellitus.

14.1.2 Retention phenomena

Placental changes following intrauterine fetal demise are a combination of cessation of fetal circulation and ongoing maternal circulation. Early changes of retention are morphologically seen in the fetal vessels and the villous stroma. Later retention changes are seen in the chorionic epithelium and are indirectly related to the maternal blood circulation.

Morphological placental changes following fetal demise in the villi

Fetal vessel changes
- Acute luminal collapse of the stem villous vessels and microcirculatory system.
- Endothelial edema and endothelial necrosis in the stem villous vessels.
- Collapse sclerosis, concentric constriction, and eventual obliteration of the stem villous vessels
- Thickening of the basal membrane and luminal loss in arterioles and venules; as well as capillaries of the intermediate and terminal villi.

Stromal changes
- Condensed ground substance in the terminal and intermediate villi.
- Proliferation of the connective tissue cells.
- Proliferation of collagenous fibres.
- Karyorrhexis and complete nuclear loss in stromal cells.

Vessel and stromal changes preferentially develop in pre-damaged tissue areas rather than in areas of normal placental tissue.

Table 14.2: Morphological placental changes following fetal demise-retention stages.

retention follow-ing fetal demise	chorionic epithelium	villous stroma	fetal vessels
< 1 week (stage I)	eosinophilic syncytium, increased syncytial sprouts	sparse condensation of the interstitial sub-stance, nuclear pyknosis	collapse of fetal vessel lumina
few weeks (stage II)	nuclear pyknosis and karyorrhexis of the syn-cytium, loss of cytrophoblast, increased perivillous fibrin (-oid)	collagenous edema, increased fibers, hydropic / mucoid degen-eration, nuclear pyknosis	endothelial desquama-tion, obliteration of vascular lumen, vessel wall fibrosis in stem villi
several weeks (stage III)	epithelial desquamation, increased perivillous fibrin (-oid), fibrinous obliteration of the intervillous space	mucoid or hyaline trans-formation, fibrosis, cellular loss	loss of endothelium obliteration of vascular lumen

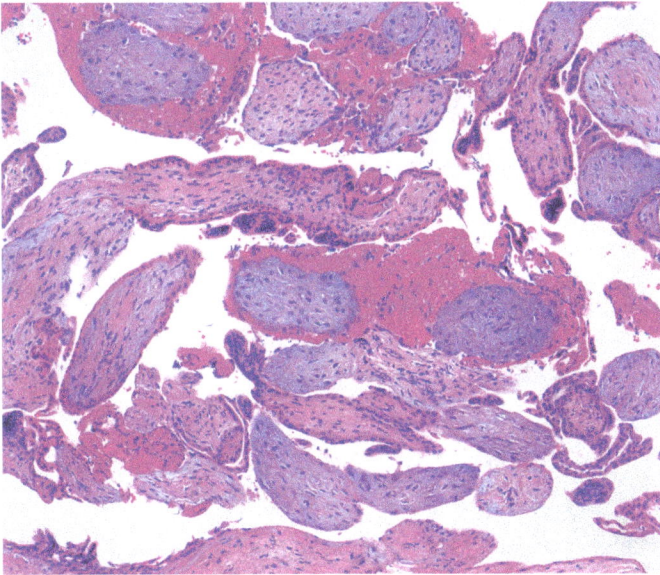

Fig. 14.1: Retention stage I. Eosinophilic syncytium, increased syncytial sprouts, sparse condensa-tion of the interstitial substance, nuclear pyknosis, collapse of fetal vessel lumina.

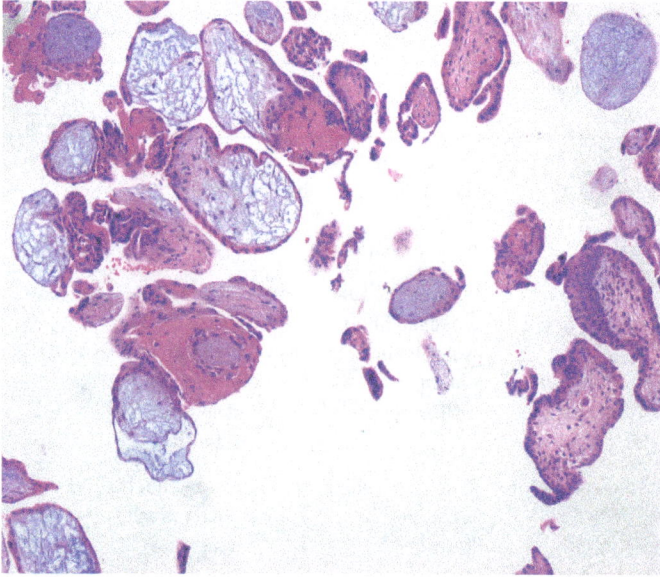

Fig. 14.2: Retention stage II. Nuclear pyknosis and karyorrhexis of the syncytium, loss of cytrophoblast, increased perivillous fibrin (-oid), hydropic / mucoid degeneration, nuclear pyknosis, fibrosis in stem villi.

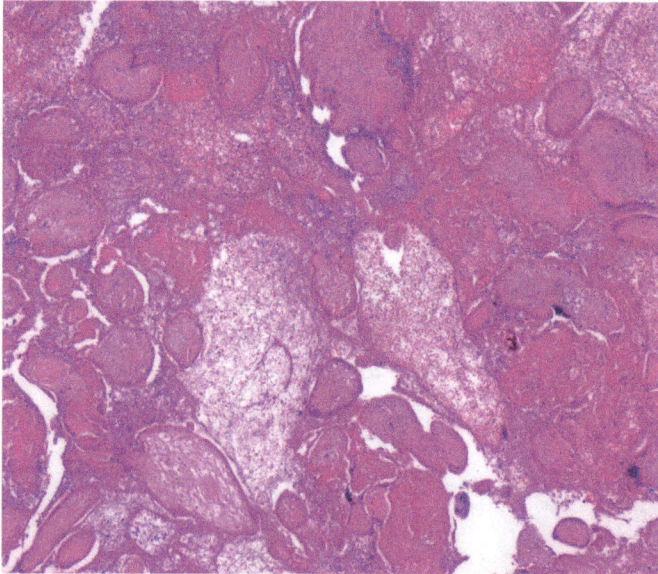

Fig. 14.3: Retention stage III. Epithelial desquamation, increased perivillous fibrin (-oid), fibrinous obliteration of the intervillous space, mucoid or hyaline transformation, fibrosis, cellular loss, loss of endothelium, obliteration of vascular lumen.

Chorionic epithelial changes
- Aggregation of nuclear sprouts on the villous surface.
- Regressive nuclear knots with karyorrhexis and focal epithelial loss.
- Secondary fibrin deposition on the villous surface.

Ghost Villi: Stillborn placentas are still surrounded and oxygenated by maternal blood, and so villous morphology can be maintained for several days and weeks. Regressive changes, with formation of necrotic ghost villi, start in the villous axis, after the loss of a direct connection to the maternal blood supply due to isolation by fibrin deposits [10].

Well demarcated infiltrates along the basal chorionic plate were seen in ca. 66 % of intrauterine fetal deaths with maceration grade II and III [11]. The aggregates were composed of maternal granulocytes and are considered to be related to maternal immunoreactions, due to ineffective oxygenation and tissue acidosis of the chorionic tissue.

Calcification

Placentas from stillbirths may show considerable calcification on macroscopy and histology:
- granular calcification of the basal membrane, in the chorionic epithelium and in the fibrillary structures of the villous tree,
- microcalcification.

Deposits of calcification may be focal or generalized and can be partly associated with depositions of iron salt.

Microcalcification and calcification of the basal membrane are more often reported in placentas from stillbirths and fetal and embryonic abortions. They may also be seen, focally, in placentas from live births with associated chronic maternal vascular malperfusion, endangiopathia obliterans and villous stromal fibrosis. Deposits are not considered to be part of a specific placental dysfunction but reflect regressive changes of the chorionic villi [11]. Usually they do not affect fetal nutrition. Decreased fetal blood flow increases calcium deposits in the local tissue, even though the chorionic epithelium is unaffected. Due to local acidosis the calcium remains soluble but following necrosis and increased amounts of amphoteric protein the pH becomes alkaline and lime salt precipitates.

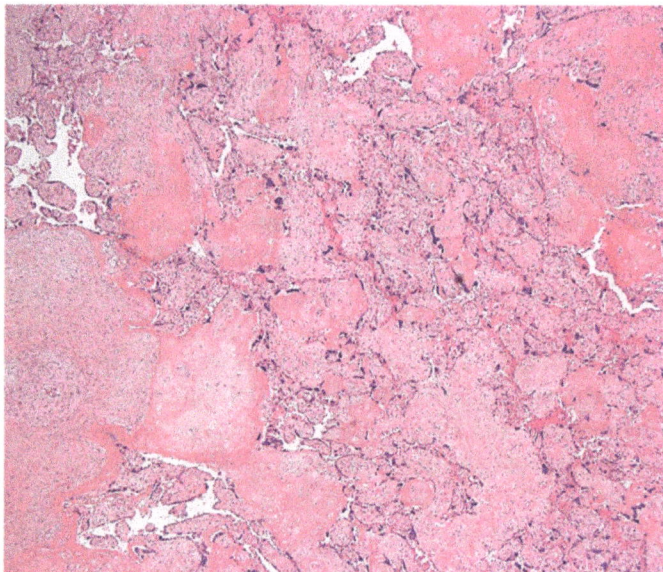

Fig. 14.4: Degenerative villous changes: Placental villi, close to the basal membrane and surrounded by fibrin, with an eosinophilic stroma and a chorionic epithelium with regressive nuclear sprouts. Placenta in Gestational Week 38.

14.1.3 Placental changes associated with sudden unexpected death (SIDS)

In a retrospective study of placentas from sudden unexpected newborn deaths, placental growth disorder and chronic circulatory disturbance was seen as often as in controls. Chorioamnionitis was seen in 17 %, morphological changes due to a restricted diffusion capacity were seen in ca. 33 % and changes due to fetal hypoxia, such as meconium phagocytosis in the amniotic stroma and/or chorionic plate, were seen in 33 %. However, perinatal asphyxia was clinically documented in only 7 of 24 SIDS cases (sudden unexpected infant death) 3 newborns required intensive care treatment while 4 were without any symptoms [6].

Acute chorioamnionitis in SIDS children was interpreted as a primary disease in 35 % of pre-term and 25 % of term deliveries with multiple episodes of neonatal apnea [12,13]. Amniotic infections, villous maturation disorders with limited diffusion capacity and hypoxia are possible clues to early intrauterine injury. Pathogenic evidence; however, is still missing [14].

14.2 Placental changes in pre-terms

Pre-term birth is defined as delivery before gestational week 37, and in Europe this accounts for 6–8 % of all pregnancies. Approximately 1 % of pre-terms are born with a weight less than 1500 g, and of these ca. ⅓ with a weight between 500 and 999 g [15].

The most frequent placental changes are:
–   villous maturation disorders: 89 %,
–   implantation disorders: 70 %,
–   circulatory disorders: 67 %,
–   amniotic infections: 38 %,
–   placental growth restriction: 26 %.

The characteristic and pathogenic changes of pre-term placentas are villous prematurity and amniotic inflammation.

Pre-term accelerated villous maturation was seen in more than 60 % of pre-term placentas and may be subdivided into:
–   pre-term (accelerated) villous maturation: 51 %,
–   deficiency of intermediate villi 11 % (Fig. 14.2).

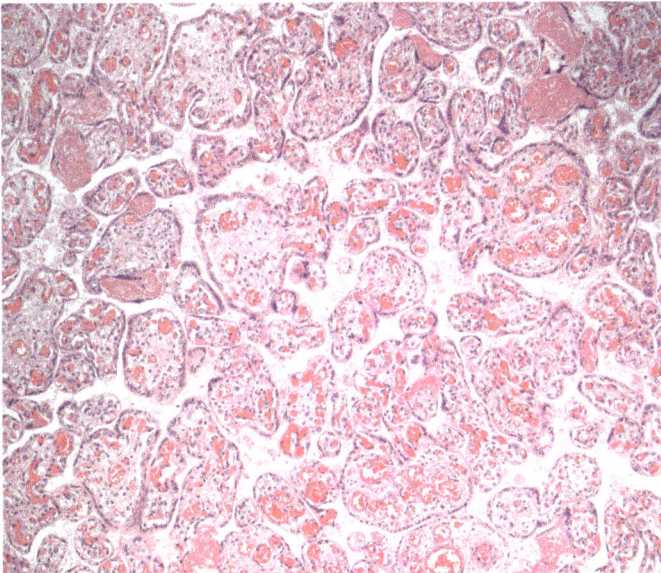

Fig. 14.5: Accelerated villous maturation. Placenta in Gestational Week 27.

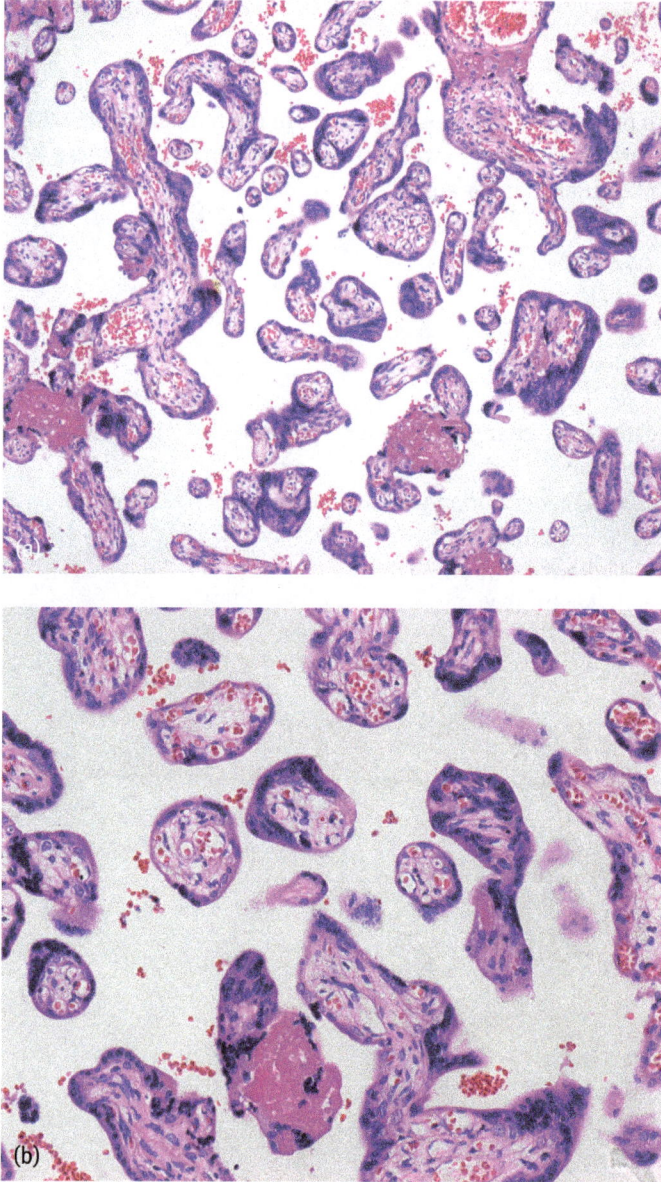

Fig. 14.6: (a) Deficiency of intermediate villi (MPF). Branching into intermediate villi of the central and peripheral type is not seen. Unexpected IUFD in Gestational Week 40 + 2. (b) Deficiency of intermediate villi (HPF). Reticular stroma with a varying degree of fibres and capillaries. Chorionic epithelium with dense nuclei and rare vasculosyncytial membranes.

Pathogenesis of pre-term (accelerated) villous maturation
- Primary placental growth restriction,
- secondary placental growth restriction due to chronic circulatory disturbance.

Primary growth restricted placentas are seen in more than 90 % of pre-term placentas and are associated with variable grades of accelerated villous maturation. This may be due to a decreased maternal heart volume and insufficient placental bed perfusion, which may be associated with maternal physical constitution during pregnancy, chronic maternal heart disease and occupational exposure of the pregnant woman [16,17]. Reduced perfusion of the implantation bed in the uterus and reduced perfusion of the intervillous space causes a reactive and compensatory accelerated villous maturation which restricts placental growth. Pre-term villous development may cause pre-term birth. In 20 % of these placentas a partial placental abruption was seen [18]; a placentogenous pre-term delivery.

Another pathogenic cause of primary placental growth restriction is placental bed injury due to: uterus malformation, leiomyoma, mucosal scars and placental location. This may cause a relatively reduced intervillous perfusion and lead to an accelerated villous maturation.

Accelerated villous maturation in *secondary growth restricted placentas* is seen in cases of normal growth for gestational age with secondary microfibrin deposition (gitterinfarcts and massive infarcts) due to uteroplacental malperfusion. Areas of villous sclerosis and loss of functionality stimulate a compensatory response, accelerated villous maturation with vasculosyncytial membrane formation, in other areas to ensure continued placental function and fetal survival. Why fetal growth restriction persists in pre-terms despite an adaptive placental enlargement to fetal remains unexplained. .

Ascending amniotic inflammation is a frequent finding in pre-term placentas. Approximately every 10th delivery shows a high grade inflammation as a possible cause of pre-term delivery. It is often associated with cervical insufficiency and pre-term rupture of the membranes.

Pathophysiology of pre-term delivery (Ch. 9)
The pathophysiology of pre-term delivery with labor pain and preterm cervical maturation is still not completely understood in detail. Oxytocin, estrogen, progesterone and prostaglandins are all suggested as possible/contributing causes. Hormonal and biochemical factors in the decidua and membranes are supposed to cause increased secretion of cytokines, which in turn stimulate prostaglandin production and secretion. Local cervical inflammation and premature rupture of the membranes seems to be a trigger for this production and secretion of cytokines. Correlation between villous maturation and prostaglandin activation is hypothesized but not proven.

14.3 Placental changes in post-terms

Post-term delivery is defined as delivery occurring 7–10 days after the calculated date of birth. No single or associated change was characteristic for post-term placentas after gestational week 42 [19]. Post-term placentas demonstrated:
- *Circulatory disorders*, small and focal, in 40.4 %. More often seen as gitterinfarcts, subchorionic pseudoinfarcts and intervillous thrombi.
- *Inter- and perivillous microfibrin depositions* (grade 2 and 3) in 28 %,
- *Villous maturation disorders* in 70 %; only 7.5 % showed a widespread retarded villous maturation which posed a serious threat, due to decreased diffusion capacity, to the fetus. Small or medium sized foci were seen in 90 % of cases,
- *Syncytial sprouts and nuclear knots* in 32 %, increased in mature placental areas,
- *Deposits of calcification* in 30.5 %, occurring in villi and extravillous islands. Without pathological significance,
- *Amniotic inflammation* in 15 %, with high grade inflammation in 5.3 %,
- *perivillitis/villitis* in 2.2 %.

According to Becker [11] villous immaturity (maturitas retardata) is one of the main placental findings in clinically diagnosed post-term pregnancies and is explained by a placental inability to adapt during delivery *("relative placental insufficiency")*. Hirschhold et al. [20] studied the placentas of 253 newborns, between gestational week 41 and 43, and found normal maturation according gestational age in ca. 54 % and retarded villous maturation, of varying degrees, combined with infarcts in 46 %. A worsening degree of maturation disorder correlated with higher resistance values on Doppler Flow measurements of the umbilical cord artery. Placentas with pathological flow resistance showed villous retardation/immaturity in 60 %, while placentas with normal blood flow only showed villous immaturity in 6 %. 50 % of placentas with a normal weight for gestational age with villous retardation and infarction (more than 20 % of the villous volume) were delivered by cesarean section to prevent fatal fetal asphyxia. 5 % of these placentas displayed normal villous maturity on histological examination.

14.4 Placental changes in Fetal Growth Restriction (FGR)

Fetal growth restriction is defined as fetal weight and/or fetal length less than the 10th percentile of reference measurements for "small for date infants". It may be classified as:
- harmonized or proportional type: weight and length below the 10th percentile,
- disharmonic type or disproportional type: weight below the 10th percentile but with a normal length.

Fetal growth restriction in term deliveries is 1.6x more often of the disharmonic type than the harmonic. FGR affects ca. 7 % of live births but risk factors are present in 20 %

Morphological placental changes in growth restricted pre-term and term deliveries are seen in more than 80 % of cases. The severity/extent of the changes varies and may be seen in combination with: placental growth restriction, focal or diffuse chronic circulatory disturbances, maturation disorders, villous stromal fibrosis, endangiopathia obliterans and perivillitis/villitis [21,22].

Placental growth disorders were seen as a decreased weight (69 %) and a decreased size of the basal plate (66 %). Rarely (2.7 %) the basal plate was enlarged. Placentas over the 90th percentile (macrosomic) are only very rarely seen with fetal growth restriction with:
– partial moles,
– diffuse trophoblast islands in the placenta without molar development,
– diffuse intervillous decidual islands,
– multiple chorangiomas, seen in chorangiomatosis.

Circulatory disorders due to *maternal vascular malperfusion* were seen in ca. 80 % of placentas from growth restricted newborns. These were chronic disorders in 50 %, combined with other changes in 25 % and acute in ca. 5 %. Morphological changes were, in the majority of cases, focal and small; only 25 % had involvement of more than 10 % of the total placental parenchyma:
– Gitterinfarct: 72 %
– subchorionic pseudoinfarct: 36 %
– massive infarct and cotyledon infarct: 27 %
– intervillous thrombi: 17 %

Inter- and perivillous fibrin deposition was seen in 45 %, 20 % of which was grade 3 microfibrin deposition. Villous maturation disorders were seen in 75 % and in 66 % several different maturation disorders occurred in combination. In detail:
– peripheral villous immaturity: 36 %
– retardation of villous maturation: 23 %
– arrest of villous maturation: 9.5 %
– chorangiosis type I: 8 %
– chorangiosis type II: 11 %
– pre-term accelerated villous maturation: 25 %
– villous stromal fibrosis: 21 % (large foci in 33 %)
– endangiopathia obliterans: 9.5 %
– perivillitis/villitis: 8 %

Pathogenesis
Fetal growth restriction is influenced by fetal, maternal and placental factors.

Fetal factors
- genetic: primary restricted fetal growth potential, chromosomal abnormalities, syndromes, multiple pregnancy,
- reduced utilization of nutrients due to fetal organ and cell damage,
- fetal vascular malperfusion.

Maternal factors
- reduced nutrient availability due to nutrient deficiency in the maternal blood,
- maternal vascular malperfusion.

Placental factors
- reduced villous surface area,
- decreased nutrition transport due to chorionic epithelial injury.
- hypoperfusion of the intervillous space,
- hypoperfusion of the umbilical cord and villous vessels,
- placental mosaic.

Placental changes in detail
- placental changes due to large tumors, partial moles and conjoined twins in multiple pregnancies,
- placental changes leading to fetal deficiency; fetal growth restriction correlated with chronic morphological placental insufficiency in 60 % of cases [23],
- multiple changes leading to a decrease in the total absolute villous surface area (to less than the 10th percentile for gestational age) [24]. There are three different causes of reduced villous surface area:
  - decreased placental growth without compensatory accelerated villous maturation,
  - chronic vascular malperfusion,
  - peripheral villous immaturity without compensatory placental growth.

Laurini et al. correlated histological placental changes to Doppler Flow results in 37 growth restricted fetuses. The placentas showed: infarcts, massive perivillous fibrin deposition, ischemic villitis, thrombi close to stem villous vessels and hemorrhagic endovasculopathy. Infarcts and reduced flow close to the umbilical cord arteries and descending fetal aorta correlated significantly with morphology [25].

14.5 Fetal anemia

Fetal anemia may occur during the intrauterine period or during delivery. It may be caused by fetal blood loss, hemolysis or absent erythrocyte neogenesis.

In cases of fetal blood loss placental examination is part of the initial investigation and, even in cases of hemolytic anemia, placental morphology may help to explain underlying causes.

Hemorrhage may be acute or chronic and with a small or severe volume loss. The fetus may present with a wide range of symptoms; from hypovolemic shock to chronic intrauterine anemia. An acute blood loss of 30–50 ml may lead to hypovolemic shock and if the hematocrit decreases below 25 %, the risk of perinatal mortality increases from 20 to 50 %.

Three sources of hemorrhage are observed:
- large fetal vessels,
- feto-maternal transfusion,
- feto-placental transfusion.

14.5.1 Hemorrhage from large vessels

Bleeding from large placental vessels (umbilical cord vessels and membranes) directly into the amniotic sac is usually acute and has a high mortality risk to the fetus. It is only rarely seen.

Other sources of hemorrhage:
- vasa previa in a velamentous umbilical cord insertion,
- vasa aberrantia in the placental margin or membranes,
- vessel bridges in an accessory placenta or placenta bi/multipartita.
- rupture of the umbilical cord vessels in cases of varicosis, thin cord complex, short umbilical cord, furcate umbilical cord insertion,
- varicosis of the chorionic plate.

Unexpected hemorrhage may be seen in combination with premature rupture of the membranes with variable CTG decelerations.

14.5.2 Feto-maternal transfusion

Feto-maternal transfusion means an acute or chronic transfusion of fetal blood cells from the fetal villous vessels and capillaries into the maternal intervillous space or the retroplacental space (Fig. 14.7).

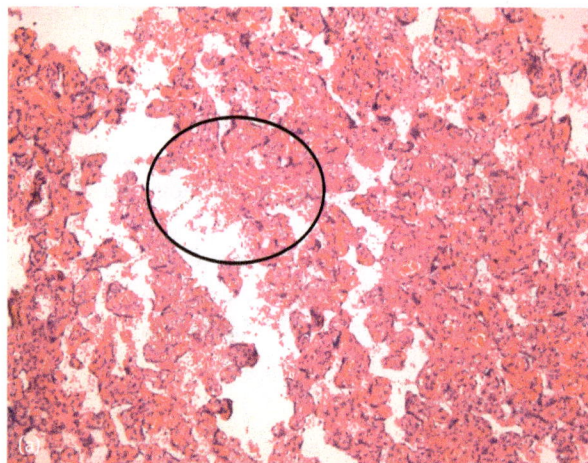

(b)

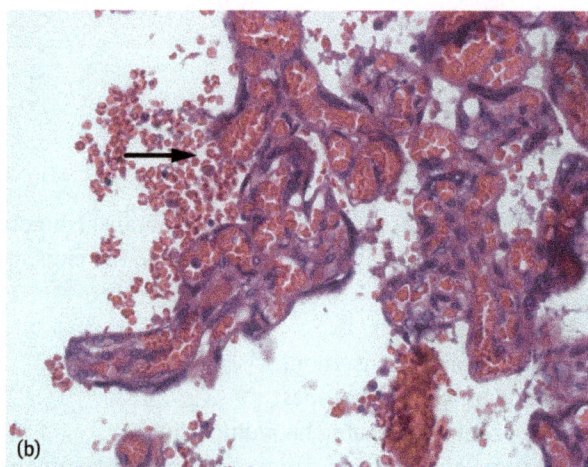

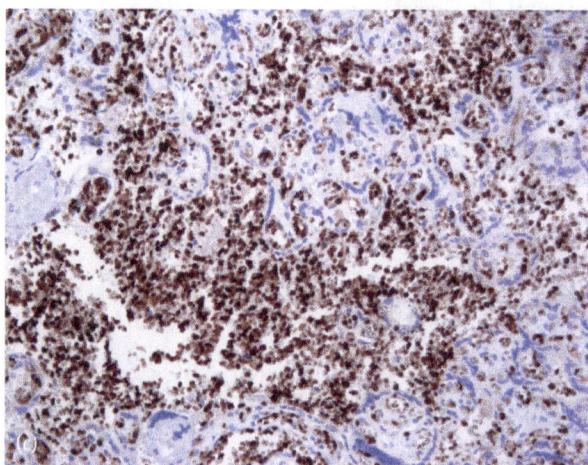

Fig. 14.7: (a) Feto-maternal microtransfusion. A focal lack of chorionic epithelium and a deficient fetal endothelium (circle) enables the entry of fetal blood into the maternal intervillous space. Placenta in Gestational Week 39 + 2, unexpected anemic fetus. (b) Feto-maternal microtransfusion (HPF) with fetal blood cells in the intervillous space (arrow). (c) Fetal erythrocytes. Positive immunoreaction on hemoglobin F (HbF).

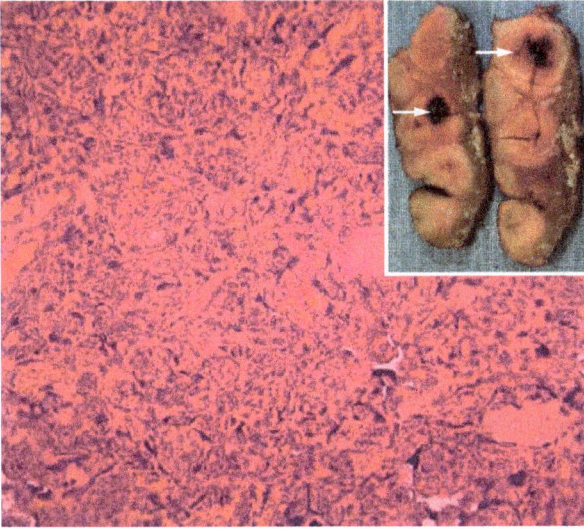

Fig. 14.8: Acute hemorrhagic infarction: Massive villous congestion with acute bleeding. Inlet: Cotyledon infarct.

Extremely small numbers of fetal blood cells enter the maternal circulatory system:
– in the last trimester,
– during delivery,
– following abortion,
– after diagnostic amniocentesis and chorionic biopsies in early pregnancy,
– after oxytocin therapy for labor induction.

Morphologically, an erosion of the chorionic epithelium with an overlying thin fibrin coat is seen. This may facilitate microtransfusion into the intervillous space.

Feto-maternal macrotransfusion (> 25 ml fetal blood) into the intervillous space or the retroplacental space with resultant fetal circulatory blood loss may be caused by:
– placenta previa/deep placental implantation,
– pre-term placental rupture of a normally implanted placenta,
– cesarean section with an anteriorly implanted placenta,
– chorangioma.

However, a detailed morphological placental examination may not always identify a source of hemorrhage. Associated changes which may be seen are:
– acute intervillous bleeding, congestion and thrombi.
– acute hemorrhagic infarction.

Definitive evidence of a feto-maternal blood transfusion is the identification of fetal erythrocytes, or fetal hemoglobin, in the maternal circulation or in the retroplacental hematoma [26].

Aside from acute feto-maternal macrotransfusion, a few cases of chronic feto-maternal transfusion with fetal anemia and without a known source of bleeding are reported [27,28].

A feto-maternal macrotransfusion progresses, usually, without complication until an acute and fatal fetal decompensation. A diagnostic umbilical cord puncture enables diagnosis prior to a therapeutic intrauterine transfusion [29].

14.5.3 Feto-placental transfusion

An acute and life threatening fetal anemia can be caused by blood congestion in the peripheral fetal microcirculation and is clinically interpreted as a placental shock.

Possible causes are: maternal bleeding with reactive hemorrhagic blood congestion in the placenta fetalis, PROM, marginal sinus bleeding in normally implanted placenta, placenta previa and vena cava compression syndrome. A fetal cause may be cardiac insufficiency but further studies are required to confirm this.

Other types of anemia
–   fetal hemolytic anemia
–   feto-fetal transfusion

14.6 Hydrops fetalis et placentae (Hydrops fetalis)

Definition and pathogenesis (Ch. 11)
Increased extravascular fluid, due to an imbalance of intra- and extravascular (interstitial) exchange, it is seen in:
–   hydrostatic pressure change (valvular heart defect),
–   oncotic pressure change (congenital nephrotic syndrome),
–   capillary permeability change (hypoxia, anemia, infection),
–   lymphatic flow change (jugular lymphatic obstruction sequence).

Causes
–   immunohemolytic hydrops: Rh-incompatibility, ABO-incompatibility and incompatibility with irregular antibodies,
–   non immunohemolytic hydrops (NIHF): includes diseases of different causes and pathogeneses (Table 14.3)

In 10 % of hydrops fetalis no etiology can be identified, even following a thorough examination of both the fetus and the placenta:
–   idiopathic hydrops fetalis (et placentae).

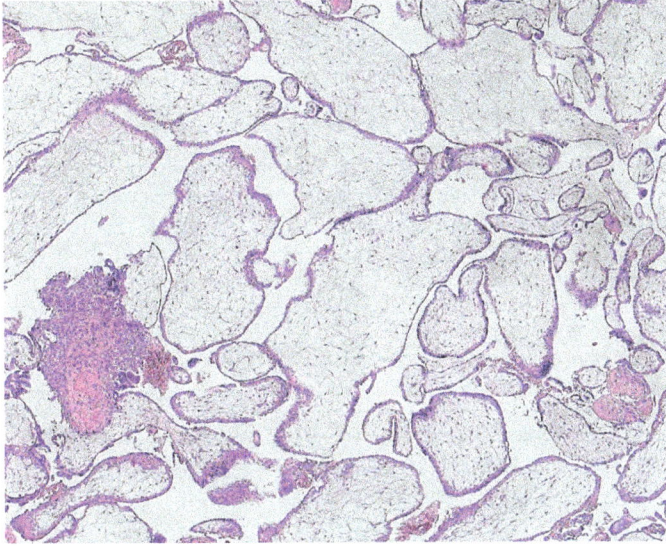

Fig. 14.9: Placental villi with hydropic stroma, scant capillaries and a flat chorionic epithelial layer.

Hydrops placenta (Examples)

Macroscopy: the placenta is enlarged (macrosomic) for gestational age, often weighing more than 1,000 g and on cut section shows a pale and edematous surface with bullous and distended villi morphologically. (Ch. 11 late abortion)

Morphology:
- arrest of villous maturation,
- stem villous vessel hypoplasia,
- less capillaries,
- flat villous syncytiotrophoblast.
- adaptive changes:
- chorangiosis (capillary hyperplasia) in single villi or villous groups,
- intravascular erythroblastosis; a hallmark of a compensatory increased erythropoiesis, also seen in chronic anemia or viral infection.

Table 14.3: Causes of hydrops universalis.

chronic anemia	– immune hemolytic anemia (RH-incompatibility) Hemoglobinopathy (Homozygous α thalassemia) – chronic TTTS – chronic feto-maternal transfusion syndrome – disseminated intravascular coagulation (DIC) microangiopathic hemolytic anemia – glucose-6-P-dehydrogenase deficiency
placental changes	– chorangioma – chorangiosis type 1 – chorionic venous thrombosis – umbilical cord vein thrombosis
fetal hypoproteinemia	– congenital nephrotic syndrome (finnish type) bilateral hydronephrosis – kidney vein thrombosis – congenital hepatitis / cirrhosis – hemangioma in the liver
cardiovascular fetal diseases	– fetal heart malformation – intrauterine obliteration of the foramen ovale arteriovenous anastomosis – fetal tachyarrhythmia – fetal heart insufficiency – cardiac tumor complete AV-block
fetal cardiac-pulmonary malformation	– cardiomegaly / lung hypoplasia with bilateral hydrothorax – adenomatoid cystic lung malformation – bilateral pulmonary lymphangiectasia
chronic intrauterine infection	– cytomegaly – parvovirus B19 – toxoplasmosis – congenital Syphilis (Lues connata) – leptospirosis – chagas disease
maternal and fetal diseases	– poorly controlled diabetes mellitus – chronic maternal kidney disease – preeclampsia – chromosome anomaly (trisomy 13, 18, 21; X = -monosomy, triploidy) – fetal neuroblastoma – fetal nephroblastoma – congenital myeloid leukemia – sacral teratoma – epignathus – skeletal dysplasia (achondrogenesis) – metabolic diseases (Morbus Gaucher)

14.6.1 Idiopathic non-immunological hydrops

Approximately 15 % of children with non-hemolytic hydrops (NIHF) are of the idio-pathic type, in which neither cause nor characteristics of the diseases are known [30].

In a study of 300 fetuses with NIHF, 12 % were designated idiopathic. An immu-nological basis for idiopathic hydrops was considered if mothers showed reduced im-munization against paternal HLA-antigens in increased parental histiocompatibility of several HLA-characteristics [31].

14.7 Congenital nephrotic syndrome (Finnish type)

The majority of congenital nephrotic syndrome cases arise in Finland with ca. 130 affected families. Additionally 24 cases, with 40 affected children, are reported from USA and single case reports have been published from Central America [32].

Morphology
–   enlarged and pale placenta, up to 2000 g net weight,
–   large villous groups with maturation arrest and focal stromal edema [33,34].

Pathogenesis
Genetic factors determine metabolic glycoprotein disorders with subsequent develop-mental defects of the basal membrane in the kidneys and, probably, in the placenta. Placental enlargement is not only due villous hydrops, but also a consequence of vil-lous immaturity and increased villous growth.

Clinical information
Maternal hypertensive disease during pregnancy is increased with fetal congenital nephrotic syndrome.

Alpha-fetoprotein is increased in amniotic fluid and in maternal serum.

Children are usually pre-term and low in weight (extreme increase in the fe-tal-placental quotient).

14.8 Morbus hemolyticus neonatorum (hemolytic disease of the newborn)

Definition
Morbus hemolyticus neonatorum is an immune mediated hemolytic fetal and newborn anemia and is caused by maternal erythrocyte antibodies that cross the placenta. In most cases a rhesus incompatibility is diagnosed.

Incompatibility is not only associated with the development of maternal antibodies. The fetus can be rhesus negative from a heterozygote rhesus positive father. A rhesus negative mother will not develop antibodies in the 1st pregnancy, if not immunized before; she can be sensitized by earlier intra- and extrauterine pregnancies or by blood transfusion. In the two first months of pregnancy IgM antibodies which are unable to cross the placental barrier can be detected in maternal blood (iso-agglutinins). A new antigen exposure stimulates maternal IgG-iso-antibody development in the 2nd pregnancy. These iso-antibodies pass the placental barrier and cause intrauterine hemolysis, anemia, hydrops universalis (fetus and placenta) and extrauterine icterus graviditatis.

Anti-D immunoglobulin prophylaxis reduces prenatal lethality by factor of 10, from 0.5–1:1,000 live births to 0.05–0.1:1,000 live births.

Macroscopy
– placentomegaly, more than 1,000 g, with a pale cut surface and edema,
– high grade intrauterine embryonic damage and development of hydrops universalis fetus et placentae (diagnosis and follow up by ultrasound),
– non hydropic placenta is neither heavy nor edematous,
– intervillous thrombi.

Morphology
Histologically the condition is characterized by villous maturation disorders and increased fetal erythroblastosis in the villous capillary lumen (Fig. 14.10), additionally edema in the large villi may be seen.

Histology of villous maturation disorders:
– retardation of villous maturation in 53 %,
– arrest of villous maturation with stromal edema in 33 %,
– chorangiosis type I in 31 %.

Villous maturation disorders were seen in both middle and high grade diseases [35] and arrest of villous maturation was often seen in fetal deaths.

In low grade disease, or rhesus incompatibility without illness, retardation of villous maturation or chorangiosis type I is seen in small foci in 20 % of placentas.

ABO-incompatibility, with or without antibody detection, is not associated with placental changes. Fetal disease is often first diagnosed after delivery.

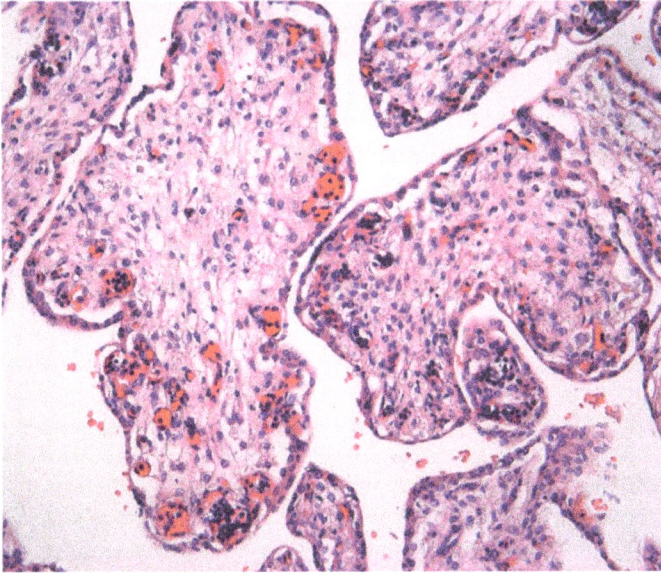

Fig. 14.10: Rhesus erythroblastosis. Placental villi with fetal vessels filled with immature erythrocytes in Gestational Week 27.

Pathogenesis of placental changes

The most serious type of morbus hemolyticus neonatorum is diagnosed in hydrops universalis fetus et placentae; assumed to be caused by early transplacental antibody transfusion in the 1st trimester with subsequent manifestation of embryonic villous maturation disorders [21,36]. This early onset of villous maturation disorders is compensated by villous growth and placental enlargement. As pregnancy progresses the tendency for hydrops increases.

Placental changes seem to not depend solely on early antibody transfusion, time is also important for the development of tissue injury. Even in severe cases, placental changes only manifest in the middle to late fetal developmental period.

No placental change is detectable before gestational week 25, even if the clinical diagnosis of morbus hemolyticus neonatorum has already been made by serum examination and amniotic fluid spectrometry. In cases of late antibody transfusion to the fetus, the mature placenta shows only low grade villous maturation disorders or no maturation deficiency at all. The quantity of transfused antibodies may play a role in the severity of the disease.

14.9 Alpha-thalassemia

Alpha-thalassemia is an autosomal inherited hemoglobinopathy caused by lack, or impaired production, of the α-globin chains of hemoglobin. It is often due to alpha-gene deletion. In homozygote α-thalassemia, the α-globin chains which are normally identifiable in 1st trimester are missing. Due to this, a high grade intrauterine anemia and hydrops fetalis, with intrauterine fetal death or death in the newborn period, may occur. This type of anemia corresponds to geographical malaria exposure and has been suggested as a protective measure against severe malarial infections [37].

Morphology of the placenta
Placentomegaly
- Villous maturation arrest associated with chorangiosis type I,
- High grade erythroblastosis,
- Villous stromal edema of different grades, up to and including hydrops placentae,
- Diagnosis with antenatal DNA analysis by amniocentesis or chorionic biopsy [38].

14.10 Fetal storage disorders

Storage phenomena in the placenta are rare and described only in case reports as:
- fetal manifestations of lysosomal storage disease
- fetal storage disorder due to maternal hydroxyethyl infusion

The storage cells of the placenta are the trophoblast cells, stromal cells and endothelial cells of the villi. These cells may be seen on light microscopy and confirmed by immunohistochemistry and electron microscopy. Prenatal diagnosis of enzyme defects are made from amniotic or placental cell cultures taken after amniocentesis or chorionic biopsy [39].

Placental involvement is reported in following storage diseases:
- Generalized type of GM1-gangliosidosis; an autosomal recessive storage disorder due to a deficiency of β-Galactosidasis.
- GM2-gangliosidosis type I (Tay-Sachs) and type II (Sandhoff).
- Congenital sialidosis, characterized by lack of neuraminidase activity.
- Fetal galactosialidosis; an autosomal recessive lysosomal storage disorder with inactivity of α-neuraminidase and β-galactosidasis.
- Mucolipidosis type II (I-cell disease) and type IV; autosomal recessive storage diseases causing an intracellular increase in mucopolysaccharide breakdown products and glycolipids.

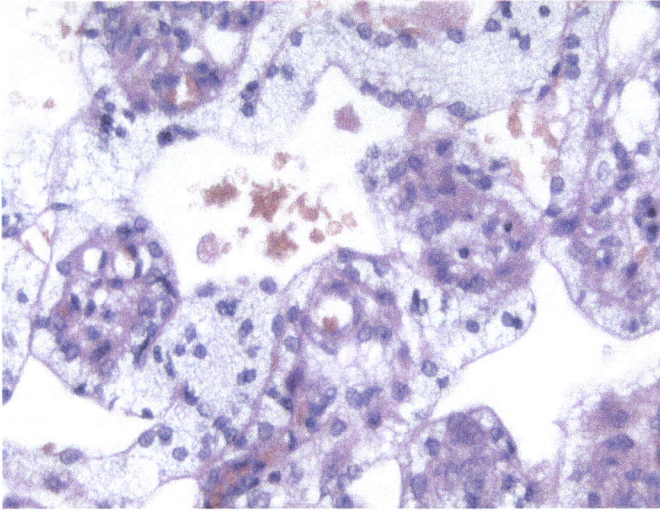

Fig. 14.11: Storage vacuoles in the syncytiotrophoblast after Hydroxyethyl infusion (by courtesy of Dr. N. Sarioglu, Department of Pediatric Pathology and Placentology, Charité, Berlin, Germany).

– Mucopolysaccharidosis type I (Hurler), type IV (Morquio) and type VI (Maroteaux-Lamy); caused by disturbances of glycosaminoglycan breakdown.
– Fetal morbus Gaucher; autosomal recessive storage disease with defective glucocerebrosidase activity and an accumulation of glucocerebrosides in the monocytic-phagocytic-system (MPS) and stromal cells of the chorionic villi.
– Sphingomyelinosis (Niemann-Pick) with sphingomyelin accumulation in the cyto- and syncytiotrophoblast, endothelial cells, stromal cells and Hofbauer cells.
– Glycogenosis type II (Pompe) with massive glycogen deposition in the cytotrophoblast and stromal cells of the chorionic villi [40].

The different storage cells may be visualized after infusion of hydroxyethyl glycogen.

Maternal hydroxyethyl is infused to optimize uteroplacental circulation in fetal growth restriction (hemodilution). Storage of macromolecular substances in the trophoblast, stromal and endothelial cells of the chorionic villi depends on duration of infusion and the quantity. Storage cells in the chorionic villi could be identified multiple weeks post infusion [41]. Placental dysfunction due to lysosomal storage disease or hydroxyethyl infusion is not reported.

14.11 Diabetes mellitus

The prevalence of diabetes mellitus is increasing worldwide and figures from the WHO estimate an increase in those with the condition from 347 million in 2013 to 439 million in 2030. Type 1 (TDM1) accounts for ca. 10 % and type 2, and subgroups, (TDM2) for ca. 80–90 % of these figures. Furthermore, the WHO states ca. 1–11 % of all pregnancies to be complicated by gestational diabetes (GDM) [42].

Therapeutic insulin has decreased infertility in diabetic mothers to 2 % and deliveries by diabetic women are reported to be between 0.1 to 0.5 % of all deliveries; however, glucose intolerance in pregnancy is reported in 2 % of all deliveries each year [43].

The fetal risk of malformations (embryopathia diabetica), perinatal mortality and morbidity, as well as perinatal risk to the newborn depends on metabolic control and normoglycemia during pregnancy [44]. Another diabetic disease of the newborn and frequently seen in inadequate metabolic control is fetal hyperinsulinemia. It is assumed to be the cause of fetopathia diabetica: fetal Cushing's disease, macrosomia, organomegaly (specifically splanchnomegaly) with hypoglycemia and insufficient metabolic adaption due to structural and functional organic immaturity.

Historically, perinatal mortality has decreased from 10 % (1969–1973) to 1.9 % (1979–1983) and fetopathia diabetica has decreased from 18 % to 9.8 % [45].

14.11.1 Definition and classification of Diabetes Mellitus in pregnancy (GDM)

There are different diabetes classifications regarding fetal prognosis and quality assessment. Gestational diabetes mellitus and pre-gestational diabetes can be differentiated:
- in *gestational diabetes mellitus* the metabolic imbalance has its onset in pregnancy and ends with pregnancy
- in *pre-gestational diabetes the* metabolic imbalance exists prior to conception and remains after pregnancy; with or without complications such as retinopathy, nephropathy and macroangiopathy.

Metabolic control is subcategorized as:
- well controlled,
- uncontrolled [44].

Clinically, the White classification defines the grade and duration of GDM (Table 14.4).

Table 14.4: Classification of diabetes mellitus in pregnancy, according to White [46].

A	– abnormal glucose tolerance test. – no symptoms – diet regulated normoglycemia – no exogenous insulin use
	insulin regulated diabetes
B	onset at 20 years of age or duration less 10 years
C	onset between 10 and 19 years of age or duration between 10 and 19 years
D	onset before the age of 10 or duration of more than 20 years or benign retinopathy
E	calcification of pelvic arteries
F	glomerulosclerosis
R	proliferative retinopathy
RF	glomerulosclerosis and proliferative retinopathy
G	history of recurrent abortion, IUFD
H	coronary arteriosclerosis
T	post kidney transplantation

Placental morphology

Placental morphology may be suggestive for diabetes; however, due to optimized diabetes control over the last five decades, a diagnosis should be made with caution. Placental macroscopy and microscopy shows variable findings in diabetes and the findings depends on the duration and metabolic control of the disease [21,47,48]. Clinical and morphological correlation is important for evaluation of the stages in manifest diabetes mellitus, latent glycogenic intolerance disorders and gestational diabetes [49].

14.11.2 Placental changes in manifest diabetes mellitus

Typical macroscopic and morphological findings are:
- enlarged placenta,
- arrest of villous maturation,
- peripheral villous immaturity

A combination of these findings was called "Placopathia diabetica" [50], and was diagnosed in 50 % of pregnancies with manifest diabetes in the last century [51]. These findings are now rare due to advances in the management of diabetes in pregnancy [45].

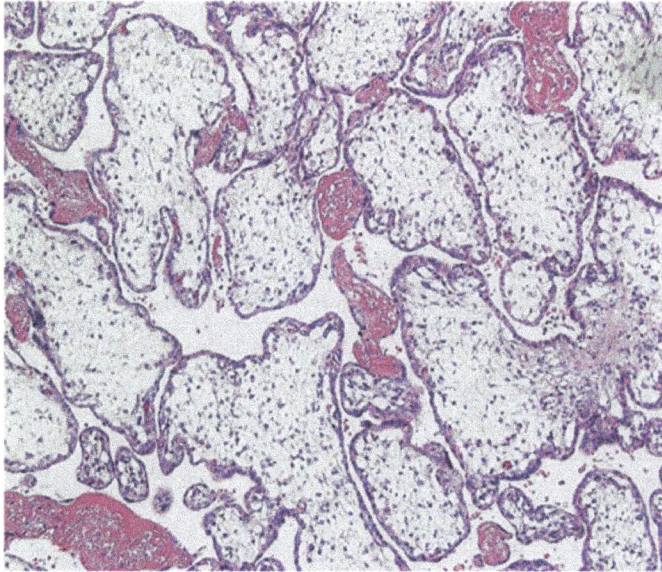

Fig. 14.12: Arrest of villous maturation: Group of enlarged villi with embryonic stroma, irregular and flat villous trophoblast layer and scant capillaries. GDM.

An *enlarged macrosomic placenta is* defined as a placental weight and basal plate above the 90th percentile for a given gestational age, and it represents White stages without vessel complications; A, B and C.

Arrest of villous maturation is seen focally as impaired branching, enlargement of the central type of intermediate villi, a persisting embryonic stroma and an incomplete transformation of the stem villi. The stem villous vessels have a narrow caliber and an incompletely developed paravascular contractile sheath [52]. Grouping of enlarged villi is characteristic.

Peripheral villous immaturity (Ch. 8) is classified as a low grade maturation disorder and characterized by normal branching and a focally coarsely meshed 'edematous' reticular or mesenchymal stroma with only few capillaries. The villous trophoblast is single-layered focally, without nuclei and with only a very few vasculosyncytial membranes. The term "villous edema", which is used in the literature for this disorder of maturation, is, in our opinion, inadequate and confusing. We agree with Kaufmann [53] that these changes represent a "persisting villous immaturity" in only small foci of the placenta.

Placentas with arrest of villous maturation and peripheral villous immaturity were frequently seen in combination with uncontrolled metabolic disorders and were completely absent in pregnancies with normoglycemia and controlled diabetes, with serial glycosylated hemoglobin values (HbA1) less than 7 %. [54]. Villous maturation arrest and the persistence of embryonic villous structures, previously seen in 50 %

of placentas from diabetic women, has decreased to less than 39 % [55]. Maturation disorders in particular have decreased, from 35 % to less than 10 %. Diabetic control seems to normalize placental maturation in placentas from diabetic mothers to that of placentas without glycogenic disorders [56].

Adaptive changes

Histology in placentas from clinically manifest diabetes may be affected by associated diseases and complications, such as:
- pregnancy induced hypertension and preexisting chronic maternal hypertension with kidney disease.
- diabetic angiopathy.

In these cases the histology is characterized by normal maturation or accelerated villous maturation. Diabetogenic maturation disorders are only seen focally or not at all. Increased villous capillarization (chorangiosis type II) and the following changes are seen:
- multiple nuclear sprouts and regressive nuclear knots on the villous surface,
- inter- and perivillous microfibrin deposition and microinfarcts,
- focal villous stromal fibrosis and endangiopathia obliterans, more frequently seen in White stages D, R and H.

In placentas of pre-term deliveries, villous maturation may show pre-term changes or may even be appropriate for gestational age.

Thrombi in the chorionic plate vessels or stem villous arteries, as well as acute funiculitis, were infrequently found [57].

14.11.3 Placental changes with latent Diabetes mellitus

In general, the changes in latent diabetes mellitus are the same as in insulin controlled diabetes mellitus. Peripheral villous immaturity may show persistent embryonic villous structures, not only in the central area but also in the periphery of the feto-maternal unit, surrounded by normal mature villi.

Focal circumscribed villous maturation arrest in one high power field was seen in 37 % of women with latent diabetes mellitus and in 10 % it was found with a maturation disorder with disseminated and persistent embryonic stromal structures. Normal mature villi according to gestational age were seen in 50 %.

Villous maturation disorders were seen in ca. 50 % of placentas from GDM women and in more than 33 % of placentas from women with borderline glucose tolerance (IGT); therefore, women with IGT should be as closely followed up as women with GDM [58,59]. Arrest of villous maturation and small foci of persistent embryonic villous structures are not sufficiently specific for the diagnosis of disorders due to glucose metabolism but they do warrant further investigations to exclude the presence of such disorders.

Pathogenesis of placental changes

Correlation between the grade of maturation disorder and the duration and metabolic control of the disease is shown by several histological and morphological studies. The placental parenchyma and villous surface in insulin controlled diabetic placentas is 20 % and 50 % larger, respectively, when compared to non-diabetic placentas [60]. The grade of villous immaturity increases with increasing White stages A–C [61–63]. Supplementary oxygen therapy seems to not only reduce the grade of villous maturation retardation but also demonstrates a normalization of maturation following therapy [64].

In White stages D, R and H the absolute villous surface area is significantly smaller, and in cases of retinopathy the microfibrin density ratio is significantly increased compared to other diabetic placentas; possibly due to pre-pregnancy vascular disorders, diabetic arteriopathy or hypertension [54]. Histologically these placentas often show accelerated villous maturation and chorangiosis-like vessel hyperplasia with adequate metabolic membrane development; interpreted as a compensatory villous reaction due to chronic intervillous malperfusion. This interpretation is supported by the combination of mature villi and villi with increased numbers of capillaries seen in these placentas, often with regressive chorionic epithelium changes, microfibrin depositions in the intervillous space and small foci of villous stromal fibrosis.

In diabetic maturation disorders the villi are typically enlarged, elongated and have less branches than expected for normal longitudinal and total growth. Additionally, characteristic findings of inhibited mesenchymal maturation are seen: persistence of embryonic stromal structures, vessel wall hypoplasia in the stem villi and capillary deficiency in the villous periphery. Differentiation disorders of the chorionic epithelium show a single-layered syncytiotrophoblast with a variable nuclear density and an incomplete cytotrophoblast. The lack of villous maturity in diabetic placentas facilitates increased villous growth and the exhaustion of chorionic epithelium's ability for cell regeneration. As a consequence, the villous surface increases at the expense of villous diameter, tissue maturation, vessel development and chorionic epithelial differentiation.

Increased growth and fetal macrosomia, associated with retarded maturation, is assumed to be a response to maternal hyperglycemia and fetal hyperinsulinemia. Of note, insulin receptors are only found on the maternal side of the syncytiotrophoblast, not on the fetal side [65].

Consequences for the fetus

The structural changes in the placental parenchyma due to large foci of villous maturation arrest may limit placental perfusion capacity. Large foci of villous maturation
arrest are often associated with:

- fetal macrosomia: 48%,
- intrauterine/subtotal hypoxia: 38%,
- IUFD: 9%,
- neonatal mortality: 5%.
- embryopathia diabetica
- fetopathia diabetica

14.12 Hypertensive diseases in pregnancy

Classification

Preeclampsia is a specific symptom complex in the 2nd trimester, and it encompasses
arterial hypertension, proteinuria and edema. Additionally, there may be associated CNS symptoms: headache, visual disorders, hyperreflexia, spasms and coma. The
symptoms usually cease after delivery. Preeclampsia may be classified using the following, commonly used systems: International society for the study of hypertension
in pregnancy (Table 14.5) and the Organization of Gestosis (Table 14.6). Grading system is additionally listed in Table 14.7.

Table 14.5: Hypertensive diseases in pregnancy, International society for the study of hypertension
in pregnancy.

gestational hypertension	diastolic blood pressure beyond 90 mmHg
gestational proteinuria	proteinuria more than 0.5 g/l in 24-h-urine
eclampsia	chronic hypertonia (high blood pressure before gesta-tional week 20 without proteinuria)
chronic kidney disease	diagnosed kidney disease before pregnancy, disease continues 40 days after delivery
chronic hypertension with "pfropf"-eclampsia (late onset)	increased arterial pressure before gestational week 20 and proteinuria

Table 14.6: Gestosis classification.

	symptoms	pathogenesis	onset of 1st EPH-gestosis
1.	monosymptomatic EPH gestosis: edema (E) or proteinuria (P) hypertonia (H)	"pfropf"-gestosis vascular disease before pregnancy renal disease before pregnancy	antepartum (related to gestational week)
2.	polysymptomatic EPH-gestosis combination of 2 or 3 symptoms	gestosis transitoric gestosis essential gestosis	intrapartum
3.	life threatening eclampsia subjective illness, progressive coma	unclassified gestosis	postpartum
4.	eclampsia EPH-gestosis with convulsion		

Table 14.7: Hypertensive diseases in pregnancy.

low grade hypertensive disease	– diastolic blood pressure 90–110 mmHg – systolic blood pressure 140–160 mmHg – proteinuria 0.5-5g/l in 24-h-urine
high grade hypertensive disease	– diastolic blood pressure above 110 mmHg – systolic blood pressure above 160 mmHg – proteinuria above 5 g/l in 24-h-urine – oliguria (under 400 ml/24 h)

The frequency of hypertensive diseases in pregnancy varies in the reported literature. According to Dudenhausen, pathologically increased blood pressure above 135/85 mmHg is expected in 4–5% of all pregnancies and proteinuria with protein elimination in 24 h urine above 0.5 g/l is expected in 2% of all pregnancies. Eclampsia frequency is reported as 0.1% of all deliveries and the proportion of these with "pfropfgestosis" at 30–40%; however, it even higher in those pregnant over the age of 30 in multiple pregnancy [66].

Morphology
Pathology in basal and spiral arteries of the placental bed with vessel wall changes is characteristic, but not specific, for hypertension [67]:
– acute atherosclerosis,
– hyperplastic arterio/arteriolopathy.

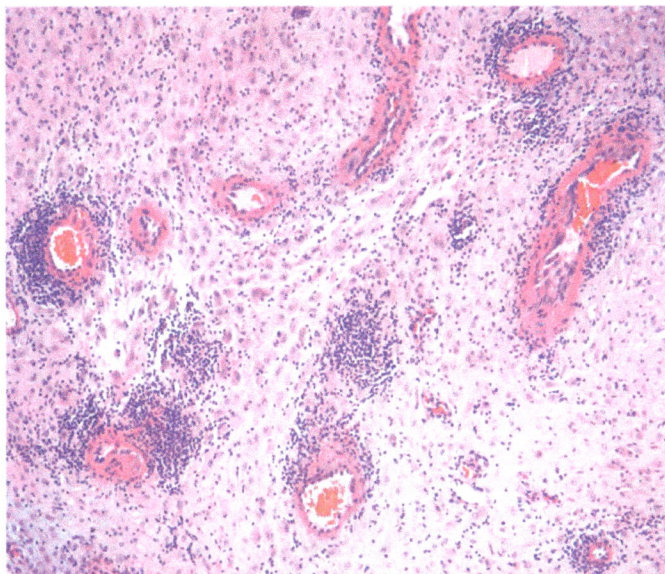

Fig. 14.13: Implantation bed, periarteriolar inflammatory, dominating lymphocytic infiltration. Tight vascular lumen. Acute atherosis in preeclampsia with vessel wall inflammation (s. Fig. 14.14).

Acute arteriosclerosis is characterized by the accumulation of foamy lipophages in the vessel wall (Fig. 14.14b), transmural fibrinoid necrosis of varying intensity and extent and intravascular thrombi. Vessel lumina show extensive constriction or total occlusion. A lympho-monocytic cellular infiltrate in the affected vessel is frequently seen.

Affected are:
– spiral arteries at the endomyometrial transition of the pre-placental bed,
– basal arterioles below the placental bed,
– the intradecidual course of the spiral arteries along the placental margin and outside the placental bed.

Hyperplastic arterio/arteriolopathy: a partly concentric and partly eccentric constriction of the vessel lumen by intimal hyperplasia with a well preserved tunica media.

Hyperplastic vasculopathy is more frequently seen in chronic hypertension and maternal preeclampsia, whereas acute arteriosclerosis is more often seen in pregnancy related hypertension and preeclampsia.

Placental pathology: There is no specific placental change in preeclampsia. Any other cause of stenosis in the arteries or arterioles of the pre-placental vascular bed may cause similar changes in the placenta.

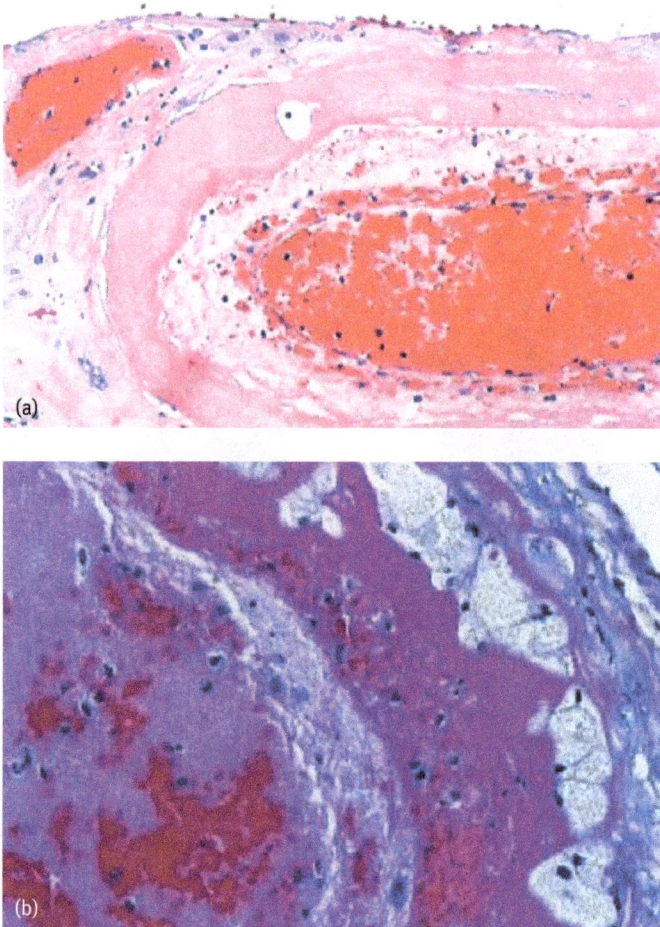

Fig. 14.14: (a) Extended fibrinoid transformation of the vessel wall. (b) Acute atherosis with fibrinoid necrosis and foamy macrophages (HPF). Partial thrombosis.

Circulatory disturbances

Focal or generalized circulatory disturbances are seen in 66 % of placentas. Of 485 placentas from hypertensive and normotensive pregnancies with late onset gestosis, ca. 80 % of placentas from hypertensive pregnancies showed circulatory disorders and ca. 33 % proteinuria [7]. Morphological changes caused by circulatory disorders were of low grade, in 70 % of placentas with gestosis and involved less than 5 % of the total placental tissue volume. Circulatory disturbance was seen in 5–20 % of placentas and 5 % showed infarction of more than 20 % of the placenta (infarcted placenta).

Chronic circulatory disturbance was predominantly seen as gitterinfarcts, intervillous thrombi, cotyledon infarcts and massive infarcts. It was seen with associated acute changes in 33 % of the placentas.

Acute circulatory disturbance was seen as intervillous thrombi, cotyledon infarcts- and massive infarcts. Signs of premature placental abruption were found in 11 % of preeclampsia placentas.

Approximately 50 % of the placentas showed macroscopic signs of circulatory disorders, the remaining placentas had histologically diffuse circulatory disorders, such as:

- inter- and perivillous microfibrin depositions,
- fibrinoid villous degeneration,
- syncytial sprouts,
- perivillitis.

Inter- and perivillous microfibrin depositions are more than twice as frequently seen in placentas with gestational hypertension and preeclampsia when compared to placentas from normotensive gestational proteinuria (60:27.5 %). The microfibrin density ratio was 3.6 in hypertension, which was 3-times increased compared to the normotensive group [24]. The highest values for microfibrin density were found in preeclampsia with a ratio of 6.2 and a microfibrin surface area of 2.8 m^2, compared to 0.6 m^2 in the control group.

Appositional growth of inter- and perivillous microfibrin causes fibrin bridging of neighbouring terminal villi and alters flow pathways in the intervillous space. The entrapped villi undergo regressive changes, up to and including total necrosis, and this pathological process is analogous to that of microinfarct formation.

Fibrinoid villous degeneration primarily affects the villous subepithelial stroma (Fig. 14.15) and leads to a partial or complete loss of the blood barrier function. Increased transfusion of maternal macromolecules into the villous stroma may cause fibrinoid villous necrosis. The villous architecture remains preserved and the homogenous amorphic stroma is covered by extremely immature chorionic epithelium.

Higher grades of primary perivillous fibrin deposition cannot be differentiated from primary fibrinoid villous degeneration. Both are seen as components of microinfarcts.

Increased syncytial knots and regressive syncytial sprouts were seen in every case of gestational hypertension. These solid nuclear aggregations were seen on the villous surface and affected more than 50 % of villi in each MPF (Fig. 14.16), with morphometrically measured 25 % nuclear sprouts and knot participation on the surface [68].

Due to chorionic epithelium degeneration and necrosis *perivillitis* can be found with loss of the epithelium in small villous conglomerates. Fibrin and the villous stroma are infiltrated, to a varying degree, by maternal granulocytes and monocytes. Stromal connective tissue cells proliferate and there are increased collagenous fibres. Perivillitis is probably a localized expression of the focal destruction of the immune barrier between the mother and the child.

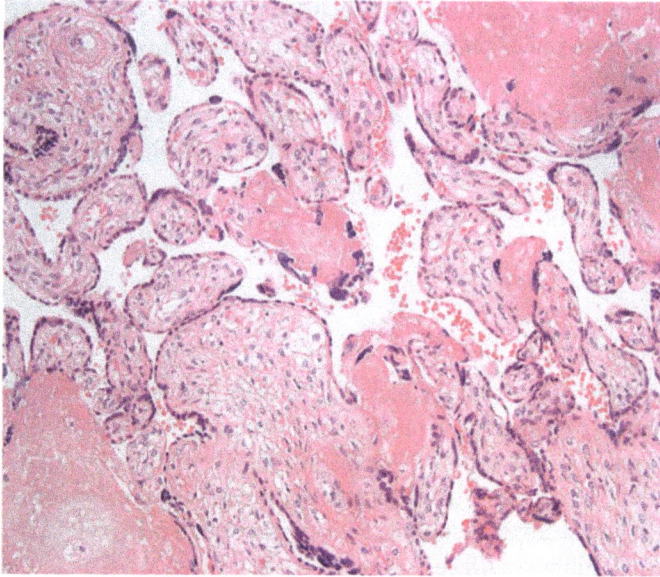

Fig. 14.15: Perivillous microfibrin deposition with fibrinous obstruction of the intervillous space and necrosis of the villi. Preeclampsia with placenta in Gestational Week 38.

Placental growth restriction

Placental growth restriction was seen in 33 % of the placentas from hypertensive women and in 20 % of placentas with monosymptomatic proteinuria of pregnancy. Placentas from perinatal deaths, after a late onset of maternal gestosis, showed absolute and/or relative growth restriction in 66 % of cases [69].

Villous maturation disorders

50 % of placentas with clinical gestosis showed villous maturation according to gestational age; as well as partially accelerated villous maturation. These findings were seen in both hypertensive and non-hypertensive women. A phase contrast microscopic examination study found an increased number of mature for gestational age placentas in preeclampsia [70].

Peripheral villous immaturity was seen in 20 % of the placentas and was independent of hypertension. It was frequently associated with villous stromal fibrosis. A further ca. 4 % of the placentas showed *embryonic villi* or patchy arrest of villous maturation; consistent with findings seen in hyperglycemia. Maternal late onset gestosis and diabetes mellitus should be evaluated in the context of hypertensive pregnancy disorders, persistent embryonic villi and fetal hypertrophy.

Deficiency of intermediate villi was seen in ca. 10 % of placentas associated with hypertension.

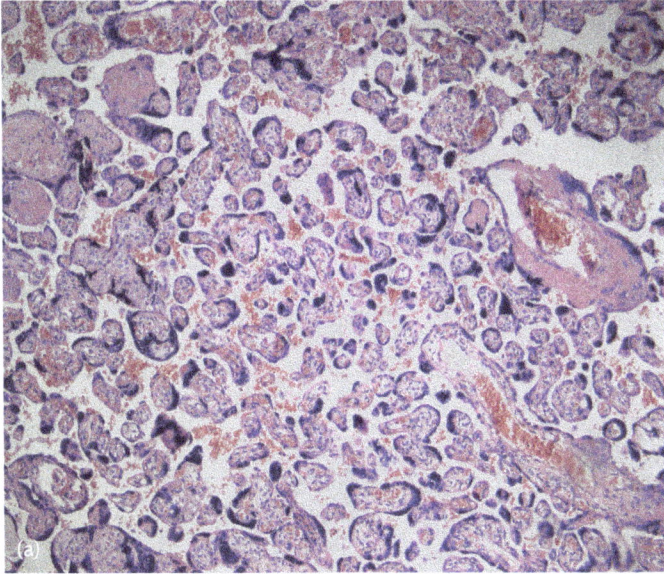

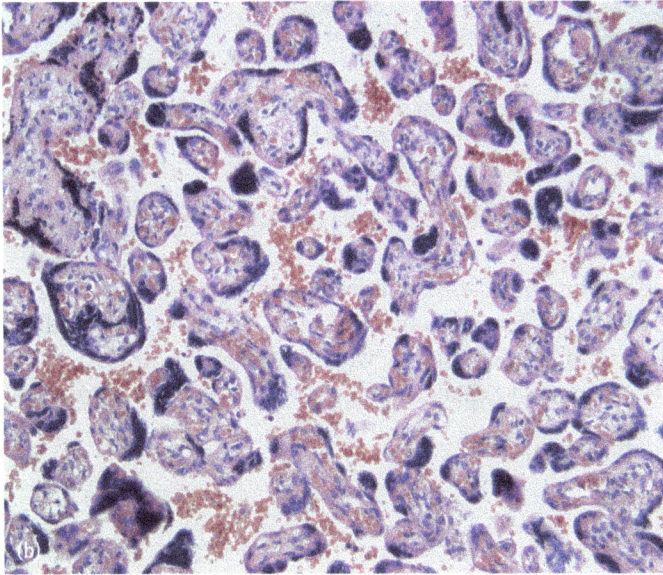

Fig. 14.16: (a) Tenney Parker phenomenon. Supernumerary nuclear knots. (b) HPF.

Accelerated villous maturation was the main finding in placentas of pre-term deliveries with preeclampsia. "Pfropf"gestosis was seen in ca. 70 % of the placentas and was associated, in less than 33 %, with distal villous hypoplasia.

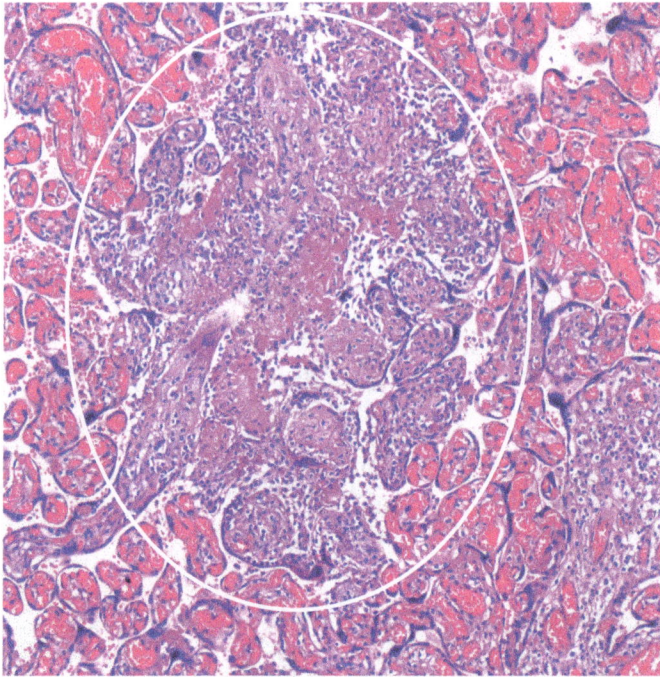

Fig. 14.17: Perivillitis. Villous group (circle) with a lymphoid cell infiltrate, knots of the chorionic epithelium and fibrin deposition. Placenta in Gestational Week 37.

Accelerated maturation and deficient intermediate villi were seen in fetal abortion in the early 2nd trimester.

When diagnosing and estimating placental functionality in pre-terms, a pre-term villous maturation disorder may be masked. In these cases the villous tree displays immature branches and a fibrotic villous stroma with only few fetal capillaries. The chorionic epithelium shows regressive changes and has few/absent vasculosyncytial membranes.

Villous stromal fibrosis

In a study, villous stromal fibrosis was seen in more than 15 % of placentas from hypertensive women, but in only 2.5 % of those with only proteinuria. Fox found villous fibrosis in late onset gestosis in 11.1 % of placentas, prior to gestational week 38, and in 17.5 % at a later gestational age [71]. An unpublished study (Department of Pediatric Pathology and Placentology, Charité Berlin, Germany) showed villous fibrosis in less than 50 % of each MPF and a diffuse distribution in only 5 % of placentas. Generally, fibrosis increases if associated with inter- and perivillous microfibrin deposition and develops into high grade in areas adjacent to perivillitis. In these cases villous fibrosis is often associated with endangiopathia obliterans of the peripheral stem villous arteries.

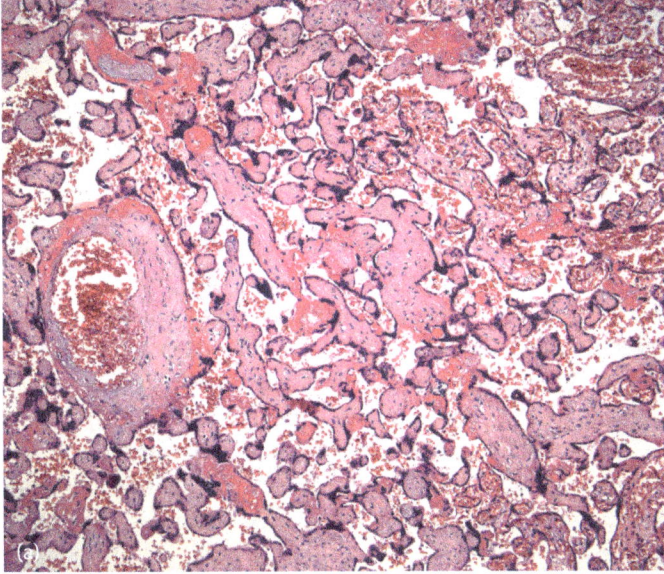

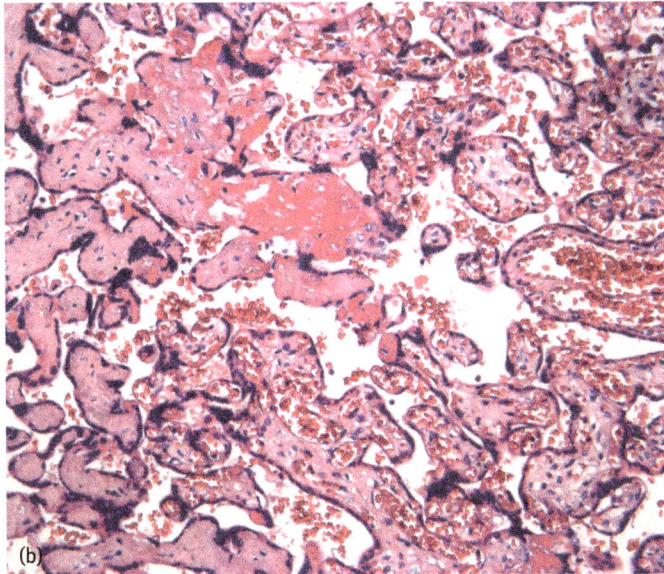

Fig. 14.18: (a) Focal villous fibrosis. Well vascularized villi in the neighbourhood. (b) MPF.

Pathogenesis of placental changes

An important preceding factor for the development of arteriosclerosis and hyperplastic vasculopathy in the pre-placental uterine bed is the lack of spiral artery remodelling [67]. Between gestational week 14 and 22 trophoblasts migrate from the placental base into the intradecidual spiral arteries. They break down the musculoelastic wall elements and convert the vessel lumina into funnel shaped dilated channels from the endomyometrial transition zone into the intermediate villous space. If the vessel walls are not structurally altered there will be persistence of smooth muscle fibers, elastic fibers and adrenergic receptors after gestational week 20.

The pathogenesis of hypertension in pregnancy is somewhat controversial. It is suggested to be a defective response to the formation of the maternal and uteroplacental circulatory system. Prostacyclins, mainly expressed in the vessel wall cells, may play a central role in this process. During pregnancy the volume in the maternal circulatory system increases, caused by: increased plasma volume, increased maternal cardiac ejection fraction and decreased vessel sensitivity to blood pressure and flow resistance. In the uteroplacental circulation the remodelled spiral arteries lack the ability to react to vasoactive stimuli, which results in reduced flow resistance and inhibition of thrombocyte aggregation. These features of the spiral arteries lead to increased uteroplacental circulation, from ca. 50 ml up to 500 ml per minute until delivery.

Lacking this ability to adapt is considered to be a result of an imbalance between prostacyclin and thromboxane A2. Thromboxane is expressed in the thrombocytes and has, in contrast to prostacyclin, a constrictive effect on the vessels and increases blood platelet aggregation. An imbalance of thromboxane over prostacyclin may cause thrombi development in the peripheral maternal vessels and thrombosis in the placental vessels. In the absence of spiral artery remodelling increased circulation in the uteroplacental vessel bed does not occur and the vessels retain sensitive to vasopressin, retaining their resistance to blood flow. Placental changes may be interpreted as a result of a reduced blood supply into the intervillous space and secondary malperfusion [11,21,72,73].

These following changes are seen:
- Hypoxia related proliferation and secondary regressive changes of the chorionic epithelium.
- Local coagulopathy causing microfibrin deposition on the villous surface. Plasmaprotein PP5 is expressed in the syncytiotrophoblast and has antithrombin activity [74]. Hypoxia related injury of the syncytiotrophoblast may cause loss of antithrombin activity and lead, in combination with a thromboxane favouring imbalance, to localized coagulation.
- Dysfunction of the chorionic epithelial blood barrier may cause increased villous deposition of macromolecules with fibrinoid degeneration and stromal necrosis.
- Decreased intervillous perfusion may cause villous stromal fibrosis and endangiopathy in the peripheral stem villi.

Hypertension in pregnancy is usually seen after gestational week 26, with the exception of mothers with "pfropf" preeclampsia in chronic hypertension or kidney disease. Additionally, single case reports have been published of early onset pregnancy related hypertension in proliferating trophoblast diseases:
- complete hydatidiform mole,
- trophoblast island hyperplasia with variable infiltration of extravillous trophoblast islands in macrosomic placentas, sometimes completely encasing the stem and peripheral villi. Foci of fibrinoid degeneration alternate with intact cells. The proportion of syncytiotrophoblasts is relatively low and this differentiates island hyperplasia from reactive syncytial chorionic epithelial hyperplasia in hypertension during the last trimester
- chorangioma.

Consequences of placental changes for pregnancy and follow up
Postpartum diagnosis of placental infarction or placental growth restriction with inter- and perivillous microfibrin deposition (grade 3) shows a statistically significant correlation with pre- and antepartum Doppler Sonography [75]. Characteristically, a diastolic flow reduction approaching zero in the maternal preplacental vessels is seen. Stromal fibrosis and endangiopathy of the peripheral stem villous vessels, as well as accelerated villous maturation and distal villous hypoplasia, correlate with flow reduction or zero flow in the fetal umbilical artery [76].

Consequences for the fetus
Fetal risk is determined by the grade of disease. Risk is seen as:
- increased pre-term delivery rate,
- intrauterine fetal growth restriction,
- increased perinatal mortality.

Fetal hypotrophy was seen in 41% of women with preeclampsia or "pfropf"-preeclampsia and in only 18% of mothers with gestational proteinuria.

Perinatal mortality was 13.4% with high grade disease, and it was reported between 3 and 12% in preeclampsia and between 8 and 27% in eclampsia [15].

Doppler Flow analysis may show a more obvious relationship between hemodynamics and fetal welfare, than between hemodynamics and intrauterine growth restriction in some cases [77].

Placental function is dependent on placental architecture and deficiencies may limit maternal-fetal gas and metabolic exchange, leading to:
- Decreased perfusion capacity caused by stenosis and occlusion of blood vessels.
- Limitation of diffusion capacity caused by an increased diffusion distance in poorly developed villous vessels and a reduced surface area of the vasculosyncytial membranes (ca. 2.8m^2 in hypertensive diseases compared to 4.8m^2 in healthy

controls). A decrease of the nuclear free epithelium in gestosis is supported by other authors.
–   A combination of chronic circulatory disorders and a reduced membrane exchange surface may cause a progressively worsening placental dysfunction, up to and including chronic placental insufficiency with fetal growth restriction.
–   Acute uteroplacental malperfusion and pre-term placental abruption are mainly responsible for the acute risk to the fetus.

14.12.1 HELLP syndrome

A form of preeclampsia which can be described as a triad of [78]:
–   H = Hemolysis
–   EL = Elevated Liver enzymes
–   LP = Low Platelet counts

Often a progressive disease with increased maternal and fetal risk.

Placental changes
–   growth restriction,
–   intervillous malperfusion,
–   accelerated villous maturation with regressive chorionic epithelial changes.

Acute malperfusion with intervillous thrombosis, marginal hematomas and premature placental abruption are also seen [79]. In a single case, sparse cytotrophoblast invasion in the spiral arteries and walls of vessels in the endomyometrial transition zone with acute atherosis and partial vessel occlusion was seen [80].

Cases have been reported without any of the above changes; clinically supported by observations of mothers with HELLP without any fetal findings.

14.13 Maternal hypotension

Hypotension is defined as a systolic blood pressure below 100 mm Hg after gestational week 28 and is reported in 5–10 % of pregnancies [81]. Hypotension is associated with orthostatic dysregulation in 80 %. It may result in abortion, pre-term delivery and FGR [82].

Morphology
Systemic studies of the placenta in maternal hypotension have not been performed. Our observations describe nonspecific low grade placental malperfusion with only low grade placental dysfunction [7].

From unpublished research, 35 % of placentas had a subchorionic granulocytic infiltration and/or meconium phagocytosis, and this may indicate a transitory hypoxia prior to labor or during delivery (Department of Pediatric Pathology and Placentology, Charité, Berlin, Germany).

Pathogenesis
A decrease in maternal arterial blood pressure results in a uteroplacental malperfusion, caused by reduced and refractory uterine vessel resistance [83]. Uteroplacental perfusion reduction in hypotension may be measured using radioisotopics [84]. Dysregulation of intervillous perfusion is assumed to be due to orthostatic dysregulation with an imbalanced arterial blood pressure and cardiac frequency.

14.14 Maternal nicotine abuse

Maternal smoking is defined regular use of 10–15 cigarettes per day in pregnancy and includes nicotine use before pregnancy [85].

Morphology
Placentas from smokers show changes uncharacteristic of gestosis; however, it is not possible to relate the changes to smoking without clinical information. Placental weight and area are often of a normal size for gestational age. The placenta has the same proteomic and DNA profiles as placentas of non-smokers [86]. Placental weight over the 50th percentile, from smokers over a 6 year or more period, shows the following histology [87]:
– peripheral villous immaturity,
– villous stromal fibrosis,
– increased nuclear sprouts and knots of the syncytiotrophoblast,
– increased inter- and perivillous microfibrin depositions.

Peripheral villous immaturity: villi are regularly branched but show an increased number of intermediate villi of the peripheral type with reduced fetal vessel development and few vasculosyncytial membranes [88]. Placentas from both smokers and non-smokers showed increased villous branching but decreased capillary volume density in the villous periphery and an increased volume stromal density. Vasculosyncytial membranes were decreased in smokers but the relative volume density of the trophoblast was the same in both groups (percentage of the total tissue).
Villous stromal fibrosis: was seen in only small foci and of low grade. Increased vessel lumen obliteration in the stem villi was not seen [89].
Electron microscopy shows a thickened basal lamina near the chorionic epithelium and a fragmented basal lamina near the fetal capillaries [90]. Degenerative chang-

es close to the capillaries with loss of cellular organelles and an increased thickness of the basal lamina are reported [91].

Increased nuclear sprouts and knots: were seen in more than 50 % of the peripheral villi in a single MPF. Nuclear sprouts with hormonal activity or regressive nuclear knots with loss of endocrine activity on immunohistochemistry are reported. Increased nuclear sprouts of the syncytial trophoblasts are not supported by other studies [92]. Necrosis of the syncytiotrophoblast on electron microscopy is believed to cause a reduced Human chorionic gonadotropin synthesis and increases permeability of the chorionic villi for alpha-fetoprotein, which can be identified in smokers in gestational weeks 13–27 [88,91,93].

Inter- and perivillous microfibrin depositions: microscopic microfibrin deposition is primarily seen in peripheral portions of the feto-maternal circulatory unit; infrequently these deposits merge and form microinfarcts. Macroinfarcts are frequently seen in placentas from women with nicotine use prior to pregnancy (7 cigarettes or more a day for more than 6 years) and is associated with pre-term placental abruption and placenta previa [85].

Pathogenesis of the placental changes
Placental changes are interpreted as result of hypoxic and/or toxic injury to the chorionic tissue. Placental impairment is partly due to an intervillous malperfusion brought about by the vasoconstrictive effects of nicotine on preplacental vessels. An acute decrease of intervillous flow is reported after a single cigarette [94]. Associated changes are proliferative and regressive syncytiotrophoblast changes, including: focal cellular necrosis, increased microfibrin depositions in the intervillous space, increased collagen production and reduced sinusoidal dilatation of the fetal capillaries. The hypoxic effect of intervillous malperfusion may be triggered by increased carbon monoxide in the blood.

The toxic effect on chorionic epithelium is believed to be caused by polycyclic aromatic hydrocarbons and cadmium, which are of relatively high concentrations in tobacco. The concentration of cadmium is increased in the placentas of smokers and seems to have degenerative effect on the cytotrophoblast, stromal cells and fetal endothelial cells; however, these findings are not consistently reported across studies. The detailed pathological mechanisms behind the placental changes remain unknown [90].

Consequences for the fetus
From the literature an increased rate of intrauterine growth restriction and perinatal mortality is reported. Isolated morphological findings in the placenta, as an explanation of a deficiency of materno-fetal nutrition and gas exchange should be considered carefully and additional supportive evidence sought prior to diagnosis.

14.15 Maternal heroin and cocaine abuse

Approximately 33 % of heroine dependent women in Germany are of fertile age. Pregnancy is at risk due to non-pregnancy related risk factors and specific pregnancy complications, such as: increased abortion rate, increased amniotic infection after premature membrane rupture, hypertension, abnormal placental implantation, preterm delivery and intrauterine underdevelopment [95,96].

Morphology
In placentas with associated heroin use, only a few characteristics may be found:
-   pre-term accelerated villous maturation
-   increased syncytiotrophoblast nuclear sprouts and knots,
-   increased inter- and perivillous microfibrin depositions,
-   hypoxic changes.

Pre-term accelerated villous maturation: villous branching is not altered. Many of the intermediate and terminal villi in the periphery are capillary rich, which increases the vascularization ratio in placentas when compared to controls at the same gestational age

Morphologically, no significant difference in the villous surface or metabolic exchange membranes could be identified when compared to controls; however, the structural density ratio of syncytial knots and microfibrin deposits were significantly increased in placentas from women with heroin use [95,96].

Pathogenesis of the placental changes
Placental changes are non-specific. Short term heroin use has no direct or specific effect on the placenta. The histological findings of villous maturation disorders increased nuclear sprouts and knots of the syncytiotrophoblast with microfibrin depositions are a consequence of intervillous malperfusion; analogous to changes in placentas from smokers and those with pregnancy induced hypertension.

Heroin induces a parasympathetic hypertension and vasoconstriction, and even small amounts cause respiratory depression with an increase of CO_2 and decrease of O_2 in the maternal blood [97]. Chorionic epithelial changes and microfibrin deposition are signs of tissue hypoxia. Increased villous vascularization may point to a compensatory chorionic tissue reaction, due to transient intervillous malperfusion and hypoxia.

Changes indicating hypoxia: stromal meconium macrophages in the chorionic plate and membranes and increased subchorionic granulocytes are indicators of placental hypoxia. Hypoxic changes may develop in intrauterine heroin withdrawal and due adulteration with other agents. It may result in increased fetal movements and increased fetal oxygen demand. IUFD due to withdrawal is widely reported [98,99].

Consequences for the fetus
– pre-term delivery,
– increased intrauterine fetal death (IUFD),
– intrauterine hypoxia,
– intrauterine growth restriction (FGR),
– withdrawal (intrauterine and postpartum).

The hypertensive and vasoconstrictive effect of *cocaine* on the maternal vessels is well known and abuse in pregnancy may lead to maternal hypertension and preeclampsia, pre-term delivery and fetal growth restriction. Several authors report cases of pre-term placental abruption as a direct consequence of cocaine use in pregnancy [100].

Findings in placentas are varying due to coexisting maternal abuse of heroin- and cocaine (polytoxicomania).

14.16 Alcohol abuse

Alcohol abuse in pregnancy causes well known fetal malformations, such as embryo- and fetopathy by passing the placental barrier. Specific placental changes correlating with chronic maternal alcohol abuse and different degrees of "fetal alcohol syndrome" could not be found.

Morphology
– growth restricted placenta in 60 % of children with 'fetal alcoholic syndrome,
– small foci of chronic circulatory disturbance in 50 %,
– chorioamnionitis in 30 %, predominantly pre-terms [101].

These changes indicate direct damage to the embryo/fetus by maternal alcohol abuse. Experimental studies in rats show that chronic alcohol exposure inhibits transplacental transport of amino acids [102].

14.17 Systemic lupus erythematosus (SLE)

Pregnancy in systemic lupus erythematosus increases fetal risk due to transmission of anti-nuclear antibodies to the fetus. Neonatal lupus syndrome with placental, dermal and myocardial involvement (complete cardiac block) is well known [103]. In 1,045 pregnancies the SLE associated abortion rate was 16.8 % and the intrauterine fetal death rate 7.65 % [104].

Lupus anticoagulant and anticardiolipin antibodies are believed to cause fetal risk [105,106] and are identified in ca. 20 % of SLE cases [107]. Abortion rates in SLE pregnancies with detected Lupus anticoagulant antibodies are higher (58.7 %) than in patients without detectable antibodies (24.7 %).

Morphology

In approximately half of the placentas from SLE mothers the placental changes are similar to those of hypertensive pregnancies; however, in contrast to preeclampsia, SLE can result in fetal death in mid pregnancy and placentas may show:
- placental growth restriction with low weight and low basal area,
- massive gitterinfarcts macroscopically, massive chronic and subacute cotyledon infarcts (up to and including infarction of the placenta; > 20 % placental area involved),
- microscopically diffuse and extensive microfibrin deposition with fibrin rich obliteration of the intervillous space, perivillitis and villous stromal fibrosis,
- acute atherosis, fibrinoid vessel wall necrosis and thrombotic obliteration of the lumina in the spiral arteries of the placental bed.

IgM, as well as C3, deposits in the vessel wall of the spiral arteries can be seen with immunofluorescence microscopy.

Pathogenesis

Nuclear antibodies show anti-trophoblastic activity at the basal membrane of the villi [108].

Lupus anticoagulant is an immunoglobulin which reacts with phospholipids secreted by thrombocytes. Formation of the prothrombin activator complex is blocked causing an increased partial thromboplastin time (PTT) and prothrombin time (PT). Clinically, thrombopathy in the arteries and veins is the primary cause of hemorrhage in SLE during pregnancy. The pathogenic mechanism of these thrombi is not completely understood. Placental anticoagulation protein-1 may be a possible trigger of arterial thrombosis [109].

14.18 Scleroderma / dermatomyositis / chronic polyarthritis

The above diseases are rarely seen in pregnancy, but when present, abortion and still-birth are more frequent and fetuses show a deficiency of development for a given gestational age.

Placentas are small for gestational age and macroscopic sections show gitterinfarcts, subchorionic pseudoinfarcts and maternal floor infarction.

Histologically examination shows: microfibrin deposition in the intervillous space, regressive chorionic epithelial changes of the villous surface and patchy focal villous stromal fibrosis. Multiple cysts and an expansive extravillous trophoblastic cell (X-cell) proliferation may characterize the placenta of mothers with scleroderma [108].

References

[1]   International statistical classification of diseases and related health problems ICD-10, 10th revision [Internet]. World Health Organization. 2004. [cited 2004].

[2]   Leisher SH, Teoh Z, Reinebrant H, et al. Classification systems for causes of stillbirth and neonatal death, 2009–2014: an assessment of alignment with characteristics for an effective global system. BMC Pregnancy Childbirth. 2016;16:269.

[3]   Smith GC. Screening and prevention of stillbirth. Best practice & research Clinical obstetrics & gynaecology. 2017;38:71–82.

[4]   Smith GC, Fretts RC. Stillbirth. Lancet. 2007;370(9600):1715–1725.

[5]   Carberry AE, Gordon A, Bond DM, et al. Customised versus population-based growth charts as a screening tool for detecting small for gestational age infants in low-risk pregnant women. The Cochrane database of systematic reviews. 2014(5):CD008549.

[6]   Vogel M. Atlas der morphologischen Plazentadiagnostik. 2 ed. Berlin: Springer; 1996.

[7]   Vogel M. Atlas der morphologischen Plazentadiagnostik. 1. ed. Berlin: Springer; 1992.

[8]   Völker U. Gewichts- und Grössenvergleich von Plazenten und Feten bei intrauterinem Fruchttod. PerinatMed. 1992;4:8–16.

[9]   Hegele-Döhring M. Intrauterine Fetal death. Results of kyematopathological basic studies to estimate the cause of death.: Free University; 1983.

[10] Roeckelein G, Kobras G, Becker V. Physiological and pathological morphology of the umbilical and placental circulation. Pathology, research and practice. 1990;186(1):187–196.

[11] Becker V, Schiebler TH, Kubli F. Allgemeine und spezielle Pathologie der Plazenta. Die Plazenta des Menschen. Stuttgart: Thieme; 1981. p. 251–393.

[12] Naeye RL. Placental abnormalities in victims of the sudden infant death syndrome. Biology of the neonate. 1977;32(3–4):189–192.

[13] Naeye RL, Ross SM. Amniotic fluid infection syndrome. Clin Obstet Gynaecol. 1982;9(3):593–607.

[14] Stoltenburg-Didinger G, Franke D, Vogel M. Störung der Gliareifung bei akuter und chronischer Plazentainsuffizienz. Der Pathologe. 1987;108.

[15] Dudenhausen JW. Prakische Geburtshilfe. Berlin: DeGruyter; 1989.

[16] Raiha CE. Relation of maternal heart volume in pregnancy to prematurity and perinatal mortality. Bull World Health Organ. 1962;26:296–300.

[17] Raiha CE. Prematurity, Perinatal Mortality and maternal Heart Volume. Guys Hosp Rep. 1964;113:96–110.

[18] Vogel M. Plazentamorphologische Aspekte zur Formalgenese Frühgeborener und untergewichtiger Neugeborener. In: Dudenhausen JW SE, editor. Perinatale Medizin. IV. Stuttgart: Thieme; 1973. p. 343–346.

[19] Han T. Überreifegrad des Kindes und Morphologie der Plazenta. Berlin: Free University (FU); 1990.

[20] Hitschold T, Weiss E, Berle P, Muntefering H. [Histologic placenta findings in prolonged pregnancy: correlation of placental retarded maturation, fetal outcome and Doppler sonographic findings in the umbilical artery]. Z Geburtshilfe Perinatol. 1989;193(1):42–46.

[21] Kloos K, Vogel M. Pathologie der Perinatalperiode. Stuttgart: Thieme; 1974.

[22] Theuring F, Kemnitz P. [Electron microscopic observations of placentas in fetal intrauterine growth retardation (so-called small-for-dates-babies) (author's transl)]. Zentralbl Allg Pathol. 1974;118(1):82–89.

[23] Emmrich P, Lassker G. [Morphologic changes of placentas in cases of intrauterine growth retardation]. Pathol Microbiol (Basel). 1971;37(1):57–72.

[24] Vogel M. Plazentagrösse und -struktur als Voraussetzung für den Wachstumsstand des reifgeborenen Kindes bei der Geburt, mit besonderer Berücksichtigung der Plazentationsstörungen. Berlin: Freie Universität (FU); 1975.

[25] Laurini R, Laurin J, Marsal K. Placental histology and fetal blood flow in intrauterine growth retardation. Acta Obstet Gynecol Scand. 1994;73(7):529–534.

[26] Martius G, Look W. Blutungen in der zweiten Schwangerschaftshälfte. In: Martius GS, Gollwitzer M, editor. Differentialdiagnose in Geburtshilfe und Gynäkologie. Stuttgart: Thieme; 1984. p. 283–289.

[27] Neeb U. [Feto-maternal transfusion with severe fetal anaemia. A case report (author's transl)]. Geburtshilfe Frauenheilkd. 1982;42(3):213–214.

[28] von Criegern T, Gille J. [Feto-maternal transfusion with severe fetal anemia. A case report (author's transl)]. Geburtshilfe Frauenheilkd. 1981;41(1):52–54.

[29] Salfelder A, Kochanowicz J, Spenner R, Hickl EJ. [Fetomaternal macrotransfusion--a cause for decreased fetal movements. 2 cases]. Zeitschrift fur Geburtshilfe und Neonatologie. 1995;199(2):86–89.

[30] Jauniaux E, Van Maldergem L, De Munter C, Moscoso G, Gillerot Y. Nonimmune hydrops fetalis associated with genetic abnormalities. Obstetrics and gynecology. 1990;75(3 Pt 2):568–572.

[31] Mallmann P, Gembruch U, Mallmann R, Hansmann M. [A possible "immunologic" origin of idiopathic non-immunologic hydrops fetalis and initial results of preventive immunotherapy of subsequent pregnancies]. Z Geburtshilfe Perinatol. 1989;193(4):161–166.

[32] Spitzer A, Edelmann CM Jr, Boichis H et al. The kidney and urinary tract. In: Fanaroff AA, editor. Neonatal-perinatal medicine. 4 ed. St.Louis: Mosby; 1987. p. 981–1015.

[33] Faulk WP, van Loghem E, Stickler GB. Maternal antibody to fetal light chain (Inv) antigens. The American journal of medicine. 1974;56(3):393–397.

[34] Fox H, Sebire NJ. Pathology of the placenta: Saunders Elsevier; 2007.

[35] Busch W, Vogel M. [The placenta in hemolytic disease of the newborn]. Z Geburtshilfe Perinatol. 1972;176(1):17–28.

[36] Hörmann G. [An attempt to systematize disorders of placental development]. Geburtshilfe Frauenheilkd. 1958;18(4):345–349.

[37] Flint J, Hill AV, Bowden DK, et al. High frequencies of alpha-thalassaemia are the result of natural selection by malaria. Nature. 1986;321(6072):744–750.

[38] Monni G, Ibba RM, Olla G, Rosatelli C, Cao A. Chorionic villus sampling by rigid forceps: experience with 300 cases at risk for thalassemia major. American journal of obstetrics and gynecology. 1987;156(4):912–914.

[39] Weaver DD. Catalogue of prenatally diagnosed conditions. Baltimore: John Hopkins Clin Press; 1989.

[40] Jones CJ, Lendon M, Chawner LE, Jauniaux E. Ultrastructure of the human placenta in metabolic storage disease. Placenta. 1990;11(5):395–411.

[41] Unger M, Jimenez E, Vogel M, et al. Morphologische Plazentaveränderungen nach Hydroxyäthylstärke-Infusion. In: Dudenhausen JW SE, editor. Perinatale Medizin. XIII. Stuttgart: Thieme; 1991.

[42] Shaw JE, Sicree RA, Zimmet PZ. Global estimates of the prevalence of diabetes for 2010 and 2030. Diabetes Res Clin Pract. 2010;87(1):4–14.

[43] Weiss PA, Hofmann H, Winter R, Purstner P, Lichtenegger W. Amniotic fluid glucose values in normal and abnormal pregnancies. Obstetrics and gynecology. 1985;65(3):333–339.

[44] Jovanovic L, Peterson CM. Optimal insulin delivery for the pregnant diabetic patient. Diabetes Care. 1982;5 Suppl 1:24–37.

[45] Semmler K, Emmrich P. [Morphology of the placenta in relation to glycemia status in pregnancy in diabetes mellitus]. Z Geburtshilfe Perinatol. 1989;193(3):124–128.

[46] White P. Diabetes mellitus in pregnancy. Clin Perinatol. 1974;1(2):331–347.

[47] Semmler K, Emmrich P, Fuhrmann K, Godel E. [Placental maturation disorders in relation to the quality of metabolic control during pregnancy in insulin-dependent and gestational diabetes]. ZentralblGynakol. 1982;104(23):1494–1502.

[48] Werner C, Schneiderhan W. [Placental morphology and placental function in relation to the control of diabetes in pregnancy]. Geburtshilfe Frauenheilkd. 1972;32(11):959–966.

[49] Stoz F, Schuhmann RA, Schebesta B. The development of the placental villus during normal pregnancy: morphometric data base. Arch Gynecol Obstet. 1988;244(1):23–32.

[50] Hormann G. [Classification of placental pathology in man]. Arch Gynakol. 1958;191(3):297–344.

[51] Vogel M, Kloos KF. Diabetes in der Schwangerschaft; neue morphologische Befunde an Plazenta und Fet. In: Dudenhausen JW SE, editor. Perinayale Medizin. VI. Stuttgart: Thieme; 1975.

[52] Graf R, Schönfelder G, Muhlberger M, Gutsmann M. The perivascular contractile sheath of human placental stem villi: its isolation and characterization. Placenta. 1995;16(1):57–66.

[53] Benirschke K, Burton G, Baergen RN. Pathology of the human placenta. 6 ed. New York: Springer; 2012.

[54] Steldinger R, Weber B, Jimenez E, Vogel M. Morphologische Untersuchungen von Plazenten bei Typ I Diabetes mellitus. In: Dudenhausen JW SE, editor. Perinatale Medizin. XIII. Stuttgart: Thieme; 1991.

[55] Vogel M. [Plakopathia diabetica. Developmental disorders of the placenta in diabetes mellitus of the mother]. Virchows Arch Pathol Anat Physiol Klin Med. 1967;343(1):51–63.

[56] Semmler K, Emmrich P. [Morphology of the placenta in relation to glycemia status in pregnancy in diabetes mellitus]. ZGeburtshilfe Perinatol. 1989;193(3):124–128.

[57] Yampolsky M, Salafia CM, Shlakhter O, et al. Centrality of the umbilical cord insertion in a human placenta influences the placental efficiency. Placenta. 2009;30(12):1058–1064.

[58] Schafer RG, Bohannon B, Franz M, et al. Translation of the diabetes nutrition recommendations for health care institutions. Diabetes Care. 1997;20(1):96–105.

[59] Schafer-Graf UM, Dupak J, Vogel M, et al. Hyperinsulinism, neonatal obesity and placental immaturity in infants born to women with one abnormal glucose tolerance test value. J Perinat Med. 1998;26(1):27–36.

[60] Boyd PA, Scott A, Keeling JW. Quantitative structural studies on placentas from pregnancies complicated by diabetes mellitus. British journal of obstetrics and gynaecology. 1986;93(1):31–35.

[61] Haust MD. Maternal diabetes mellitus--effects on the fetus and placenta. Monogr Pathol. 1981(22):201–285.

[62] Stoz F, Schuhmann RA, Schmid A. Morphometric investigations of terminal villi of diabetic placentas in relation to the White classification of diabetes mellitus. J Perinat Med. 1987;15(2):193–198.

[63] Teasdale F. Histomorphometry of the placenta of the diabetic women: class A diabetes mellitus. Placenta. 1981;2(3):241–251.

[64] Salafia CM. the fetal, placental and neonatal pathology associated with matrnal diabetes mellitus. In: Reece EA CD, editor. Diabetes mellitus in pregnancy Principles and practice. New York: Livingstone; 1988.

[65] Whitsett JA. Specializations in plasma membranes of the human placenta. The Journal of pediatrics. 1980;96(3 Pt 2):600–603.

[66] Dudenhausen JW. Praktische Geburtshilfe. Berlin De Gruyter; 1989.

[67] Robertson WB, Brosens I, Dixon HG. Uteroplacental vascular pathology. In: Brosens JA DG, Robertson WB., editor. Human placentation. Amsterdam: Excerpta Medica; 1975.

[68] Schlief-Pflug E. Morphometrische Plazentauntersuchungen bei EPH-Gestose. Berlin: Free university (FU); 1984.

[69] Kloos K, Luckschus B, Vogel M. [Placental changes in perinatal death (functional-kyematopathological analysis for the initiation of preventive measures)]. Zeitschrift fur Geburtshilfe und Gynakologie. 1967;166(2):149–158.

[70] Werner CH, Schwartz G. Plazentabefunde bei EPH Gestose, eine phasenkontrastmikroskopische Untersuchung. In: Rippmann ET, editor. EPH Gestosis. Berlin: De Gruyter; 1972.

[71] Fox H. Fibrosis of placental villi. J Pathol Bacteriol. 1968;95(2):573–579.

[72] Perrin EVDK. Pathology of the placenta. Churchill Livingstone: New York; 1984.

[73] Fox H. Pathology of the placenta in maternal diabetes mellitus. Obstetrics and gynecology. 1969;34(6):792–798.

[74] Meisser A, Bischof P, Bohn H. Placental protein 5 (PP5) inhibits thrombin-induced coagulation of fibrinogen. Arch Gynecol. 1985;236(4):197–201.

[75] Jimenez E, Vogel M, Arabin B, Wagner G, Mirsalim P. Correlation of Ultrasonographic Measurement of the Utero-Placental and Fetal Blood Flow with the Morphological Diagnosis of Placental Function. In: Kaufmann P, Miller RK, editors. Placental Vascularization and Blood Flow: Basic Research and Clinical Applications. Boston, MA: Springer US; 1988. p. 325–334.

[76] Arabin B, Jimenez E, Vogel M, Weitzel HK. Relationship of utero- and fetoplacental blood flow velocity wave forms with pathomorphological placental findings. Fetal Diagn Ther. 1992;7(3–4):173–179.

[77] Vetter K. Considerations on growth discordant twins. J Perinat Med. 1993;21(4):267–272.

[78] Weinstein L. Syndrome of hemolysis, elevated liver enzymes, and low platelet count: a severe consequence of hypertension in pregnancy. American journal of obstetrics and gynecology. 1982;142(2):159–167.

[79] de Dycker RP, Neumann RL. [HELLP syndrome: a life-threatening form of pre-eclampsia]. Geburtshilfe Frauenheilkd. 1987;47(2):128–130.

[80] Friedmann W, Vogel M, Unger M, Martius G. [Fatal outcome in HELLP syndrome]. Zentralbl Gynakol. 1990;112(14):925–929.

[81] Kirchhoff R. [Catastrophe medicine in general practice]. Fortschr Med. 1981;99(23):887–889.

[82] Goeschen K, Schmoldt V, Pluta M, Saling E. [The effect of low blood pressure on venous function during and outside of pregnancy and therapeutic consequences]. Geburtshilfe Frauenheilkd. 1985;45(8):525–533.

[83] Moll W, Kunzel W. [The uteroplacental circulation (author's transl)]. Z Geburtshilfe Perinatol. 1974;178(1):1–18.

[84] Grunberger W, Leodolter S, Parschalk O. [Pregnancy hypotension and fetal outcome]. Fortschr Med. 1979;97(4):141–144.

[85] Naeye RL. The duration of maternal cigarette smoking, fetal and placental disorders. Early human development. 1979;3(3):229–237.

[86] Picone TA, Allen LH, Olsen PN, Ferris ME. Pregnancy outcome in North American women. II. Effects of diet, cigarette smoking, stress, and weight gain on placentas, and on neonatal physical and behavioral characteristics. Am J Clin Nutr. 1982;36(6):1214–1224.

[87] Agrawal P, Chansoriya M, Kaul KK. Effect of tobacco chewing by mothers on placental morphology. Indian Pediatr. 1983;20(8):561–565.

[88] van der Velde WJ, Copius Peereboom-Stegeman JH, Treffers PE, James J. Structural changes in the placenta of smoking mothers: a quantitative study. Placenta. 1983;4(3):231–240.
[89] Lohr J, Dehnhard P, Wehler V, Ardelt W. [Proceedings: Morphology of placenta in smokers]. Arch Gynakol. 1975;219(1–4):376–377.
[90] van der Velde WJ, Peereboom-Stegeman JH, Treffers PE, James J. Basal lamina thickening in the placentae of smoking mothers. Placenta. 1985;6(4):329–340.
[91] van der Veen F, Fox H. The effects of cigarette smoking on the human placenta: a light and electron microscopic study. Placenta. 1982;3(3):243–256.
[92] Spira A, Philippe E, Spira N, Dreyfus J, Schwartz D. Smoking during pregnancy and placental pathology. Biomedicine. 1977;27(7):266–270.
[93] Cuckle HS, Wald NJ, Densem JW, et al. The effect of smoking in pregnancy on maternal serum alpha-fetoprotein, unconjugated oestriol, human chorionic gonadotrophin, progesterone and dehydroepiandrosterone sulphate levels. British journal of obstetrics and gynaecology. 1990;97(3):272–274.
[94] Lehtovirta P, Forss M. The acute effect of smoking on intervillous blood flow of the placenta. British journal of obstetrics and gynaecology. 1978;85(10):729–731.
[95] Köpp W, Vogel M. [Heroin disease. Its significance during pregnancy and the early development of the child]. MMW Muench Med Wochenschr. 1982;124(42):915–917.
[96] Köpp W, Vogel M. [Histologic and morphometric findings in placentas of heroin addicts (author's transl)]. Z Geburtshilfe Perinatol. 1982;186(1):37–40.
[97] Hauschild F. Pharmakologie und Grundlagen der Toxikologie. Leipzig: Thieme; 1973.
[98] Finnegan LP, Reeser DS, Connaughton JF Jr. The effects of maternal drug dependence on neonatal mortality. Drug Alcohol Depend. 1977;2(2):131–140.
[99] Rementeria JL, Nunag NN. Narcotic withdrawal in pregnancy: stillbirth incidence with a case report. American journal of obstetrics and gynecology. 1973;116(8):1152–1156.
[100] Little BB, Snell LM, Klein VR, Gilstrap LC 3rd. Cocaine abuse during pregnancy: maternal and fetal implications. Obstetrics and gynecology. 1989;73(2):157–160.
[101] Lindner C, Spohr H, Vogel M, et al. Cartographer Alterations in the placenta of children with fetal alcoholic syndrome. Marburg: Tedum; 2001.
[102] Fisher SE, Atkinson M, Burnap JK, et al. Ethanol-associated selective fetal malnutrition: a contributing factor in the fetal alcohol syndrome. Alcohol Clin Exp Res. 1982;6(2):197–201.
[103] Provost TT, Watson R, Gammon WR, et al. The neonatal lupus syndrome associated with U1RNP (nRNP) antibodies. The New England journal of medicine. 1987;316(18):1135–1138.
[104] Cecere FA, Yoshinoya S, Pope RM. Fatal thrombotic thrombocytopenic purpura in a patient with systemic lupus erythematosus. Relationship to circulating immune complexes. Arthritis Rheum. 1981;24(3):550–553.
[105] Firkin BG, Howard MA, Radford N. Possible relationship between lupus inhibitor and recurrent abortion in young women. Lancet. 1980;2(8190):366.
[106] Kentenich H, Schwerdtfeger R, Vogel M. [Lupus anticoagulant in pregnancy]. Geburtshilfe Frauenheilkd. 1986;46(7):467–469.
[107] Averbuch M, Koifman B, Levo Y. Lupus anticoagulant, thrombosis and thrombocytopenia in systemic lupus erythematosus. Am J Med Sci. 1987;293(1):2–5.
[108] Benirschke K, Burton GJ, Baergen RN. Pathology of the Human Placenta. 6 ed. Heidelberg, NY, London: Springer; 2012.
[109] Triplett DA. Antiphospholipid antibodies and thrombosis. A consequence, coincidence, or cause? Arch Pathol Lab Med. 1993;117(1):78–88.

15 Morphological diagnosis of placental insufficiency

Placental insufficiency is clinically defined as any disorder of exchange between mother and child, it may be classified as, either acute and chronic. Acute placental insufficiency is characterized by changes that occur within minutes and hours of fetal hypoxemia, hypoxia and acidosis: *acute respiratory placental insufficiency*.

Chronic nutritional placental insufficiency shows changes which occur over weeks and months and that cause, primarily, fetal developmental disorders. Chronic placental insufficiency may be complicated by disorders of acute gas exchange during onset of labor, *global placental insufficiency*. A presumed placental dysfunction may be clinically diagnosed by ultrasound, CTG, amnioscopy and fetal blood analysis.

The pathological-anatomical definition of placental insufficiency is an overly broad one, encompassing placental, maternal and fetal disorders and as such, does not provide insight into the actual causes of an acute or chronic lack of fetal blood supply [1,2].

Placental insufficiency is, pathologically defined as an imbalance of exchange due to morphologically identifiable organ damage [3]. However, the morphological characteristics of placental insufficiency are somewhat controversial [4]. Many disorders, which traditionally have been interpreted as a result of placental insufficiency, are related to maternal circulatory disorder without evidence of causal relationship to placental insufficiency. It must be taken into account that placental changes are partly caused by vessels outside the placenta [5,6].

However, examples in general pathology show that a macroscopically observed disorder in the organ may be interfered by adaptive responses and compensatory changes in the organ. More obvious than in the placenta are morphological findings in the coronary arteries and myocardium related to functional defects and cardiac failure. Principally, morphology describes structural changes as a precondition or expression of disorders of organ function, but it is not possible to assess hemodynamic or biochemical adjustments to the anatomical condition.

Of importance in *morphological placental diagnosis* is not only a qualitative assessment of particular pathological changes but also a quantitative evaluation with identification of additional findings which may have negative functional impact. A comparative analysis of a large series of defined pathological patterns and the presenting clinical symptoms in acute and chronic fetal lack of supply may permit morphological assessment of placental insufficiency [7].

Morphological description of structural placental findings due to fetal hypoxia or acidosis may help to explain, why the fetus is in some cases of hypertension at high risk or growth restricted in others. In unknown diseases, morphological evidence of placental insufficiency may give a formal pathogenetic explanation for IUFD or perinatal fetal risk, or even a hint to a not yet manifested disease.

https://doi.org/10.1515/9783110452600-015

Agreement on normal values of organ size, villous maturation, villous chorionic surface, exchange surface of the fetal vessels and their location and extent of micro-fibrin deposits is the precondition for the diagnosis of placental insufficiency. In routine diagnostics, criteria are used semiquantitativly and are expressed in stage and grade, following morphometric study results.

Structural placental changes affecting placental function appear as change of:
- placental growth
- placental maturation
- placental circulation

Placental function constantly adapts to fetal demand and these characteristics of the placenta are essential for normal fetal growth, development and maturation, which in turn influence hormonal and enzymatic placental development and function.

Morphologically, normal placental growth and villous maturation, according to gestational age, correspond to the functionality of the chorionic tissue and the exchange surface between the mother and child.

Furthermore, adequate placental circulation/perfusion with sufficient nutritive maternal supply for fetal demands in the feto-maternal unit is required. Disorders stimulate compensatory mechanisms. If compensation is absent, reduced placental function and fetal maldevelopment is the result.

Compensatory mechanisms are intra and extraplacental. In the first instance, maternal and fetal perfusion increases. If the disorder persists, histological features become apparent. If villous maturation is retarded, a compensatory increased villous growth with increased placental growth, which increases villous surface and intervillous volume, is seen. Additionally, in growth restricted or chronic vascular malperfused placentas, compensatory increased villous maturation, which increases intra-villous vessel volume and reduces diffusion distance is found.

The placenta is the organ with an immense ability to adapt to exogenous stimuli and so even placentas from normal, healthy children, without any known risk factors, may show low grade pathological changes. *"Even a pathological placenta is not insufficient, as long as fetal development and homeostasis is normal"* [8].

The compensatory ability of the placenta is limited by the grade of pathology, time of onset and duration. If the compensatory threshold of the placenta is exceeded, morphological changes and placental function derangement will occur.

Typical morphology in manifested compensations is:
- Increased placental growth with increase of the organ size and increase of the feto-maternal exchange surface, in:
  - villous maturation arrest;
- accelerated villous vasculogenesis, in:
  - primary placental growth restriction (in premature villous maturation in preterm placentas),

- accelerated villous maturation, or
- chorangiosis type II in secondary placental decrease, with the aim to increase intravillous fetal vessel volume and to decrease diffusion distance due to chronical circulatory disturbances in the villous parenchyma (in preeclampsia, chronic maternal kidney- or vessel disease).

Table 15.1: Qualitative and quantitative placental changes correlating with placental dysfunction.

growth disorders	– low weight – Reduced maternal area
villous maturation disorder	– preterm accelerated – villous immaturity – chorangiosis type I
circulatory disturbance	– acute and chronic – microfibrin depositions
endangiopathy obliterans	
villous fibrosis	
placentitis parenchymatosa	
chorangioma	

Morphological findings depend on the severity of the imbalance between supply and demand in placental exchange. The following changes may be seen:
- decreased exchange surface
- increased intravillous diffusion distance
- constriction of maternal and/or fetal vessels.

Pathological size and structural changes in delivered placentas show a significant correlation with antenatal Doppler Flow examination of the uteroplacental and fetal vessels [9–11]. This indicates that a single change in the placenta can potentially cause hemodynamic disorders in changes of high grade. Multiple combined changes may lead to a limitation of placental function.

Following this we suggest a *subclassification of placental function*, including grade of individual an associated findings (Table 15.2).

Quantity of single changes, as well as changes with similar negative functionality in combination should be interpreted.

Table 15.2: Subclassification of functional placenta function [12,13].

changes without effect on placental function	latent insufficient placental function	manifest placental insufficiency
no change / normal	restriction of diffusion capacity	chronic
minimal changes	restriction of perfusion capacity	acute

15.1 Placental findings without functional significance

Macroscopical and microscopical studies of placentas from eutrophic newborns without any risk factor may have following findings in combination:
– normal weight but small areas of abnormal villous maturation or villous fibrosis
– small for age placenta but normal villous maturation
– large for age placenta with appropriate maturity of the villi, or fibrosis
– normal weight placenta with appropriate villous maturation, but multiple microfibrin deposits

Additionally to each associated findings of minimal changes like small areas of chronic infarcts less 10 % of the total organ volume, or acute infarcts less 5 %, as well as abnormalities in placental shape and pathological umbilical cord insertion can be seen [14].

Fetal consequences
Both, normal and minimal changes showed clinically rate of intrauterine fetal asphyxia. Stillbirth rate in normal placental findings was 1.07‰, in minimal changes 1.37‰.

15.2 Placental changes with reduced diffusion capacity

Morphology
Reduced diffusion capacity often is caused by villous maturation disorders with decreased development of vasculosyncytial membranes and in placental growth disorder:
– Large areas with villous maturation retardation/arrest (grade 3) in normal and enlarged placentas.
– Medium grade developed villous maturation retardation/arrest (grade 2) and decreased placental growth.
– Large foci with Chorangiosis type 1.

Pathogenesis
In villous maturation retardation grade 3:
- Number of fetal capillaries and vasculosyncytial membranes is reduced by more than 50 %.
- Intravillous diffusion distance is increased compared to normal mature placentas according gestational age (20–50 μm).
- The villous surface is normally developed.

In chorangiosis type 1, increased intravillous diffusion distance is caused by deficient development of vasculosyncytial membranes.

Consequences for the fetus
Term pregnancies are mainly affected. Structural limitation of diffusion capacity may cause *chronic fetal hypoxia* during the final weeks of pregnancy and the unique hemo-dynamic conditions shortly before and d*uring delivery* may cause *acute fetal hypoxia and anoxia*. This may explain the high incidence of stillbirths in this group, and the high number of newborns transferred to intensive care units.

Table 15.3: Morphological placental findings and fetal outcome [12].

fetal outcome:				
placental morphology	intrauterine asphyxia (clinically)	IUFD	preterm delivery	fetal growth restriction
1. normal (n = 1858)	11.0 %	1.07‰	8.4 %	5.3 %
2. minimal (n = 1453)	16.0 %	1.37 ‰	13.6 %	7.9 %
3. deficient diffusion (n = 494)	43.0 %	5.7 %	23.1 %	8.2 %

15.3 Placental changes with reduced perfusion capacity

Reduced perfusion capacity is caused by placental growth disorders associated with chronic malperfusion and accelerated villous maturation/distal villous hypoplasia [15].

Morphology
- placental growth restriction with generalized accelerated villous or maturation or distal villous hypoplasia, grade 2,
- placental growth restriction with increased microfibrin depositions, grade 3, or chronic infarcts, less than 20 % of the placental volume,

-   chronic placental vessel obliteration with villous stromal fibrosis or villous imma-
    turity, grade 2, and microfibrin depositions, grade 2, (in normal sized placenta)

Pathogenesis

A limitation in the circulatory placental capacity may be caused by decreased maternal and/or fetal blood compartments in a growth restricted placenta, chronic circulatory disturbances and/or maturation disorders.

In *preterm born* children the majority of placentas show:

-   *Growth and circulatory disturbances associated* with *accelerated villous matura-
    tion*. This is considered to be a compensatory structural response *to* a chronic vas-
    cular malperfusion due to organic growth restriction or placental size reduction,
    secondary due to chronic circulatory disturbance. These placentas show preterm
    mature peripheral villi, increased intravillous vessel surface area, but reduced
    development of vasculosyncytial membranes by ca. 25 % compared to mature ter-
    minal villi. Degeneration of the syncytiotrophoblast is proportionally increased
    accelerated villous maturation, up to 59 %, and show by immunohistochemistry
    a decrease or loss of HPL and SP 1 positivity.
-   *Distal villous hypoplasia* is characterized by loss of medium sized villi ("deficien-
    cy of intermediate villi"). Terminal villi are extremely elongated and can contain
    many stromal vessels or with marked fibrosis. Loss of intermediate villi and defi-
    cient vessel development in terminal villi cause a significant reduction of vessel
    volume, which leads to limited perfusion capacity in the placenta.
-   *Increased microfibrin depositions* in the intervillous space and macroscopic in-
    farcts are a consequence of reduced uteroplacental vascularization and limited
    placental perfusion capacity.

Fetal Consequences

Table 15.4: Fetal outcome in reduced placental perfusion capacity.

preterm and term births are affected	
fetal growth restriction	55 %
intrauterine hypoxia (live borns)	44 %
stillbirths	1.7 %

15.4 Placental findings with manifested acute placental insufficiency

Acute placental insufficiency is caused by acute circulatory disturbance, followed by dysfunction and failure of maternal-fetal gas exchange. Manifestation of the functional disorder depends on the severity of circulatory disturbance and structural placental pathology.

Morphology
Three types can be distinguished:
1. large foci with acute circulatory disturbances in more than 20 % of the placenta without prior pathological changes,
2. small foci of acute circulatory disturbances (more than 5 %) of the placenta with preexisting structural pathology, such as primary reduced functional capacity,
3. acute circulatory disturbances with primary chronic placental insufficiency (global insufficiency).

Pathogenesis
Disorder and failure of maternal-fetal gas exchange is seen as morphology fulfilling the criteria of acute circulatory disturbance, possibly caused by large infarcts or preterm placental abruption. Small foci are of high significance if the placentas show preexisting changes.

Fetal Consequences

Table 15.5: Fetal outcome in manifested acute placental insufficiency.

fetal growth restriction	32 %
preterm deliveries	65 %
intrauterine hypoxia (live borns)	63 %
stillbirths	37 %

Fetal and Newborn mortality and morbidity depend on preexisting placental pathology [16]. Mortality in acute placental insufficiency without preexisting pathology was relative lower than in those with preexisting placental pathology. Newborns discharged from hospital after transitory hypoxia or after maternal postpartum depression, were highly represented in the first group. This may be interpreted as high grade placental pathology causing high grade mortality and less postpartum adaptation in the newborn.

15.5 Placental findings with manifested chronic placental insufficiency

The most significant changes associated with chronic placental insufficiency are placental growth restriction, chronic maternal vascular malperfusion, villous immaturity, fetal vascular malperfusion and villous fibrosis.

Morphology

Significant associated findings can be classified into 3 groups:

1. Chronic maternal vascular malperfusion (more than 20 % placental volume)/ diffuse increased inter and perivillous microfibrin depositions *(infarct placenta)*; associated placental growth restriction and villous immaturity/villous fibrosis grade 2–3.
2. Placental growth restriction and villous immaturity grade 3.
3. Endangiopathia obliterans and villous fibrosis grade 3 (normal and low weight placentas), associated with microfibrin depositions and chronic villitis.

Pathogenesis

Chronic placental insufficiency is associated with varying morphology. In general, individual changes may cause restricted placental diffusion or perfusion capacity. Associated findings may cause additional negative effects on villous surface area and intraplacental perfusion, which affect fetal demands and fetal supply.

Fetal Consequences

Table 15.6: Fetal outcome in manifested chronic placental insufficiency.

fetal growth restriction	97 %
preterm deliveries	24 %
intrauterine hypoxia (live borns)	46 %
stillbirths	10,8 %

In a retrospective study of 255 placentas with morphological chronic placental insufficiency: Fetal weight of 170 newborns was less than 3rd percentile: 75 newborns weighted less than 10th percentile and 10 newborns less than the 25th percentile (weight adjusted for gestational age).

Fetuses with associated placental pathology were at a high hypoxic risk while intrauterine [17].

References

[1]   Gille J. Kritische Gedanken zur 'Plazentainsuffizienz'. MedKlin. 1985;80.
[2]   Kuss E. [What is the placental insufficiency syndrome?]. Geburtshilfe Frauenheilkd. 1987;47(9):664–670.
[3]   Becker V, Schiebler TH, Kubli F. Allgemeine und spezielle Pathologie der Plazenta. Die Plazenta des Menschen. Stuttgart: Thieme; 1981. p. 251–393.
[4]   Gruenwald P. Fetal deprivation and placental pathology: concepts and relationships. Perspectives in pediatric pathology. 1975;2:101–149.
[5]   Fox H. Pathology of the Placenta. London: Saunders; 1978.
[6]   Vogel M. Morphological placental findings and fetal outcome. In: Merten UP LJ, editor. Pathology, a medical speciality. Cologne: News Bull World Assoc Soc Pathol. 1979:72–75.
[7]   Vogel M. Plazentagrösse und -struktur als Voraussetzung für den Wachstumsstand des reifgeborenen Kindes bei der Geburt, mit besonderer Berücksichtigung der Plazentationsstörungen. Berlin: Free University of Berlin; 1975.
[8]   Kubli F, Wernicke K. Plazentainsuffizienz. In: Becker V, Schiebler TH, Kubli F, editor. Die Plazenta des menschen. Stuttgart: Thieme; 1981. p. 395–470.
[9]   Arabin B, Jimenez E, Vogel M, Weitzel HK. Relationship of utero- and fetoplacental blood flow velocity wave forms with pathomorphological placental findings. Fetal Diagn Ther. 1992;7(3–4):173–179.
[10] Jimenez E, Vogel M, Arabin B, Wagner G, Mirsalim P. Correlation of Ultrasonographic Measurement of the Utero-Placental and Fetal Blood Flow with the Morphological Diagnosis of Placental Function. In: Kaufmann P, Miller RK, editors. Placental Vascularization and Blood Flow: Basic Research and Clinical Applications. Boston, MA: Springer US; 1988. p. 325–334.
[11] Arabin B, Siebert M, Jimenez E, Saling E. Obstetrical characteristics of a loss of end-diastolic velocities in the fetal aorta and / or umbilical artery using Doppler ultrasound. Gynecol Obstet Invest. 1988;25(3):173–180.
[12] Vogel M. [Histological stages of development of the chorionic villi in the embryonal and early fetal period (5th to 20th week of pregnancy)]. Pathologe. 1986;7(1):59–61.
[13] Vogel M. Morphological placental findings and fetal outcome. In: Merten UP LJ, editor. Pathology, a mediacal speciality. Cologne: News Bull World Assoc Soc Pathol; 1979:72-75.
[14] Vogel M. Morphology of placenta dysfunction: a contribution to the recognition of pathogenic factors in intrauterine hypoxia and fetal growth restriction. In: Grauel EL S-RJ, Wauer RR., editor. Research in Perinatal Medicine. Leipzig: VEB Thieme; 1986. p. 292–299.
[15] Vogel M. Wachstums- und Reifestörungen sowie Durchblutungsstörungen der Plazenta. In: Dudenhausen JW, editor. Praxis der Perinatalmedizin. Stuttgart, New York, : Thieme; 1986. p. 422–430.
[16] Vogel M, Schmittert J. Morphologie der akuten Plazentainsuffizienz und Schicksal des Kindes. BerPathol. 1987;108,240ff.
[17] Passmann M. Chronische Plazentainsuffizienz (Ergebnisse eines Vergleichs der Plazentamorphologie mit dem klinischen Zustand des Kindes). Berlin: Free University; 1994.

Appendix

Table A1: Reference values of placental net weight and placental area.

gestational week	placental net weight in g			placental area in cm^2		
	percentile					
	P10	P50	P90	P10	P50	P90
15 or 16	45	70	115	25	45	70
17	50	100	125	32	50	85
18	65	105	155	38	55	94
19	90	125	160	54	67	102
20	105	140	165	54	84	103
21	110	145	215	54	101	138
22	115	165	230	71	103	143
23	120	180	240	76	104	146
24	120	205	250	82	105	152
25	145	210	300	75	121	142
26	155	230	300	90	135	155
27	165	220	305	103	142	165
28	170	255	345	103	150	188
29	185	295	350	115	158	211
30	225	285	375	122	164	211
31	230	335	420	125	176	223
32	265	320	400	133	178	216
33	295	370	465	146	187	253
34	285	365	490	141	197	240
35	300	390	495	153	211	266
36	340	435	555	169	226	283
37	345	470	550	173	226	293
38	375	460	605	186	235	296
39	395	490	620	200	251	310
40	405	500	625	200	253	314
41	415	515	650	200	266	314
42	410	495	625	221	266	314

Table A2: Ratio placental weight – placental area related to gestational week.

gestational week	placental weight-placental area ratio		
	percentile		
	P 10	P 50	P 90
15 and 16	1.55	1.80	2.64
17	1.54	1.90	2.66
18	0.96	1.85	2.76
19	1.37	1.71	2.22
20	11.36	1.85	2.51
21	0.93	1.60	2.44
22	0.75	1.67	2.60
23	1.01	1.55	2.44
24	1.18	1.79	2.64
25	1.20	1.81	3.40
26	1.41	1.74	2.16
27	1.31	1.65	2.23
28	1.08	1.78	2.17
29	1.42	1.72	2.02
30	1.14	1.80	2.57
31	1.27	1.87	2.77
32	1.28	1.88	2.42
33	1.28	1.93	2.75
34	1.28	1.99	3.19
35	0.97	1.94	3.19
36	1.19	1.97	3.10
37	1.21	2.04	3.41
38	1.27	2.02	3.45
39	1.09	2.00	3.58
40	0.96	2.03	3.67
41	1.30	2.03	3.24
42	1.29	1.95	2.98

TableA3: Placental weight and fetal weight ratio [1].

gestational age	placental weight-fetal weight ratio		
	percentile		
	P10	P50	P90
15–16	0.90	1.16	1.57
17	0.61	0.78	0.95
18	0.53	0.63	0.76
19	0.46	0.55	0.64
20	0.43	0.48	0.57
21	0.38	0.44	0.52
22	0.35	0.40	0.47
23	0.32	0.37	0.43
24	0.30	0.35	0.38
25	0.26	0.33	0.36
26	0.25	0.30	0.34
27	0.23	0.25	0.29
28	0.20	0.22	0.27
29	0.18	0.21	0.25
30	0.16	0.19	0.23
31	0.15	0.18	0.21
32	0.14	0.18	0.22
33	0.13	0.17	0.21
34	0.13	0.16	0.19
35	0.13	0.15	0.19
36	0.12	0.14	0.18
37	0.12	0.14	0.16
38	0.11	0.13	0.15
39	0.11	0.13	0.15
40	0.11	0.122	0.14
41	0.12	0.13	0.15

Table A4: Fetal weight-placental weight ratio [2].

gestational age	fetal weight-placental weight ratio
15	0.80
16	1
17	1.29
18	1.63
19	1.78
20	2.23
21	2.54
22	2.78
23	2.96
24	3.11
25	3.28
26	3.47
27	3.72
28	3.97
29	4.19
30	4.38
31	4.58
32	4.78
33	4.97
34	5.28
35	5.56
36	5.81
37	6.04
38	6.37
39	6.65
40	7.23

Table A5: Umbilical cord length, reference values [3].

gestational week	cm
20–21	32.4 ± 8.6
22–23	36.4 ± 9.0
24–25	40.1 ± 10.1
26–27	42.5 ± 11.3
28–29	45.0 ± 9.7
30–31	47.6 ± 11.3
32–33	50.2 ± 12.1
34–35	52.5 ± 11.2
36–37	55.6 ± 12.6
38–39	57.4 ± 12.6
40–41	59.6 ± 12.6
42–43	60.3 ± 12.7

Table A6: Gestational sac diameter opened size (P10–P50) in complete gestational product and embryo without macroscopic malformation, and embryonic size in mm.

gestational week	gestational sac (mm diameter)	embryo CRL (mm)
6	13–23	3–6
7	14–29	5–12
8	20–40	12–22
9	24–47	19–29
10	31–55	26–32
11	39–68	28–41
12	54–83	38–55
13	63–90	55–67
14	69–108	69–82

Table A7: Fetal weight and length from week 15 to 27.

gestational week	percentile					
	weight (g)			crown-foot length (cm)		
	P10	P50	P90	P10	P50	P90
15	50	60	100	13.0	14.5	16.0
16	65	95	120	14.0	16.0	18.5
17	95	120	160	16.0	18.0	22.0
18	135	165	205	18.0	20.5	23.5
19	175	210	250	19.5	21.5	24.0
20	200	260	325	21.5	23.5	26.0
21	250	325	400	22.5	26.0	28.0
22	320	405	490	24.0	27.5	30.5
23	355	505	580	26.0	29.0	31.0
24	400	550	670	27.5	30.5	33.0
25	500	625	780	28.5	31.5	34.0
26	605	720	875	30.5	33.0	35.0
27	650	810	985	32.0	34.5	36.5

References

[1]   Vogel M. Morphologie der Plazenta. In: Vogel M, editor. Atlas der morphologischen Plazenta-diagnostik. 2 ed. Berlin: Springer Verlag; 1996. p. 1–29.
[2]   Molteni RA, Stys SJ, Battaglia FC. Relationship of fetal and placental weight in human beings: fetal/placental weight ratios at various gestational ages and birth weight distributions. The Journal of reproductive medicine. 1978;21(5):327–334.
[3]   Naeye RL. Umbilical cord length: clinical significance. J Pediatr. 1985;107(2):278–281.

Index

www.ingramcontent.com/pod-product-compliance
Lightning Source LLC
Chambersburg PA
CBHW081500190326
41458CB00015B/5294

* 9 7 8 3 1 1 0 4 4 9 9 7 6 *